GW00871144

A Pocket Guide to
DIFFERENTIAL DIAG

A Pocket Guide to
DIFFERENTIAL DIAGNOSIS

R. D. EASTHAM
MD(Cantab), FRCP(Lond), FRCPath
MRC Psych, DCP, Dipl. Path

Consultant Pathologist
to the Frenchay Group of Hospitals, Bristol

Bristol
John Wright & Sons Ltd
1980

R. D. Eastham MD, Department of Pathology, Frenchay Hospital, Bristol BS16 1LE.

BY THE SAME AUTHOR

Biochemical Values in Clinical Medicine
Clinical Haematology
A Laboratory Guide to Clinical Diagnosis
Clinical Pathology in Mental Retardation
(R. D. Eastham and J. Jancar)

British Library Cataloguing in Publication Data

Eastham, Robert Duncan
A pocket guide to differential diagnosis.
1. Diagnosis, Differential
I. Title
616.07'5 RC71.5

ISBN 07236 0542 4

Printed in Great Britain by
John Wright and Sons Limited
at The Stonebridge Press, Bristol

Preface

I began with *Biochemical Values in Clinical Medicine* and in this pocket book and in my second one, *Clinical Haematology,* I have listed the many laboratory investigations that are available today and how they are affected by diseases, by physiological changes and by drugs. In the *Laboratory Guide to Clinical Diagnosis* I have attempted to provide guidance on those tests that are most useful in the diagnosis and subsequent treatment of different diseases. Those books have had a good reception and have gone into several editions.

I am hoping, therefore, that this new *Pocket Guide* will prove to be as popular. While the aphorism 'Common conditions are common' is commonly true, it is also true that unless rare conditions are thought of in problem cases, even if only briefly, the correct diagnosis will not always be made.

The initial section is a general list of signs and symptoms. It is followed by twenty specific sections under headings that are generally found in textbooks of medicine. There is a list of contents at the head of each section and there are over 800 lists of the different causes of various signs, symptoms and disease processes. It would not have been useful to provide a comprehensive index or cross reference system.

Since the incidence of different diseases varies throughout the world, the commonest causes do not necessarily appear at the top of each list. If it is known that only a few cases of a particular condition have been reported then [R] is placed against it. When the inheritance of a disease or deficiency state is known this is shown as (D, AD, AR or XR) against the entry.

I hope that this book will be useful to doctors in clinical practice, especially when a patient presents with symptoms that suggest a condition outside the specialty within which the particular clinician is experienced. It should also be useful for quick revision before examinations, for the reassessment of a diagnosis already made, and especially when large comprehensive textbooks are not available.

I am grateful to my wife, Joan, for her help in the preparation of the manuscript and in subsequent proof reading, and I am also grateful to John Wright & Sons for their usual support.

November 1979 R. D. E.

Contents

In the text [R] stands for 'Rare', and also (D) stands for Dominant, (AD) Autosomal Dominant, (AR) Autosomal Recessive and (XR) Sex-linked Recessive.

GENERAL SIGNS AND SYMPTOMS

Pyrexia
 Pyrexia following exposure to external heat
Shock
Compulsive sighing
Sense of smell
Swelling in the groin
Swelling in the scrotum
Syncope
Taste: disorders of taste
Tetany
Vertigo *see* CNS Section
Vomiting
Yawning

ABDOMEN

Swollen Abdomen

General obesity
Ascites
Tympanites
Ovarian cyst
Gravid uterus with increased amniotic fluid
Distended bladder
Abdominal cyst
Hydronephrosis, pyonephrosis
Distended stomach
'Phantom tumour'

Ascites

Diseases of peritoneum
- malignant ascites
- tuberculous ascites

Cardiac
- constrictive pericarditis
- right-sided cardiac failure

Hepatic
- hepatic venous obstruction (Chiari's syndrome)
- cirrhosis – with reduced albumin synthesis
- portal vein thrombosis – obstruction to hepatic venous outflow increases the formation of hepatic sinusoidal fluid

Renal nephrosis
- reduced glomerular filtration rate results in sodium retention
- increased circulating aldosterone results in sodium retention
- natriuretic response by kidney, with expansion of extracellular fluid by 3rd factor

Haemodilution – results in low plasma albumin levels
Chylous ascites

Plain Abdominal X-ray Appearances

Normal gas pattern
- Abnormalities which may be seen
  - dilatation of small bowel
  - dilatation of large bowel
- Abnormal gas pattern
  - abnormal outline to gas within bowel lumen
    - severe mucosal oedema associated with infarction
    - ulcerative colitis
    - Crohn's disease
  - gas in abscess or abscesses
  - gas in peritoneal cavity
  - intramural gas
    - pneumatosis cystoides intestinalis
    - hiatus streaks
    - gallbladder wall
    - bladder wall
  - gas in the biliary tract
- Calcification: *see next list*

Radio-opacities on plain X-ray of Abdomen

Opaque tablets swallowed by the patient
Phleboliths
- mesenteric glands
- haemangioma

Lymph nodes
Blood vessels
- calcification in abdominal aneurysms
  - aorta
  - splenic artery

Adrenal glands – calcification may occur in –
- post-haemorrhage into adrenal
- post-tuberculosis of adrenal
- unknown cause, often bilateral calcification
- adrenal carcinoma
  - phaeochromocytoma
  - neuroblastoma
  - ganglioneuroma
- benign cysts (very rare)

Liver
- hepatic calcification, e.g. in hepatoma

Biliary tract
- 'limey bile'
- gallbladder wall calcification
- gallstone

Pancreas
- calculi
- calcification in area of fat necrosis following pancreatitis

Intestine
- Diverticula of colon and appendix
- Appendolith
- Rarely in mucin-secreting carcinoma
  - stomach
  - colon
- Retroperitoneal
  - calcification of tuberculous psoas abscess
  - tuberculosis of spine
  - retroperitoneal sarcoma
- Faecolith

Genito-urinary tract
- Renal calcification
  - nephrocalcinosis
  - hypernephroma
  - renal cyst
  - chronic glomerulonephritis } linear cortical calcifications parallel with renal outline
  - renal cortical necrosis } linear cortical calcifications parallel with renal outline
  - renal tubular acidosis
  - secondary to hypercalcaemia
  - sponge kidney
  - polycystic kidneys
  - tuberculosis
  - calculi
- Ureter: calculi
- Calculi in pelvis, ureter, bladder or urethra –
  - calcium phosphate } opaque
  - calcium oxalate } opaque
  - magnesium ammonium phosphate – moderately opaque
  - cystine – faintly opaque
  - uric acid, xanthine and matrix not opaque, and therefore not seen
- Bladder calcifications
  - calcification of bladder tumour
  - Bilharzial bladder
  - bladder calculi
- Prostate
- Dermoid: bone or teeth
- Calcified fibroid
- Ovarian masses
- Fetus

Soft tissues
- Buttock injections, e.g. bismuth salts
- Parasitic infestation – cysticerci with calcification

BLUSH – FLUSH

Physiological
  normal
  menopausal 'hot flushes'
Drugs
  histamine
  nicotinic acid
  meprobamate
Insects
  bee sting } in 'sensitive' people
  wasp sting }
Pathological
  intestinal carcinoid tumour
  urticaria pigmentosa (histamine over-production)
  hypertension
  medullary thyroid carcinoma
  neuroblastoma
  tumours of the endocrine pancreas (some)

CHYLOTHORAX

Thoracic duct cut during surgery
Thoracic duct torn
  wounding
  acute hyperextension of the neck
  blunt injury
  blast injury
  violent coughing
  violent vomiting
Widespread intrathoracic lymphatic obstruction
  lymphoma
  malignant pleural disease
  retroserous tumours
Rarely chylothorax occurs in
  Noonan's syndrome [R]
  pulmonary lymphangiomyomatosis [R]
  thoracic lymphangiectasis [R]

FINGER CLUBBING

Due to increased vascularity, hyperplasia of fibrous tissue and oedema

1. Bilateral
Hereditary finger clubbing
Lung disease
  bronchial carcinoma
  bronchiectasis
  lung abscess
  fibrosing alveolitis
  diffuse lung fibrosis

Circulatory system
congenital cyanotic heart disease
bacterial endocarditis
Liver disease
cirrhosis of the liver
(Hypertrophic osteoarthropathy occasionally accompanies finger clubbing)

2. Unilateral
Arterial aneurysm with arteriovenous fistula in affected arm
Disruption of ipsilateral cervical sympathetic nerves
tuberculosis at lung apex
tumour at lung apex

'COLLAPSE'

With elevated central venous pressure
acute massive pulmonary embolism
respiratory failure
tamponade, e.g. bleeding from aortic aneurysm into pericardium
chronic thrombo-embolic pulmonary hypertension
With low central venous pressure
haemorrhage
Gram-negative septicaemia
With acute dyspnoea
pneumothorax

COMA

With focal signs
Supratentorial
cerebral haemorrhage
massive cerebral infarction with oedema
subdural haematoma
extradural haematoma
brain tumour
Brainstem lesion
infarction
pontine haemorrhage
cerebellar haemorrhage
tumour
secondary pressure from cerebral tumour
Diffuse intracranial disorders
encephalitis
subarachnoid haemorrhage
head injury
hypertensive encephalopathy

Without focal signs
Metabolic

anoxia
diabetic ketosis
hypoglycaemia
respiratory failure
cardiac failure
liver failure
kidney failure
hypothyroidism
hypoadrenalism
hypothermia

Drug overdose
alcohol (with or without head injury)
morphine and related drugs
barbiturates
aspirin
etc.

Diffuse intracranial disorders
meningitis
encephalitis
subarachnoid haemorrhage
head injury
cerebral malaria
trypanosomiasis
general paralysis of the insane
epilepsy

Severe infections
typhus
typhoid
cholera
etc.

(Psychogenic unresponsiveness, hysterical coma, catatonic stupor)

CONFUSIONAL STATES, ESPECIALLY IN THE ELDERLY

Cerebral
cerebral infarction
thrombosis
embolism
haemorrhage
transient cerebral ischaemia
cerebral hypoxia
cerebral neoplasm
primary
secondary
subdural haematoma
dementia – predominantly arteriosclerotic senile dementia
epilepsy

Toxic
infection
tissue necrosis
uraemia

dehydration
due to vomiting
due to diarrhoea
carcinoma
Endocrine
thyroid disorders – myxoedema
diabetes mellitus
Metabolic disturbances
electrolyte imbalance, especially hypokalaemia
venous thrombosis
urine retention
faecal impaction
Drugs, e.g. tranquillizers, etc.

COUGH

Lesion in
pharynx
larynx
trachea
bronchus
lung
pleura
mediastinum
subdiaphragmatic
pulmonary oedema
pulmonary congestion
'nervous tic'

CRAMPS

Normal subjects
Over-exertion, e.g. swimming cramp, strenuous exercise
Professional cramps – overuse of certain muscles
Spasms associated with elongation or stretching of certain muscles, e.g. in bed, in the foot
During the later stages of pregnancy

Pathological states
Metabolic
cramps associated with tetany
post-thyroidectomy
operative damage to remaining parathyroid glands after parathyroidectomy
rickets in infants
prolonged lactation in women
malabsorption
hypokalaemia
alkalosis, e.g. hyperventilation
aldosteronism causing hypokalaemia
hypomagnesaemia

uraemia
salt deficiency
  vitamin-B deficiency
  diabetes mellitus
Toxic
  alcoholic neuritis
  strychnine poisoning
  lead poisoning
  ergot poisoning
  cramps associated with high fevers, e.g. cholera, enteric fever and electrolyte imbalance
Circulation
  intermittent claudication } including
  impaired arterial blood supply to legs } nocturnal cramps
Osteoarthrosis, associated with nocturnal cramps
Specific muscle diseases – *see* Muscle Section
  Pain on exertion
  Pain at rest
  Muscle cramps
  Myoglobinuria

CYANOSIS

Central cyanosis
  Decreased arterial oxygen saturation due to cardiac disease
  Decreased atmospheric pressure
  Decreased atmospheric oxygen tension, e.g. faulty anaesthesia
  Impaired pulmonary function
  Anatomical shunts relating to heart and lungs
  Haemoglobinopathy with low oxygen affinity
  Haemoglobin abnormality
    methaemoglobinaemia
      primary inherited
      secondary
    secondary sulphaemoglobinaemia

Peripheral cyanosis
  Reduced cardiac output
    shock
    haemorrhage
    severe dehydration
    cardiac failure
    pulmonary embolism
    etc.
  Cold exposure
    normal response to cold
    increased sensitivity to cold – Raynaud's phenomenon
  Redistribution of blood flow to extremities, e.g. shock

Local obstruction
to arterial flow
to venous flow

DYSPNOEA

(Subjective awareness of the need for increased respiratory effort)

Due to a combination of any of –
increased work of breathing
reduction in ventilatory capacity
undue awareness by the subject of the act of breathing
Physiological
after exercise
after breath-holding
Pathological
thoracic cage or pleura abnormally rigid
lungs less distensible than normal
pleural cavities filled with air or fluid
airways obstruction
extrapulmonary causes
hypoxia
anaemia
blood pH lower than normal
thyrotoxicosis – increased metabolic rate
Severity of dyspnoea
occurring on exertion
occurring at rest
occurring when patient lies down (orthopnoea – 'upright breathing')

FALLS IN THE ELDERLY

Consequence of
change in gait – there is a different change in gait in the two sexes
gradual loss of muscle control
increasing postural instability
change to unusual environment, e.g. move to new house, etc.
pathological conditions –
generalized muscle weakness
arthritis
visual and motor inattention
orthostatic hypotension
giddiness
drug action
cardiac syncope
drop attacks

extrapyramidal dysfunction
Parkinsonism
apraxia (frontal lobe disease)

Incidence
at home 85% occur in morning and afternoon
in hospital, the majority occur at night
highest in widows, widowers, divorcees

GROWTH

Short Stature

Familial: (commonest) short children of short parents
Constitutional: the next most frequent
Delayed puberty
Low birth weight
Chromosome disorders
Chronic disease
- renal
- hepatic
- gastrointestinal
- excess steroid therapy
- others

Deprivation
- (psychosocial dwarfism)
- malnutrition

Bone dysplasia
Intra-uterine growth retardation
- Infection
  - rubella
  - syphilis
  - toxoplasmosis
  - cytomegalovirus
- Toxins
  - alcohol
  - nicotine
  - hydantoins
- Syndromes
  - Bloom [R]
  - Seckel [R]
  - Donahue [R]
  - Dubowitz [R]
  - Russel–Silver dwarfism [R]
  - de Lange [R]
  - Williams [R]

Endocrine
- hypothyroidism – growth slowed down
- corticosteroid excess – injudicious medication
- Cushing's syndrome
- growth hormone deficiency
  - short stature with retarded bone age
  - isolated human growth hormone deficiency occurs in boys

precocious puberty
pseudo-precocious puberty associated with gonadal tumour
true panhypopituitarism, e.g. following surgery for craniopharyngioma
congenital adrenal hyperplasia – speed up of growth with premature fusion of epiphyses

Short-stature Dwarfism (Short-limbed)

Achondroplasia: autosomal dominant
Achondrogenesis: autosomal recessive
Asphyxiating thoracic dystrophy: autosomal recessive
Cartilage–hair hypoplasia: autosomal recessive
Chondrodysplasia punctata: autosomal recessive
Chondro-epidermal dysplasia (Ellis–van Creveld syndrome): autosomal recessive
Conrad's syndrome: autosomal recessive
Diastrophic dwarfism: autosomal recessive
Ellis–van Creveld syndrome: autosomal recessive
Homozygous achondroplasia: autosomal dominant
Hypophosphatasia: autosomal recessive
Hypophosphatesaemic rickets: X-linked dominant
Lymphopenic agammaglobulinaemia with short-limbed dwarfism: ?
Metatrophic dwarfism: autosomal recessive
Metaphysical dysostosis: autosomal dominant
Osteogenesis imperfecta: autosomal dominant
: autosomal recessive
Spondylo-epiphysial dysplasia congenita: autosomal dominant
autosomal recessive
Thanatophoric dwarfism: autosomal recessive
drug-induced

Tall Stature

Genetic
familial
advanced development: early puberty
Nutrition: ?? overnutrition before puberty
Endocrine
growth hormone excess: pituitary eosinophilic adenoma
thyroid excess
precocious puberty
pseudoprecocious puberty
androgen excess before puberty
Specific syndromes associated with tallness
chromosome abnormalities
XYY syndrome
XXY (Klinefelter) syndrome
cerebral gigantism
Marfan's syndrome
homocystinuria

HEADACHE

Mechanism of production of pain uncertain
- migraine
- cluster headache (migrainous neuralgia)
- 'tension' headache
- 'psychogenic' headache

Muscle: contraction, spasm and fatigue
Pain-sensitive structures inside or outside skull
- traction
- inflammation
- pressure

Vasculature
- distension and dilatation of scalp vessels
- artery spasm: arteritis
- angioma
- aneurysm
- hypertension

Air sinuses: infection
- sinusitis
- blockage

Respiratory
- 'cough headache'
- blood gas changes, carbon dioxide intoxication

Infectious diseases
- viral infection
- bacterial septicaemia
- infectious fevers

Central nervous system disease
- stroke
- neoplasm
  - primary
  - secondary
- meningitis
- encephalitis
- brain abscess
- post-trauma
  - immediate, following head injury
  - chronic
    - subdural haematoma
    - post-traumatic instability
    - post-epileptic headache
    - neuralgia

Eyes: secondary to eye strain, glaucoma, etc.
Cervical arthritis, spondylosis
Other referred pain

HYPOTHERMIA

Exposure of normal individual to very severe cold
Loss of heat-regulating efficiency
- Physiological: old age

Pathological
brain damage
acute stroke
dementia
Parkinsonism
cardiorespiratory
bronchopneumonia
cardiac failure
myocardial infarction
immobilization
neurological disease
locomotor disability
drug action
barbiturates
phenothiazines
antidepressants
Hyperthermia, *see* Pyrexia

LIMBS – UPPER

Abnormalities visible in the Hand

Large and broad relative to the patient, with thickened skin and subcutaneous tissues: acromegaly
Podgy hand with coarse dry skin: myxoedema
Long hand with tapering fingers
Marfan's syndrome
homocystinuria
hypogonadism
Macrodactyly affecting one or more fingers
Paget's disease
neurofibromatosis
local arteriovenous fistula – the whole hand may be large
Polydactyly – extra digits
inherited
congenital defects – may be accompanied by ventricular septal defect
Syndactyly – joining of fingers
associated with multiple gross congenital abnormalities
occurring in otherwise normal subjects
Brachydactyly
absence of one of phalanges: (AD) inherited
short fingers of equal length: achondroplasia
shortening of metacarpals and carpals in pseudohypoparathyroidism
short fourth metacarpal: Turner's gonadal dysgenesis
short and broad fingers: cretin
stubbed fingers due to collapse of distal phalanx: hyperparathyroidism
Clinodactyly: in-curved fifth finger
inherited (AD)
Down's syndrome

Hurler's syndrome
Absent thumb: Fanconi's congenital aplastic anaemia

Wasting of the Small Muscles of the Hand

Lesions at
Hand
- old age
- muscle disease, e.g. dystrophia myotonica
- trophic
  - rheumatoid arthritis
  - ischaemia [R]
- disease atrophy (e.g. post-stroke)
- ulnar nerve damage – deep palmar branch

Wrist
- median nerve lesion
- ulnar nerve lesion

Elbow
- median nerve lesion
- ulnar nerve lesion

Upper arm
- trauma
- tumour

Brachial plexus
- trauma, e.g. Klumpke's paralysis
- cervical rib
- spondylosis
- tumour

Neuropathies: many types
Anterior horn cells
- poliomyelitis
- motor neuron disease

Spinal cord lesions, including
- syringomyelia
- tumour
- multiple sclerosis

Cortical lesion – sited in parietal lobe

LIMBS – LOWER

Disorders of Gait

Including
Psychoneurosis
Cerebral 'Palsy'
- upper motor neuron lesion
- parietal lobe lesion
- Parkinsonism

Cord lesion
- lower motor neuron lesion (e.g. poliomyelitis)
- proprioceptive disorder (e.g. tabes dorsalis)

Cerebellar insufficiency: e.g. primary cerebellar atrophy

Muscle disease
Skeletal disorder, e.g.
- congenital dislocation of hip
- osteoarthritis

Multiple sites of damage: multiple sclerosis

Leg ulceration

- Trauma
  - external agent
    - mechanical
    - thermal
    - chemical
    - ionizing radiation
  - self-inflicted
- Infection
  - acute pyogenic infections
  - granulomatous conditions
    - tuberculosis
    - syphilis
    - leprosy
    - leishmaniasis
  - mycoses
    - chromomycosis
    - blastomycosis
    - maduromycosis
- Metabolic
  - necrobiosis lipoidica diabeticorum
  - calcinosis cutis
- Endocrine
  - (rare) hyperparathyroidism
  - Klinefelter's syndrome
- Neuropathic
  - myelopathies
  - poliomyelitis
- Autoimmune diseases
  - systemic lupus erythematosus
  - systemic sclerosis
  - rheumatoid arthritis
  - dermatomyositis
  - polyarteritis nodosa
  - pyoderma gangrenosum
- Haematological disorders
  - sickle cell disease
  - congenital haemolytic anaemia
  - thalassaemia
  - leukaemia
  - macroglobulinaemia
  - cryoglobulinaemia
  - myeloma
  - polycythaemia rubra vera
- Connective tissue disorders
  - acrodermatitis atrophicans chronica

Ehlers–Danlos syndrome
Marfan's syndrome
Werner's disease
Secondary to bone disease
Neoplasia
basal cell carcinoma
squamous cell carcinoma
malignant melanoma
Kaposi's sarcoma
reticuloses
Circulatory disorders
arterial disease
venous disease
arteriovenous aneurysm
arteriolar and capillary allergic cutaneous vasculitis
hypostatic

Gangrene affecting Lower Limb

Causes include –
Physical agents
cold, freezing
heat, burns
severe electric shock
chemical burns
Trauma
direct } division or obstruction of artery
indirect }
Infection
abscess
gas gangrene
Drugs
ergot
thiopentone perivascular injection
Blood vessel disease
embolism
thrombosis
Raynaud's disease
thromboangiitis obliterans (Buerger's disease)
Complicating
diabetes mellitus }
atherosclerosis } especially in aged
severe infection }

Proximal Weakness of the Leg – Quadriceps Syndrome

Osteoarthrosis of knee and/or hip
Lumbar spondylosis
Diabetic amyotrophy
Motor neuron disease
Muscle disease – with metabolic myopathy
myxoedema
thyrotoxicosis

hypercalcaemia
osteomalacia
Cushing's disease
polymyositis
carcinomatous myopathy
(Hysteria)

In myasthenia gravis the muscles affected are usually supplied by cranial nerves. In Parkinsonism there is difficulty in movement rather than weakness

NODULES

Rheumatoid arthritis nodules
Rheumatic fever nodules
Heberden's nodules in osteoarthritis
Gouty tophi
Xanthomas
Neurofibromas
Dupuytren's contracture nodules on
- plantar aponeurosis
- palmar aponeurosis

Subcutaneous fat
- lipoma
- panniculitis

Tendons and bursae
- ganglionic swelling on tendon sheath
- infiltration of tendon sheath by –
  - oedematous or mucoid connective tissue
  - rheumatoid granulomatous tissue

OBESITY

Hypertrophic obesity
Hyperplastic obesity
Static obesity: no change in body weight, but overweight
Progressive obesity, e.g. body weight increasing by more than 10 lb every year

1. Complications of +50% overweight
   75% of these patients develop diabetes mellitus
   33% develop hypertension
   25% suffer from gallbladder and bile tract disease
   12% have hyperuricaemia
   10% will suffer from ischaemic heart disease
   The degree to which life expectancy is reduced is not known

2. Complications of bypass operation for progressive obesity
   The operation has a definite morbidity and a definite mortality
   Hyperoxaluria and renal calculi

Liver failure and cirrhosis
Chronic pseudo-obstruction
Malnutrition, necessitating repair of bypass, when abnormal weight is then regained
Metabolic (non-ion gap) acidosis

BODY ODOUR

Physiological
- Diet: curry, garlic, etc.
- Poor hygiene

Pathological
- Bladder and/or faecal incontinence
  - neurological damage, e.g. multiple sclerosis cord lesion
  - dementia
  - urethrocele, etc.
- Visible surface lesions
  - hyperhidrosis
  - hidradenitis suppurativa
  - Cuno albino Indians, unable to sweat (smell of 'swamp')
  - vagabond's disease
  - infected eczema
  - pemphigus
  - herpes zoster
  - herpes labialis
  - gangrenous feet
  - Darier's disease (keratin disturbance)
  - pediculosis
  - vaginal malodour (gynaecological lesions)
  - pressure sores
  - leg ulcer
  - ulcerating neoplasms
  - osteomyelitis
- Lung disease
  - bronchiectasis
  - lung abscess
  - ozaena
- Oral
  - gingivitis
  - tonsillitis
  - Vincent's angina
- General infections
  - typhoid
  - diphtheria
  - smallpox
  - yellow fever
- Metabolic disorders
  - diabetes mellitus
  - liver failure

scurvy
gout
scrofula
uraemia
rare
phenylketonuria
maple syrup urine disease
oast house urine disease [R]
branched chain amino-acid diseases
methionine abnormality [R]
short chain fatty acid abnormality [R]
(schizophrenia – ? odour of trans-3-methyl-2-hexanoic acid in sweat?)

OEDEMA

Local oedema
inflammation with or without infection
hypersensitivity
local obstruction
to venous return
to lymphatic flow

Generalized oedema
congestive cardiac failure
nephrosis
acute glomerulonephritis
cirrhosis
gross nutritional deficiency

OPISTHOTONOS

Contraction of the muscles of the neck, back and legs with the body held rigidly hyperextended
Tetanus
Strychnine poisoning (occurring in spasms)
Spinal meningitis
(Hysteria)

PAIN

Acute Precordial Chest Pain

Cardiovascular
acute myocardial infarction
ischaemic heart disease with angina, without infarction
dissecting aortic aneurysm
pulmonary embolism

Gastrointestinal
oesophageal disease

hiatus hernia
peptic ulcer
pancreatic disease
biliary tract disease

Pulmonary
pneumothorax

Damage to nerves or nerve roots
cervical spondylosis – root pain
cervical rib
spinal secondary deposits of carcinoma, or other malignancies

'Panic attacks'

Muscle Pain, Stiffness, Raised Erythrocyte Sedimentation Rate in the Elderly

Polymyalgia rheumatica
Neoplasm
Multiple myeloma
Leukaemia
Lymphoma
Polymyositis
Dermatomyositis
Myopathy
Giant cell arteritis

Pain in the Upper Limb

Neurological causes
cervical cord lesions, e.g. syringomyelia
cervical root syndromes
neoplastic brachial plexus lesion
cervical ribs and bands
costoclavicular compression
neuralgic amyotrophy
radial nerve palsy (may present with muscle weakness without pain)
ulnar nerve lesions at the elbow
carpal tunnel syndrome
ulnar nerve lesions at the hand

Non-neurological causes
cardiac pain
supraspinatus syndrome
'frozen shoulder'
'tennis elbow'
rheumatoid arthritis
wrist
hand
elbow

osteoarthrosis
wrist
hand
tenosynovitis and 'trigger finger'

Pain in the Neck

Including –
Cervical spondylosis
Brachial neuritis
Trauma
'whiplash' injury common in car accidents
extension injury in the aged
flexion injury in the young
Rheumatoid arthritis
subluxation
osteophytes
degeneration of ligaments

PALPITATIONS

Heart beat disorders
extrasystoles
ectopic bradycardia

Other conditions
thyrotoxicosis
anaemia
fever
hypoglycaemia
phaeochromocytoma
drugs
ephedrine
atropine
thyroid extract
alcohol
tea, coffee, tobacco
anxiety state

PRIAPISM

Continuous penile erection without associated sexual desire
injury to upper dorsal region of the spinal cord
leukaemia } associated with
sickle cell anaemia } local thrombosis
trauma with local haematoma formation
Intermittent penile erection without associated sexual desire:
associated with enlargement of the prostate

PYREXIA

Causes include –
Infection

bacteria virus fungus spirochaetes protozoa parasites	singly or in combination

Non-infectious disease
- Post-trauma
- Malignancy
  - carcinoma
  - sarcoma
  - lymphoma
  - Hodgkin's disease
  - leukaemia
- Autoimmune disease
  - polymyalgia rheumatica
  - giant cell arteritis
  - systemic lupus erythematosus
  - rheumatic fever
  - rheumatoid arthritis
  - hypersensitivity vasculitis
- Circulation
  - venous thrombosis
  - pulmonary embolism
  - myocardial infarction
- Metabolic, including
  - dehydration from almost any cause
  - familial Mediterranean fever [R]
  - hypertriglyceridaemia with acute abdominal pain
  - Whipple's disease [R]
- Gastrointestinal disease
  - regional enteritis
  - diverticulitis
- Hepatic: granulomatous hepatitis
- Central nervous system: cerebrovascular accident, especially if pons involved
- Muscle: malignant hyperpyrexia, associated with anaesthesia
- Endocrine: *see* list in Endocrine Section
- Drugs
  - sulphonamides
  - barbiturates
  - thiouracil
  - thyroid extract
  - antidepressant excess
- (von Munchausen syndrome – temperature measurement manipulated by patient)

Pyrexia following Exposure to External Heat

Heat hyperpyrexia, hyperthermia: follows exposure to intense heat
Anhydrotic heat exhaustion
Exercise-induced heat exhaustion: exposure in unacclimatized individuals to hot climate while performing excessive exercise
Water-depletion heat exhaustion: body temperature rises later
(cf. Salt-depletion heat exhaustion: body temperature normal, falling to subnormal)

SHOCK

Reduced venous return
- haemorrhage
- pancreatitis
- peritonitis
- severe burns
- trauma
- intestinal obstruction
- anaphylaxis
- cerebrovascular accident
- sepsis

Failure of the heart
- myocardial infarction

Massive pulmonary embolism

COMPULSIVE SIGHING

Healthy normal individuals
Anxiety
Depression
Chest wall injury
Diaphragm injury

SENSE OF SMELL

Loss of sense of smell: hyposmia (total loss: panosmia)
Abnormal sense of smell: parosmia
Hypersensitivity to smells: hyperosmia

Conditions in nose
- Hyposmia or Parosmia
  - common cold, and upper respiratory infections nasal polyposis

vasomotor rhinitis
Unpleasant smell sensations
nasal or sinus carcinoma
malignant granulomas
atrophic rhinitis
rhinitis sicca

Olfactory sense organ
Damage to olfactory sense organ
nasal fractures
nasal surgery
viral infections, e.g. post-influenzal anosmia
toxic chemicals
tars
heavy metals
formaldehyde
creosols
Damage to olfactory nerves
head injury
localized midline osteoma or meningioma [R]
brain surgery

Central
Intracranial tumours
temporal lobe – parosmia
frontal lobe – anosmia
optic chiasma – anosmia
Epilepsy – olfactory aura
hyperosmia
parosmia
Contusion of brain – parosmia

Psychogenic
Schizophrenia
Depressives with phobias

SWELLING IN THE GROIN

In the skin
lipoma
neurofibroma (usually multiple)
sebaceous cyst
dermoid cyst
pilonidal cyst
(angiomatous malformation)[R]

Blood vessel
femoral artery aneurysm
saphena varix (varicose swelling at the proximal end of the long saphenous vein)

Lymph nodes (usually multiple and discrete)
infection

lymphoma
secondary malignancy

Hernia
Inguinal
indirect
direct
Femoral
twice as common in women
(Psoas abscess tracking [R])

Male – testicular swelling
undescended testis
ectopic testis
hydrocele

Female – vulval swelling

SWELLING IN THE SCROTUM

Some causes include –

Testis
Congenital appendix of testis
Inflammation
orchitis
syphilitic gumma
Neoplasm

Epididymis
Congenital appendix of epididymis
Cysts
containing sperms – spermatocele
not containing sperms – epididymal cyst
Inflammation
'non-specific'
tuberculosis
Neoplasm

Cord
Congenital
hydrocele of cord
torsion
Varicocele
Neoplasm – lipoma

Tunica vaginalis
Congenital primary hydrocele
Secondary hydrocele
Hematocele

Scrotum
Sebaceous cyst

Idiopathic scrotal oedema
Secondary scrotal oedema
Swelling arising outside scrotum – hernia

SYNCOPE

Reflex syncope
Postural syncope
Anoxic syncope
Syncope following pain or emotional disturbance
Micturition syncope
Cough syncope
Carotid sinus syncope
Areflexic syncope
Cardiac disease causing syncope
- congenital heart disease
- rheumatic heart disease
- aortic stenosis
- cardiac arrhythmia
- heart block (Stokes–Adams attacks)

Basal migraine
Vertebro-basilar ischaemia caused by atherosclerosis
Circulatory causes
- inadequate vasoconstrictor mechanisms
- hypovolaemia
- reduced venous return
- reduced cardiac output
- arrhythmias

Altered state of blood to brain
- hypoxia
- anaemia
- diminished blood Pco$_2$ following hyperventilation (syncope rare)
- hypoglycaemia

Cerebral causes – cerebrovascular ischaemia
(Hysterical attacks)

DISORDERS OF TASTE

Loss or reduction of taste (ageusia or hypogeusia)
- Damage to chorda tympani may affect taste
- Damage to VII nucleus or VII nerve may affect taste in anterior two-thirds of the tongue
- Hypogeusia may occur after burns, or after surgery, taste returning with recovery of the patient
- Lesions of the lingual nerve
- Lesions of the glossopharyngeal nerve
- Tongue
  - coated
  - glossitis

Foul taste in mouth (cacogeusia)
- Local
  - caries
  - gingivitis
  - glossitis
  - stomatitis
  - epithelioma in mouth
  - gumma in mouth
- Gastrointestinal tract
  - gastric carcinoma
  - gastritis
  - pyloric stenosis
- Pulmonary
  - bronchiectasis
  - tuberculous lung cavity
  - lung abscess

Distorted taste (dysgeusia)
- Post-operation, or post-burns
- Bizarre tastes have been described in otherwise normal pregnancy
- Drugs
  - penicillamine
  - griseofulvin
  - lincomycin
  - diuretics
- Metabolic disorders
  - hypovitaminosis
  - hypothyroidism
  - adrenal cortical insufficiency
- Dyspepsia
- Psychosis: schizophrenic delusions

TETANY

Symptoms in order of increasing severity include –
- numbness and tingling of fingers, toes, and around mouth
- cramps in individual muscles leading to tonic contractions of muscle groups
- laryngeal stridor, crowing inspirations and dyspnoea
- gastric pain, nausea and vomiting
- grand mal convulsions
- in chronic tetanic states, cortical cataracts, and, in some cases, mental deterioration and dementia

Caused by –

Alkalosis, with normal plasma calcium levels
1. Respiratory alkalosis
2. Metabolic alkalosis
   - prolonged vomiting
   - prolonged alkali intake

Hypocalcaemia (low ionized plasma calcium)

1. Vitamin D deficiency in diet, lack of sunshine on skin
2. Malabsorption
3. Excess calcium lost in urine
   - renal tubule acidosis
4. Low plasma calcium with raised plasma inorganic phosphate
   - hypoparathyroidism
   - uraemia
   - excessive phosphate intake
5. Post-thyroidectomy, related to previous severity of hyperthyroidism

VOMITING

Neonatal
- Diet
  - overfeeding
  - excessive movement after feeding
  - excessive swallowing of mucus or amniotic fluid
  - drug withdrawal effects (addict mother)
- Infection
  - May be congenital or acquired at or after birth
  - septicaemia
  - urinary tract infection
  - respiratory tract infection
  - gastrointestinal tract infection
  - central nervous system infection
- Organic lesions of gastrointestinal tract
  - obstructive
    - congenital anomalies
    - meconium plugs
  - non-obstructive
    - hiatus hernia
    - achalasia of the cardia
- Cerebral lesions
  - birth trauma
  - anoxia
  - hypothermia
  - intracranial haemorrhage
  - meningitis
- Inborn errors of metabolism

Late newborn
- hypertrophic pyloric stenosis
- congenital adrenal hyperplasia
- hiatus hernia
- achalasia
- inborn errors of metabolism
- coeliac disease
- Hirschprung's disease
- diabetic ketosis

whooping cough
congenital lesions of the renal tract leading to uraemia

Childhood
diet
infections
organic lesions of the gastrointestinal tract
cerebral lesions
metabolic disorders
labyrinthine disease
psychomotor (e.g. car sickness)

YAWNING

Physiological
Drowsiness
Boredom
Sight or sound of another person yawning
Stuffy atmosphere

Pathological
Epileptic phenomenon
Post-encephalitis
Cerebral tumour (rarely). Posterior fossa tumours may be associated with paroxysms of yawning

BONE DISORDERS

Intrinsic diseases of bone
- Osteochondrodysplasia
- Skeletal dysplasia
- Dysmorphic syndromes with congenital skeletal dysplasia
- Dysostoses
- Idiopathic osteolyses
- Primary disturbances of growth
- Treatable conditions associated with tall stature

Bone ischaemia
Low back pain
Aseptic necrosis of the femoral head
Spinal fractures
Deformities of spine
Ochronotic pigment deposition in bone and cartilage
Bilateral bossing of the frontal bones
Discrete translucencies in X-ray of skull
Hypertrophic osteoarthropathy
Osteochondritis
Osteoporosis
Osteoporosis in childhood
Osteomalacia and rickets
Excess osteoid (unmineralized bone matrix)
Causes of phosphate depletion
Causes of bone sclerosis
Osteopetrosis

INTRINSIC DISEASES OF BONE

Osteochondrodysplasia: abnormalities of cartilage and/or bone growth and development
1. Defects of growth of tubular bones and/or spine
2. Disorganized development of cartilage and fibrous components of skeleton
3. Abnormalities of density, of cortical structure, and/or metaphysial modelling

Dysostoses: malformation of individual bones, singly or in combination
1. Dysostoses with cranial and facial involvement
2. Dysostoses with predominant axial involvement

3. Dysostoses with predominant involvement of extremities

Idiopathic osteolyses
Primary disturbances of growth
Constitutional diseases of bone with known cause
1. Chromosomal abnormalities
2. *Primary metabolic abnormalities*
   a. Disorders of calcium metabolism
   b. Mucopolysaccharidosis
   c. Mucolipidosis and lipidosis
   d. Bony abnormalities secondary to –
      endocrine disease
      neurological disease
      renal disease
      cardiopulmonary disease
      gastrointestinal disease
      haematological disease

Osteochondrodysplasia

1. Defects of growth of tubular bones and/or spine
   a. Diagnosed at birth
      achondrogenesis
      thanatophoric dwarfism
      achondroplasia
      chondroplasia punctata
      metatropic dwarfism
      diastrophic dwarfism
      chondro-ectodermal dysplasia (Ellis–van Creveld syndrome) [R]
      asphyxiating thoracic dysplasia (Jeune syndrome) [R]
      spondylo-epiphysial dysplasia congenita
      mesomelic dwarfism (Nievergelt, Langer type) [R]
      cleidocranial dysplasia [R]
   b. Diagnosed later in life
      hypochondroplasia
      dyschondrosteosis
      metaphysial chondrodysplasia
         Jansen type
         Schmid type
         McKusick type
         with malabsorption and leucopenia
         with thymolymphopenia
      spondylometaphysial dysplasia (Kozlowski) [R]
      multiple epiphysial dysplasia
      hereditary arthro-ophthalmopathy [R]
      pseudoachondroplastic dysplasia
      spondylo-epiphysial dysplasia tarda
      acrodysplasia
         rhinotrichophalangeal syndrome of Giedion [R]
         epiphysial of Thiemann [R]
         epiphysometaphysial of Brailsford [R]

2. Disorganized development of cartilage and fibrous components of the skeleton
   - dysplasia epiphysialis hemimelica
   - multiple cartilagenous exostoses
   - endochondromatosis of Ollier [R]
   - endochondromatosis with haemangioma (Maffucci) [R]
   - fibrous dysplasia
     - Jaffe–Lichtenstein syndrome
     - with skin pigmentation and precocious puberty of McCune–Albright
     - cherubism
     - multiple fibromatosis

3. Abnormalities of density, of cortical diaphysial structure and/or metaphysial modelling
   - osteogenesis imperfecta congenita: Vrolik, Porak–Durante [R]
   - osteogenesis imperfecta tarda: Lobstein [R]
   - juvenile idiopathic osteoporosis
   - osteopetrosis
     - with precocious manifestations
     - with delayed manifestations
   - pycnodysostosis
   - osteopoikilosis
   - melorheostosis
   - diaphysial dysplasia: Camurati–Engelmann
   - craniodiaphysial dysplasia
   - endosteal hyperostosis (van Buchem and other forms)
   - tubular stenosis (Kenny–Caffey) [R]
   - osteodysplasia (Melnick–Needles) [R]
   - pachydermoperiostosis
   - osteoectasia with hyperphosphatasia
   - metaphysial dysplasia – Pyle syndrome
   - craniometaphysial dysplasia [R]
   - frontometaphysial dysplasia [R]
   - oculodental osseous dysplasia [R]

Skeletal Dysplasia

Limb bud development defect: arrest of fetal bone development

Cartilage anlage development fault: abnormal size and/or shape

Chondrocyte development fault: abnormalities in matrix or reduced survival of chondrocyte

Chondrocyte proliferation: reduced cell division in proliferative zone

Chondrocyte maturation and degeneration: abnormalities leading to irregular metaphysial vascular invasion and bone formation

Epiphysial ossification: abnormalities in development of ossification centres

Membranous ossification faults: failure of fibroblasts in periosteum to transfer to osteoblasts or produce normal osteoid
Generalized ossification faults: abnormality on bone matrix composition
Calcified cartilage resorption: failure to resorb calcified cartilage
Bone resorption fault: failure to resorb cortical bone, leading to poorly modelled bones
Aberrant chondrocyte growth: erratic and excessive growth of chondrocytes disturbs the normal plate
Premature epiphysial fusion: early closure of growth plate, resulting in shortening of tubular bones

Dysmorphic Syndromes with Congenital Skeletal Dysplasia

Drugs and toxins
- fetal alcohol syndrome
- fetal aminopterin syndrome
- fetal hydantoin syndrome
- fetal thalidomide syndrome
- fetal warfarin syndrome
- fetal rubella syndrome

Genetic (include)
- chromosome abnormalities
- achondroplasia (AD)
- brachydactyly Type E syndrome
- Seckel's syndrome (AR) [R]
- diastropic dwarfism syndrome (AR) [R]
- Aarskog's syndrome (X-linked recessive) [R]
- Hunter's syndrome (X-linked recessive) [R]

Unknown aetiology
- de Lange's syndrome
- Rubinstein–Taybi syndrome
- Williams' syndrome [R]
- Russell–Silver syndrome [R]

Dysostoses

With cranial and facial involvement
- craniosynostosis
- craniofacial dysostosis: Crouzon syndrome
- acrocephalosyndactyly: Apert syndrome [R]
- acrocephalopolysyndactyly: Carpenter syndrome [R]
- mandibular hypoplasia: including Pierre–Robin syndrome
- oculomandibulo facial syndrome: Hallermann–Streiff–Francois syndrome [R]
- naevoid basal cell carcinoma syndrome

Dysostoses with predominant axial involvement
- vertebral segmentation defects – including Klippel–Feil syndrome
- cervico-oculoacoustic syndrome of Wildervanck [R]

Sprengel deformity
spondylocostal dysostosis
oculovertebral syndrome of Weyers
osteo-onychodysostosis (nail–patella syndrome) [R]

Dysostoses with predominant involvement of the extremities
amelii
hemimelia
acheiria
apodia
adactyly and oligodactyly
phocomelia
aglossia-adactyly syndrome
congenital bowing of long bones
familial radio-ulnar synostosis
brachydactyly
symphalangism
polydactyly, and syndactyly
camptodactyly
clindactyly
Laurence–Moon syndrome
popliteal pterygium syndrome
pectoral aplasia-dysdactyly syndrome of Poland
Rubinstein–Taybi syndrome
pancytopenia-dysmelia syndrome of Fanconi
thrombocytopenia-radial aplasia syndrome
orodigito facial syndrome of Papillon–Léage [R]
cardiomegalic syndrome of Holt–Oran [R]

Idiopathic Osteolyses

Acroosteolysis
phalangeal type
tarsocarpal form
with nephropathy
without nephropathy
multicentric osteolysis

Primary Disturbances of Growth

Primordial dwarfism with associated malformation
Cornelia de Lange syndrome
Bird-headed dwarfism of Virchow, Seckel syndrome [R]
Leprechaunism [R]
Russell–Silver syndrome [R]
Progeria [R]
Cockayne's syndrome [R]
Bloom's syndrome [R]
Geroderma osteodysplastica [R]
Spherophakia-brachymorphia syndrome of Weill–Marchesani [R]
Marfan's syndrome

Treatable Conditions associated with Tall Stature

Include –
Familial tall stature
Hyperthyroidism
Pituitary gigantism
Homocystinuria
Marfan's syndrome
Klinefelter's syndrome
XYY syndrome

BONE ISCHAEMIA

Trauma
Radiation damage
Dysbarism
  profuse expanding gas bubbles in bone
  fat embolism
Haemoglobinopathies: microvascular occlusion by distorted red vells
Pancreatic disease: lipase reaches the marrow
Lipid storage disease: Gaucher's disease. Gaucher cells pack the marrow, which necrose, and are replaced by fibrosis
Steroid therapy
  trabecular microfractures with secondary necrosis
  systemic fat embolism
'Idiopathic' bone necrosis. The following conditions may be associated with 'idiopathic' necrosis:
  alcoholism
  gout
  hyperuricaemia
  diabetes
  hyperglycaemia
  fat metabolism disorders
  obesity
  minor congenital hip anomalies
  systemic lupus erythematosus

LOW BACK PAIN

Inflammatory
  ankylosing spondylitis
  tuberculosis
  pyogenic infections

Metabolic
  osteoporosis
  osteomalacia

Neoplasia

Spondylitis
- Group 1 spondylolisthesis: congenital
- Group 2 spondylolisthesis: probably due to stress fracture in the pars interarticularis
- Pseudoarthrosis
- Osteoarthrosis

Intraneural lesion
- Spinal stenosis
  - congenital
    - idiopathic
    - achondroplasia
  - acquired
    - degenerative – including Group 4 spondylolisthesis
    - combined congenital and acquired, with disc herniation
    - spondylolisthesis
    - iatrogenic
      - following laminectomy
      - following anterior and posterior fusion
  - post-traumatic
  - other causes
    - Paget's disease of the bone
    - fluorosis
    - spinal dysraphism
    - arachnoiditis
    - sacral extradural cysts

Combined mechanical and intraneural
Group 4 spondylolisthesis
Lumbar disc disease
'Psychogenic' low back pain: associated with

Depression Masked depression Anxiety Hysteria Malingering	} beware of missing an actual physical lesion

Gynaecological causes
- Dysmenorrhoea
- Pelvic infection
- Malposition of uterus
- Pelvic masses
- Endometriosis and ovarian blood cysts
- Pregnancy and its after effects

ASEPTIC NECROSIS OF THE FEMORAL HEAD

Idiopathic
- Idopathic aseptic necrosis in the adult
- Legg–Perthes' disease

Trauma
 Post-fracture
  acetabulum
  intra-articular femoral fracture
 Post-reduction
  congenital dislocation of the hip
  slipped capital femoral epiphysis
 Barotrauma, e.g. caisson disease
 Post-irradiation

Systemic disease
 Haemoglobinopathies, e.g. HbS
 Storage diseases
  Gaucher's disease
  Fabry's disease
 Atherosclerosis affecting local blood supply
 Alcoholism
 Pancreatitis
 Connective tissue disorders

Steroids
 Endogenous: Cushing's syndrome
 Exogenous: during therapy
 During pregnancy and postpartum

SPINAL FRACTURES

Fractures are defined as either *Stable* or *Unstable* depending on the integrity of the posterior ligament complex, including –
 Supraspinous ligaments
 Infraspinous ligaments
 Capsules of facet joints
 Ligamentum flavum

Injury causing fractures includes –
 Flexion, especially on the lumbar region
 Combined flexion and rotation
  cervical
  lumbar
 Vertical compression
  cervical } a 'burst' fracture
  lumbar }
 Shearing: thoracic. There is gross neurological damage if the fracture is unstable
 Extension: damage to the arch of the atlas or axis

DEFORMITIES OF SPINE

Kyphosis
 Angular kyphosis: collapse of vertebra
  tuberculosis

crush fracture
metastasis, e.g. secondary carcinoma
Diffuse kyphosis (the commonest form)
muscle weakness
faulty posture
rickets
osteoporosis
osteomalacia
osteitis deformans
ankylosing spondylitis
osteoarthrosis

Lordosis
Muscle weakness
Forward projection of spine
above lumbar region = kyphosis
below lumbar spine = spondylolisthesis
Flexion deformity of the hip
Congenital dislocation of the hips

Scoliosis
Congenital
wedge-shaped deformity of a vertebra
Acquired
postural
compensatory
paralytic, e.g. post-poliomyelitis
post-rickets deformity
reflex – to relieve pain, e.g. sciatica
'hysterical'

OCHRONOTIC PIGMENT DEPOSITION IN BONE AND CARTILAGE

Alkaptonuria.
Rarely
Long-term topical contact with phenol compounds
Long-term topical contact with quinone compounds
Chlorpromazine therapy with exposure to sunlight
Malignant melanoma
Antimalarial therapy (quinacrine and related drugs)

BILATERAL BOSSING OF THE FRONTAL BONES

Achondroplasia
Rickets
Paget's disease of the bone
Congenital hydrocephalus
Gorlin's basal cell naevi syndrome [R]

DISCRETE TRANSLUCENCIES IN X-RAY OF SKULL

Myeloma
Metastatic deposits
Hyperparathyroidism
Leukaemia
Sarcoidosis
Osteomyelitis of the skull
Sickle cell disease
Rare
- Radiation necrosis
- Congenital cranial lacunae
- Histiocytosis-X

HYPERTROPHIC OSTEOARTHROPATHY

Respiratory tract
- Primary carcinoma of bronchus
- Fibrous mesothelioma of pleura
- Bronchiectasis

Gastrointestinal tract disease

Liver disease

Pachydermoperiostosis: idiopathic form, which is familial in 30%, associated with thickening of the skin of the face

(Finger clubbing nearly always present with hypertrophic osteoarthropathy)

OSTEOCHONDRITIS

Non-inflammatory, non-infectious derangement of normal bone growth occurring at the various ossification centres at the time of their greatest activity

Post-traumatic avascular necrosis
- Kienbock's disease: Avascular necrosis of lunate
- Freiburg's disease: Second metatarsal head in girls in 2nd decade
- Kohler's disease: Navicular, the last bone to ossify, at the apex of the medial longitudinal arch, which is strained in boys of 3–5 years

Avascular necrosis of unknown origin
- Perthes' disease: Femoral head affected, bilaterally in 15%, in boys : 1 girl, of 4–9 years

Avulsion injuries of epiphyses
- Osgood-Schlatter: tibial tubercle

Sinding–Larsen: lower pole of patella
Sever: calcaneum

Subarticular post-traumatic avascular necrosis
Knee
Capitellum
Talus

Juvenile discogenic disorder
Scheuermann: spine

Eosinophilic granuloma
Calvé: spine

OSTEOPOROSIS (Osteopenia or thin bones)

Primary
Idiopathic juvenile osteoporosis [R]
Post-menopausal
Post-oophorectomy
Old age

Secondary
Dietary deficiency of calcium, or calcium malabsorption
steatorrhoea
partial gastrectomy
chronic liver disease
Endocrine
hyperparathyroidism
hyperthyroidism
Cushing's syndrome
hypogonadism
Metabolic
vitamin C deficiency (+ iron overload)
pregnancy
osteogenesis imperfecta
Drugs
corticosteroids
heparin (long term)
Immobilization
generalized, e.g. space flight
localized, e.g. after fracture paraplegia
Rheumatoid arthritis
Chronic renal failure
Chronic renal dialysis
Congenital
osteogenesis imperfecta
chromosome abnormalities
i. XO
ii. XXXXY
Local
Immobilization

Sudeck's atrophy
Disappearing bone disease

OSTEOPOROSIS IN CHILDHOOD

Lifelong heritable syndrome
  Osteogenesis imperfecta
Idiopathic juvenile osteoporosis
Chronic acquired
  Biliary atresia
  Cyanotic heart disease
Acute acquired
  Immobilization
Acquired metabolic
  Thyrotoxicosis
  Cushing's syndrome
  Spontaneous
  Iatrogenic
  Calcium intake lack
  Scurvy
Neoplasia
  Leukaemia
  Primary and secondary malignancy

OSTEOMALACIA AND RICKETS

Nutritional vitamin D deficiency
  Premature infants
  Young children growing rapidly
  Adolescents
  Pregnant women
  Elderly women

Disorders of intestinal absorption of vitamin D
  Malabsorption from any cause

Disorders of vitamin D metabolism
Resistance to physiological doses of vitamin D
  Chronic renal disease
  Renal tubular hypophosphataemia
  Familial hypophosphataemia
  Multiple renal tubule defects
  Fanconi syndrome
  Uretero-colic anastomosis
  Long-term anticonvulsant therapy

EXCESS OSTEOID (UNMINERALIZED BONE MATRIX)

Vitamin D deficiency or defective metabolism
  Nutritional deficiency of vitamin D

Lack of sunlight
Chronic renal failure (renal osteodystrophy)
Vitamin-D-dependent rickets

Low plasma phosphate
Phosphate deficiency
Renal tubular disorders (vitamin-D-resistant rickets)

Chronic acidosis
Ureterosigmoidostomy
Renal tubular acidosis (proximal or distal)

High bone turnover
Fracture healing
Paget's disease
Hyperparathyroidism
Hyperthyroidism

Drugs
Anticonvulsants
Diphosphonates
Fluoride – chronic intoxication

Inherited
Fibrogenesis imperfecta ossium
Hypophosphatasia

Unexplained
Axial osteomalacia

CAUSES OF PHOSPHATE DEPLETION

Inherited renal tubular disorders
Familial sex-linked hypophosphaturia ('phosphate rickets')
Cystinosis (De Toni–Debré–Fanconi syndrome)

Acquired renal tubular defects
Hereditary tyrosinaemia } causing secondary
Hepatolenticular degeneration } renal damage
(Neurofibromatosis with associated renal tubular phosphate loss)
Mesenchymal tumours, benign, with fibroblasts, giant cells and numerous blood vessels

Prevention of intestinal absorption of phosphate
Chronic excessive ingestion of aluminium hydroxide antacids

CAUSES OF BONE SCLEROSIS

Common
Paget's disease of bone

Uraemic osteodystrophy
Osteosclerotic metastases, particularly from carcinoma of prostate and breast

Uncommon
Myelosclerosis
Myelomatosis [R] (more commonly, lytic lesions)
Sarcoidosis [R]
Primary hyperparathyroidism [R]
Infantile hypercalcaemia
Chronic vitamin D poisoning
Chronic fluoride excess
Osteopetrosis
Cretinism and adult hypothyroidism
Hereditary hyperphosphatasia
Melorheostosis
Pyrodysostosis
Osteopoikilosis
Osteopathia striata
Diaphysial dysplasia (Engelmann's disease)
Fibrogenesis imperfecta ossium
Lead poisoning

OSTEOPETROSIS

Osteosclerosis
Osteopetrosis with precocious manifestations. Autosomal recessive [R]
Osteopetrosis with delayed manifestations – Albers–Schönberg disease. Autosomal dominant delayed form
Pycnodysostosis

Craniotubular dysplasia
Metaphysial dysplasia – Pyle disease. Autosomal recessive [R]
Craniometaphysial dysplasia. Autosomal dominant
Craniodiaphysial dsyplasia
Frontometaphysial dysplasia
Dysosteosclerosis
Tubular stenosis: Kenny–Caffey syndrome [R]
Osteodysplasty: Melnick–Needles syndrome [R]

Craniotubular hyperostosis
Endosteal hyperostosis – van Buchem's syndrome. Autosomal recessive [R]
Sclerosteosis. Autosomal recessive [R]
Osteo-ectasia with hyperphosphatasia
Diaphysial dysplasia (Camurati–Engelmann syndrome) [R]
Infantile cortical hyperostosis (Caffey syndrome) [R]

Others

- Osteopathia striata, probably autosomal dominant
- Osteopoikilosis
- Melorheostasis
- Pachydermoperiostosis
- Osteitis deformans (Paget's disease)

CARDIOVASCULAR DISORDERS AND CIRCULATORY DISORDERS

General cardiac conditions
- Cardiac arrest
- Syncope
- Cardiac failure
- Chronic cor pulmonale
- Angina pectoris
- Heart disease in the elderly
- Drug-induced cardiovascular disease

Cardiac conditions in the newborn
- Cardiac malformations
- Congenital heart disease
- Congenital heart disease possibly correctable during the first year
- Common congenital heart defects found in infants
- Congenital heart defects without murmurs
- Cyanosis in newborn infant due to cardiac lesions
- Heart failure in newborn infants

Heart rhythms
- Heart block
- Cardiac arrest
- Bradycardia
- Impaired consciousness
- Tachycardia
- Arrhythmias
- Causes of arrhythmia
- Arrhythmias in acute myocardial infarction
- Sinus arrhythmia
- Atrial and junctional arrhythmia
- Ventricular arrhythmia
- Atrial ectopic beats
- Atrial flutter
- Atrial fibrillation
- Ventricular ectopic beats
- Ventricular fibrillation

Myocardium
- Ischaemic heart disease risk factors
- Myocardial infarction in young women
- Acute myocarditis
- Cardiomyopathy
- Secondary cardiomyopathy
- Rare specific myocardial disease

Coronary artery disease

Endocardium
- Infective endocarditis

Heart valves
- Innocent heart murmurs
- Mitral valve disorders
- Aortic valve disorders
- Tricuspid valve disease
- Heart valve vegetations
- Non-rheumatic valvular disease

Pericardium
- Pericarditis
- Constrictive pericarditis

Blood pressure
- Hypertension
- Miscellaneous causes of acute severe hypertension
- Renovascular hypertension
- Complications of hypertension
- Hypertensive emergencies
- Endocrine disorders associated with hypertension
- Hypotension
- Factors precipitating postural hypotension
- Drugs associated with postural hypotension

Peripheral circulatory disorders
- Aortic aneurysm
- Atherosclerosis
- Thrombosis of superior sagittal sinus and cortical veins
- Arteriovenous fistulas
- Arterial embolism
- Pulmonary embolism risk factors
- Fat embolism
- Raynaud's syndrome
- Cerebrovascular insufficiency
- Transient cerebral ischaemic attacks
- Arteritis
- Acute limb ischaemia
- Leg ischaemia
- Digital ischaemia
- High altitude disorders

GENERAL CARDIAC CONDITIONS IN ADULTS

Cardiac Arrest

Heart disease: the commonest cause
Drug errors

Massive plasma sodium, potassium, chloride, bicarbonate, pH upsets
Anaesthetic drugs
Lack of oxygen
Excess of carbon dioxide
Adrenaline excess
Embolism
- air
- blood clot
- amniotic fluid
- drug bolus

Haemorrhage
Cardiac catheterization
Electrocution
Hypothermia
Hyperthermia
Near-drowning

Syncope
Cessation of cerebral blood flow results in loss of consciousness

Cardiac output reduced
- Due to loss of fluid from the circulation, e.g. haemorrhage
- Diversion of blood flow by peripheral vasodilatation

Effort syncope
- Cardiac output reduced, and cannot be increased adequately on exercise
  - severe aortic stenosis
  - severe ventricular arrhythmias in aortic stenosis
  - pulmonary vascular disease

Circulatory obstruction
- Sudden blockage by massive pulmonary embolism
- Intermittent obstruction by left atrial tumour

Pericardial tamponade – with more gradual loss of consciousness
Obstruction of venous return
- By coughing bout
- Fallot's tetralogy
- Valsalva manoeuvre
- Weight lifting

Arrhythmia
- Asystole
- Ventricular fibrillation
- Reflex inhibition of sino-atrial node
- Complete heart block: Stokes–Adams attacks
- Cardiac infarction
- Post-cardiac surgery

Simple 'Faint'
- Increased vagal activity
- Stimulation of carotid sinus, especially in elderly

Postural
- After prolonged bed rest: loss of peripheral vascular reflex control

Patients on adrenergic ganglion blocking drugs, on standing up, or on exertion
Spontaneous in patients with peripheral autonomic neuropathies, e.g. tabes dorsalis, diabetes mellitus
Following micturition, especially after getting up during the night

Cardiac Failure

Heart muscle damage
- Myocardial infarction
- Coronary artery disease
- Cardiomyopathies

Valve damage
- Heart valve disease, e.g. mitral valve stenosis
- Bacterial endocarditis

Disorders of rhythm
- Cardiac arrhythmias
- Ventricular fibrillation
- Ventricular tachycardia
- Sick sinus node syndrome
- Atrial fibrillation
- Wolff–Parkinson–White syndrome

Pericardial disease
- Constrictive pericarditis

Chronic Cor Pulmonale

Chronic airways obstruction
- Chronic bronchitis and emphysema
- Emphysema
- Bronchial asthma

Inflammatory lung disease
- Pneumoconiosis
- Tuberculosis
- Bronchiectasis
- Extrinsic allergic alveolitis
- Cryptogenic fibrosing alveolitis
- Sarcoidosis
- Radiation fibrosis
- Beryllium disease

Pulmonary vasculature disease
- Pulmonary thrombo-embolism
- Primary pulmonary hypertension
- Polyarteritis nodosa
- Schistosomiasis

Thoracic cage disorders
- Thoracic deformities including kyphoscoliosis, resulting in alveolar hypoventilation
- Thoracoplasty
- Pleural fibrosis
- Chronic neuromuscular disorders with impairment of ventilation

Angina Pectoris

Obstructive coronary artery disease
- Atherosclerosis
- Small vessel coronary artery disease
- Coronary embolism
- Coronary artery spasm
- Arteritis
- Syphilitic ostial stenosis

Increased myocardial oxygen demand with normal or abnormal coronary arteries
- Left ventricle
  - hypertension
  - aortic valve disease: stenosis plus regurgitation
  - hypertrophic obstructive cardiomyopathy
  - hypertrophic non-obstructive cardiomyopathy
- Right ventricle
  - major pulmonary embolism
  - pulmonary stenosis
  - pulmonary hypertension
  - mitral stenosis

Extracardiac cause: thyrotoxicosis

Defective supply of oxygen to the myocardium: severe anaemia

True angina pectoris
- Coronary artery insufficiency
- Calcified aortic valve stenosis (rare)
- Attack may be produced by –
  - physical exercise
  - obstructive lesion to coronary artery supply
  - increased catecholamine drive, leading to greater velocity of heart muscle fibre shortening
  - emotion leading to greater catecholamine drive
  - night pain
    - during rapid eyeball movements in sleep, with increased oxygen requirement
    - during tachycardia
    - during bradycardia

Distinguish from
- Massive pulmonary embolism

Acute pericarditis
Dissecting aortic aneurysm
Spontaneous pneumothorax

Clinical classification
- Stable angina
  - pain related to exercise etc., recovering with rest and glyceryl trinitrate
- Unstable angina
  - recent onset
  - progressive in frequency and severity
  - pain at rest
  - pain waking patient from sleep
- (Myocardial infarction)

Heart Disease in the Elderly

Myocardium
- Ischaemic heart disease
- Hypertensive heart disease
- Senile cardiac amyloidosis
- Acute myocarditis [R]
- Tumours: rare, and of these secondary deposits occur more frequently than primary tumours

Valves
- Degenerative aortic valve calcification
- Aortic stenosis
- Degenerative mitral calcification (primarily valve ring, but may extend to cusps)
- Mucoid degeneration of mitral valve ('floppy valve')
- Mitral stenosis
- Infective endocarditis
- Non-bacterial thrombotic endocarditis (often associated with carcinoma and other 'wasting' diseases)
- Aortic incompetence

Conducting system
- Atrial fibrillation: ? due to loss of muscle in the sino-atrial node and internodal tracts
- Sino-atrial block: often associated with senile amyloidosis
- Atrioventricular block: associated with degenerative calcification of the aortic valve or mitral ring
- Bundle branch block: associated with fibrosis

Drug-induced Cardiovascular Disease

Drug-induced arrhythmia
- digitalis
  - ventricular ectopic beats
  - ventricular tachycardia
  - ventricular fibrillation
    - (atrial fibrillation)

quinidine
phenytoin
procainamide
lignocaine
adrenaline
noradrenaline
isoprenaline
halothane: ventricular arrhythmia: sensitizes myocardium to the action of catecholamines
tricyclic antidepressants: anticholinergic activity
phenothiazines: anticholinergic activity

Depressed cardiac function
beta-adrenoreceptor blocking drugs, e.g. after cardiac surgery, or in incipient cardiac failure
quinidine, procainamide, lignocaine } depress myocardial excitability, leading to heart failure and hypotension

Drug-induced disorders of cardiac muscle
alcohol cardiomyopathy not responding to thiamine therapy
cytotoxic drugs
daunorubicin, doxorubicin } cumulative dose-dependent damage
emetine: in the treatment of amoebiasis
rarely during lithium therapy
? long-term high-dosage of phenothiazines

Drug-induced hypertension
salt and water retention, with chronic hypertension
corticosteroid therapy
contraceptive steroids
carbenoxolone
phenylbutazone
acute hypertension
interaction between tricyclic antidepressants and –
guanethidine
bethamidine
debrisoquine
blockade of antihypertensive action of clonidine
action exaggerated by beta-blocking drugs
phenylpropanolamine reacts adversely with monoamine oxidase inhibitors (MAO)
monoamine oxidase inhibitors (MAO) with tyramines in foods
noradrenaline
plus monoamine oxidase inhibitors
plus guanethidine
plus reserpine
high doses of dopamine

Drug-induced hypotension
phenothiazines (alpha-adrenoreceptor blockade) especially if given with antihypertensive drugs
central depressant drugs, associated with fall in blood pressure with postural change

Peripheral artery spasm
ergot-containing preparations used in the treatment of migraine
intra-arterial injection (accidental)
barbiturates
diazepam

Thrombophlebitis and venous thrombosis
following intravenous injection, ? with venous damage
antibiotics
amphotericin B
vancomycin
high concentration of glucose
diazepam
Oral contraceptives (less risk with low-oestrogen preparations)
High doses of conjugated oestrogens

CARDIAC CONDITIONS IN THE NEWBORN

Cardiac Malformations

Incompatible with survival of the fetus
Compatible with survival of the fetus, but not with independent existence
Compatible with independent existence for months only
Compatible with survival to childhood or adult life
with severe impairment of cardiac function
with little incapacity, but risk of –
1. bacterial endocarditis
2. reduction of life expectancy following excessive strain

Congenital Heart Disease

Physiologically trivial
Acyanotic without shunt
Acyanotic with shunt
Cyanotic

Congenital Heart Disease possibly correctable during the First Year

Ventricular septal defect
Double outlet right ventricle
Primitive ventricle

Total atrio-ventricular canal
Ostium primum atrial septal defect
Ostium secundum atrial septal defect
Persistent ductus arteriosus
Truncus arteriosus
Total anomalous pulmonary venous drainage
Fallot's tetralogy
Transposition of the great arteries: the commonest cyanotic condition presenting in the first few days after birth
Tricuspid atresia
Pulmonary atresia
- with intact ventricular septum
- with ventricular septal defect

Aortic stenosis – poor prognosis when presenting in infancy
Coarctation of aorta

Common Congenital Heart Defects found in Infants

Ventricular septal defect
Persistent ductus arteriosus
Atrial septal defect
Pulmonary valve stenosis
Aortic stenosis
Coarctation of aorta
Tetralogy of Fallot
- ventricular septal defect
- pulmonary infundibulum with or without pulmonary stenosis
- overriding of aorta
- right ventricular hypertrophy

Transposition of the great vessels

Congenital Heart Defects without Murmurs

With cyanosis
- transposition of great vessels
- total anomalous pulmonary venous drainage with obstruction
- hypoplastic left heart syndrome
- pulmonary atresia, with or without ventricular septal defect
- tricuspid atresia, with or without pulmonary atresia

No cyanosis
- coarctation of aorta
- cor triatrium
- primitive ventricle without obstruction
- anomalous coronary artery
- fibro-elastosis with myocarditis

Cyanosis in Newborn Infant due to Cardiac Lesions

Reduced vascular markings on chest X-ray

tricuspid atresia
pulmonary atresia
with intact septum
with ventricular septal defect (Type 4 truncus)
critical pulmonary stenosis with right-to-left shunt
Fallot's tetralogy (Infundibular hypoplasia)
common ventricle with pulmonary stenosis or pulmonary atresia
double outlet right ventricle with pulmonary stenosis

Increased vascular markings on chest X-ray
transposition of the great vessels
common mixing situations
1. Atrial: common atrium, often with atrioventricular defect. Total anomalous pulmonary venous drainage, especially if obstructed. Anomalous systemic venous drainage. Mitral atresia
2. Ventricular
common ventricle
double outlet right ventricle
aortic atresia
3. Great vessels
truncus arteriosus

Heart Failure in Newborn Infants

Obstructive 'left-sided lesions' which impede forward flow of blood into systemic circulation
1. Mitral and aortic atresia. Soon after birth, and inevitably with closure of the ductus arteriosus, the systemic output falls, leading to irreparable shock
2. Coarctation of aorta

Anomalous drainage: Total anomalous pulmonary venous drainage

Shunts
1. Dependent: some left-to-right shunts do not present until the pulmonary vascular resistance falls and pulmonary blood flow is sufficient to cause left ventricular failure
2. Obligatory: shunts between the left ventricle and right atrium in defects of atrioventricular portion of the ventricular septum. Pressure always leads to a left-to-right shunt

HEART RHYTHMS

Heart Block

Sino-atrial block
ischaemic disease, for example acute myocardial infarction
conducting system disease
digitalis
adrenergic drugs

Atrioventricular block above division of the bundle of His
- congenital
- ischaemic heart disease
- conducting system disease

Atrioventricular block at the level of bundle branches
- ischaemic heart disease
- conducting system disease

Cardiac Arrest

Complicating
- acute myocardial infarction
- hypoxia
- chronic ischaemic heart disease
- serious disorders of cardiac conducting system, e.g. recent onset of heart block
- pulmonary embolism
  - due to vagal overactivity
  - due to circulatory standstill
- acidosis
- carbon dioxide retention
- plasma hypokalaemia or hyperkalaemia
- cardiac tamponade
- hypotension

Bradycardia

Disorders of impulse formation
- Sinus bradycardia
  1. Non-cardiac
     - trained athlete at rest
     - elderly subjects
     - post-viral infection
     - increased 'vagal tone'
       - simple syncope
       - drug sensitivity
     - obstructive jaundice
     - drugs
       - beta receptor blocking agents
       - lignocaine
       - reserpine
       - digoxin
       - tranquillizers
       - cholinergic drugs, e.g. methocholine
       - anticholinesterases, e.g. neostigmine
  2. Cardiac
     - acute myocardial infarction
     - acute nephritis with acute hypertension
     - myocarditis
     - acute or chronic myocardial ischaemia
     - myxoedema
     - phaeochromocytoma

Disorders of impulse conduction
- Sino-atrial block
- Atrioventricular block above division of bundle of His
- Atrioventricular block at level of bundle branches
  1. Right bundle branch block
     - often of little clinical significance if found in isolation
     - congenital } disease within the
     - acquired } conducting system
  2. Left bundle branch block: always clinically serious

Complete heart block
- First degree: Abnormal delay in conduction of an impulse, but no failure of transmission. The heart rate is unaffected. May precede more severe block
- Second degree: some impulses conducted with or without abnormal delay. Remaining impulses completely blocked
- Third degree: All impulses completely blocked. Control of the heart beat is taken over by a subsidiary pacemaker below the site of the block

Impaired Consciousness

Bradycardia causing Stokes–Adams attacks
Vasovagal fainting attacks
Vertebrobasilar ischaemia
Epilepsy

Tachycardia

Sinus tachycardia: (110–200 beats per minute, gradually slowing following pressure on carotid sinus)
- Non-cardiac
  - anxiety state
  - anaemia
  - fever
  - pregnancy
  - thyrotoxicosis
  - carcinomatosis
  - drugs
    - alcohol
      - acute intoxication
      - chronic intoxication
    - thyroxine
    - adrenaline
    - isoprenaline
    - atropine and analogues
- Cardiac
  - acute carditis
  - untreated cardiac failure
  - acute myocardial infarction

Supraventricular tachycardia
- Atrial tachycardia
- Atrial fibrillation
- Nodal ('junctional') tachycardia
- Paroxysmal attacks
  - idiopathic (the majority)
  - causes as for atrial ectopic beats, especially –
    - rheumatic heart disease
    - ischaemic heart disease
  - digoxin intoxication
  - pre-excitation – Wolff–Parkinson syndrome

Ventricular tachycardia
- Ventricular tachycardia
- Ventricular fibrillation

Arrhythmias

Increased rate
- sinus tachycardia
- atrial extrasystoles
- atrial tachycardia
- junctional tachycardia
- atrial fibrillation
- ventricular extrasystoles
- ventricular tachycardia
- atrial fibrillation
- paroxysmal atrial tachycardia
- paroxysmal junctional tachycardia

Decreased rate
- sinus bradycardia
- sick sinus syndrome
- slow idioventricular rhythm
- heart block

Causes of Arrhythmia

Myocardial disease
Sodium and potassium imbalance
Gaseous imbalance
- hypocapnia
- hypoxia
- respiratory alkalosis

} all associated with secondary hypokalaemia

Drugs
- digitalis
- acute and chronic alcoholism

Arrhythmias in Acute Myocardial Infarction

Sinus bradycardia
Sinus tachycardia
Supraventricular ectopic beats

Supraventricular tachycardia
Atrial flutter
Atrial fibrillation

Sinus Arrhythmia

Repetitive rhythm change
- usually related to respiration
- rarely not related to respiration

Occurring in
- young subjects
- elderly subjects
- acute myocardial infarction

Sinus tachycardia

Atrial and Junctional Arrhythmia

Atrial ectopic beats
Varying pacemaker activity
Paroxysmal supraventricular tachycardia
Atrial flutter
Atrial fibrillation
- atrial rate exceeds 360 beats per minute
- ventricular rate slower

Ventricular Arrhythmia

Ventricular ectopic beats
1. Increase in frequency of unifocal ectopic beats increases with age in healthy men
2. Increasing in frequency in patients with heart disease

Idioventricular rhythm
- acute ischaemic heart disease
- chronic ischaemic heart disease

Ventricular tachycardia
- acute ischaemic heart disease
- chronic ischaemic heart disease
- idiopathic

Ventricular fibrillation

Atrial Ectopic Beats

Idiopathic
Drugs
- caffein, alcohol, tobacco } in excess

Thyrotoxicosis
Cardiac
- mitral valve heart disease
- congenital or acquired non-rheumatic mitral valve regurgitation
- ischaemic heart disease
- atrial septal defect

Pulmonary
- acute or chronic lung disease, including carcinoma of the lung
- thoracic surgery

Atrial Flutter

(In progressive disease, atrial flutter eventually leads to atrial fibrillation)
Rheumatic heart disease: especially with mitral valve lesions
Ischaemic heart disease
Atrial septal defect
Acute or chronic lung disease
Irritation of right atrium
- extrinsic cause
- intrinsic cause

Idiopathic paroxysmal flutter attacks

Atrial Fibrillation

Established
- Rheumatic heart disease: notably with mitral valve lesions
- Thyrotoxicosis
- Lung disease
  - acute
  - chronic
- Ischaemic heart disease
- Occurring in subjects over 50 years of age, and usually due to sinus node ischaemia, reflecting coronary artery disease
- Pericarditis: including constrictive pericarditis

Self-limiting attacks of atrial fibrillation
- As in established atrial fibrillation
- Idiopathic
- Post-thoracotomy
- Acute myocardial infarction
- Acute pulmonary embolism
- Acute generalized infection
- Acute pericarditis
- Intoxication
  - alcohol
  - caffeine
  - amphetamine
  - thyroxine
  - adrenaline

Ventricular Ectopic Beats

Idiopathic
Ischaemic heart disease
- acute
- chronic

Hypertensive heart disease
Myocarditis
Associated with
- ventricular hypertrophy: any cause
- ventricular irritation: any cause

Drugs
- digoxin
- quinidine
- procainamide
- amphetamine
- caffeine
- thyroxine
- nicotine

Adrenaline excess: in phaeochromocytoma
Hypokalaemia
- excessive use of diuretics
- excessive use of biogastrone
- anoxia
- shock

Physical unfitness
Following major illness or surgery

Ventricular fibrillation

Ischaemic heart disease
Anoxia
Hypothermia
Isoprenaline
Quinidine

MYOCARDIUM

Ischaemic Heart Disease Risk Factors

The many factors increasing the incidence include
- Hypercholesterolaemia
- Hypertriglyceridaemia
- Low plasma high-density-lipoproteins (HDL)
- Diabetes mellitus
- Hypertension
- Obesity
- High plasma fibrinogen
- High haematocrit
- Stress
- Cigarette smoking
- ? Water softness
- Sedentary behaviour, lack of exercise
- Resting tachycardia
- Minimal electrocardiograph abnormalities
- Personality type
- Short stature
- (The evidence against coffee is not convincing)

Myocardial Infarction in Young Women

Rare. Less than 1% of patients admitted with myocardial infarction in the UK

Atherosclerotic in origin – majority of cases
- Associated with
  - diabetes mellitus
  - obesity
  - hypertension
- Smoking: a risk factor acting with other risk factors in a multiplicative way
- Oral contraceptives: a risk factor. 10% of users with thrombotic episodes develop anti-ethinyloestradiol antibodies
- Hypercholesterolaemia is a much lower risk factor than in males, probably due to the higher HDL levels in females

Non-atherosclerotic heart disease: less frequent
- coronary embolus
- vasculitis associated with systemic lupus erythematosus
- dissecting aneurysm of coronary artery (this may occur during pregnancy)

Acute Myocarditis

Bacterial
- Rheumatic fever – related to B-haemolytic streptococcus Group A infection
- Diphtheria: ? in 10–25% of cases
- Pneumonia: occasional. May occur associated with *Mycoplasma pneumoniae*
- Associated with bacterial endocarditis in the elderly

Rickettsia
- Rickettsia myocarditis in 50% of fatal cases of typhus
- Q-fever

Parasitic
- Trypanosomiasis: South America: Chagas' disease, due to *Trypanosoma cruzi*
- Toxoplasmosis: [R]
- Syphilis

Viral
- Fetal heart damage
  - Rubella
  - ? Mumps
- Children and adults
  - Influenza (especially Influenza A_2)
  - Poliomyelitis (myocarditis found in 40–90% of fatal cases)
  - Coxsackie (most frequently Coxsackie B)
- Less common, or rare

During generalized viral disease
Psittacosis
Echo virus (9 and 30)
Rubella: T-wave changes in up to 20% with or without 1st degree heart block
Mumps: 5–10th day, partial or complete heart block may occur
Infectious mononucleosis: abnormal ECG may be found
Varicella
Infectious hepatitis
Rabies
Fiedler's acute isolated myocarditis ? due to virus

Fungus [R]

Collagen vascular diseases, e.g. polyarteritis nodosa

Toxic substances
Emetine
Chronic alcoholism

Cardiomyopathy

Congestive cardiomyopathy
Infective myocardial damage
Acquired toxic damage
Pregnancy in some cases
Systemic hypertension in some

Hypertrophic or obstructive cardiomyopathy (HOCM) (Idiopathic hypertrophic subaortic stenosis)
Inherited genetic disorder of heart muscle, with ventricular hypertrophy and small ventricular cavity. Compliance and contractile force are reduced

Obliterative cardiomyopathy
(Endomyocardial fibrosis, EMF)
Confined almost entirely to East and West Africa

Endocardial fibro-elastosis
Left ventricular failure, associated with damage to mitral valve, and aortic valve, including coarctation of aorta, also aortic stenosis. ? a distinct disease

Löffler's fibroplastic eosinophilic cardiomyopathy
The cavity of the left ventricle is filled with thrombus and masses of eosinophilic material. Persistent marked eosinophilia

Restrictive cardiomyopathy
Infiltration or fibrosis of the endomyocardium, resulting in restricted ventricular filling. [R]

Secondary Cardiomyopathy

Infected
Brucellosis

Histoplasmosis
Pneumococcal pneumonia
Mycoplasma pneumonia
Psittacosis
Rickettsial infection
Toxoplasmosis
Trichinelliasis
Tuberculosis
Coxsackie B virus

Endocrine and metabolism
Calorie protein malabsorption
Thiamine deficiency
Thyrotoxicosis

Other
Haemochromatosis
Systemic lupus erythematosus
Sarcoidosis

Rare Specific Myocardial Disease

Infiltrations and deposits
Amyloid
Primary
causing stiffening of myocardium and hence restrictive cardiomyopathy
Secondary
chronic sepsis
myeloma
paraproteinaemia
senile amyloid
familial Mediterranean fever
Mucopolysaccharidosis, e.g. Hurler's syndrome
Glycogen storage disease
Haemochromatosis: rarely affects heart
Leukaemic infiltration

Toxic factors and drug sensitivity reactions
emetine
alcohol
isoprenaline
sulphonamides
antimony
cobalt
daunorubicin
irradiation

Deficiency states
Vitamin B_1 deficiency, beri beri

Connective tissue diseases
diffuse systemic sclerosis

scleroderma
dermatomyositis
systemic lupus erythematosus
polyarteritis nodosa
rheumatoid arthritis

Inherited neuromuscular diseases
Friedreich's disease
Dystrophia myotonia
Muscular dystrophies
Cerebellar dystrophies

Other disorders
Sarcoidosis
Acromegaly (specific growth hormone effect)
Pulmonary vascular obstruction

CORONARY ARTERY DISEASE

Acquired

1. Atheromatous coronary artery disease (commonest)
2. Non-atheromatous coronary artery disease

Embolism – Mitral stenosis (thrombus) from thrombus
in left atrium
in left ventricle
Myxoma (tumour)
Aortic stenosis (calcium)
Infective endocarditis
Valve prosthesis

Ostial stenosis
Aortitis (syphilitic)
After valve replacement
Dissection of aorta
Isolated

Coronary dissection
Marfan's syndrome
Pregnancy

Coronary thrombosis
Smokers
Spasm of coronery artery

Microvascular disease
Polyarteritis nodosa
Other connective tissue diseases
Amyloid discasc
Diabetes mellitus

Iatrogenic
Coronary artery angiography

Congenital
Ateriovenous fistulas
Anomalous origin from pulmonary artery

ENDOCARDIUM

Infective Endocarditis

Infecting organism

1. Bacterial
   Predisposed to by moderate mitral valve incompetence
   May follow bacteraemia resulting from
   a. Dental extraction
   b. Genito-urinary procedures
   c. Rectal procedures
   d. Cardiac surgery, and cardiac catheterization
   e. Contaminated intravenous injections by drug addicts
   f. Bedsores for debilitated or aged patients
   g. Invasion by opportunistic organisms during immunosuppressive or cytotoxic chemotherapy
2. Yeasts: Candida
3. Rickettsia: Q-fever

HEART VALVES

Innocent Heart Murmurs

The murmurs are of low intensity, and audible over a limited area
The murmurs are of short duration, and occur in systole (except for venous hums)
The murmurs have a coarse vibratory character
There are no other signs of heart disease

Mitral Valve Disorders

Mitral valve stenosis
- Rheumatic fever
  - commisural
  - cuspal
  - chordal
- Lutembacher's disease
- Hurler's syndrome
- Endomyocardial fibrosis (rare: regurgitation more usual)

Mitral orifice obstruction
- Left atrial tumour: usually myxoma (ball valve effect)
- Left atrial bell valve thrombus
- Cor triatrium
- Hypertrophic obstructive cardiomyopathy with obstruction to left ventricular inflow

Mitral regurgitation
- Rheumatic mitral regurgitation
- Functional mitral regurgitation

Bacterial endocarditis
Congenital mitral regurgitation (cleft mitral valve)
Hypertrophic obstructive cardiomyopathy
'Subvalvular' mitral regurgitation
Libman–Sacks syndrome (SLE)
Endomyocardial fibrosis

Floppy valve syndrome
Familial: dominant inheritance
Connective tissue disorder
Marfan's syndrome
osteogenesis imperfecta
Ehlers–Danlos syndrome
pseudoxanthoma elasticum
Atrial septal defect of the secundum type
Old age
degeneration of connective tissue of mitral ring
myxomatous degeneration
in mitral valve leaflet
in chordae tendinae
Rheumatic carditis
Bacterial endocarditis
Papillary muscle dysfunction
Chordal rupture
Cardiogenic shock
Sudden acceleration: in air pilots
Ankylosing spondylitis: aortic regurgitation more frequent than mitral fault

Aortic Valve Disorders

Aortic stenosis
valvular
subvalvular
supravalvular

Aortic regurgitation
rheumatic heart disease
incompetence of congenitally bicuspid valve
bacterial endocarditis
syphilitic aortitis
dissecting aneurysm affecting ascending aorta
Marfan's syndrome
ankylosing spondylitis
Reiter's syndrome
pseudoxanthoma elasticum
associated with supracristal ventricular septal defect
mucopolysaccharidosis
systemic hypertension
trauma (e.g. decelerating injuries)

Tricuspid Valve Disease

Tricuspid valve stenosis
Rare in isolation
Uncommon component of multivalvular disease

Tricuspid regurgitation
Congenital: usually associated with Ebstein's anomaly of the valve
Traumatic: following rupture of a right ventricular papillary muscle
Following infective endocarditis
Carcinoid syndrome
Functional – secondary to right ventricular dilatation resulting from pulmonary hypertension

Heart Valve Vegetations

Rheumatic endocarditis: small firm nodules firmly attached to the lines of closure of valves and chordae tendinae
Acute infective endocarditis
large soft friable vegetations
valve may be ulcerated, perforated, or ruptured
Subacute infective endocarditis – after evidence of previous rheumatic endocarditis
bacterial
yeasts
fungi
Atypical verrucous endocarditis (Libman–Sacks endocarditis)
Disseminated lupus erythematosus. Small warty vegetations firmly adherent to any part of the valve cusp, frequently extending to the atrial or ventricular endocardium
Endocardial tumour implants
the majority of vegetations in malignancy consist of fibrin and platelets
very rarely the vegetations contain viable tumour cells (i.e. secondary deposits)

Non-Rheumatic Valvular Disease

Mucoid degeneration: floppy valve, prolapsing posterior cusp syndrome (affecting fibrosa – central collagenous plate of valve). The mitral posterior cusp is more commonly affected. Patients are prone to both spontaneous rupture and infective endocarditis

PERICARDIUM

Pericarditis

Includes
Acute fibrinous pericarditis

Aetiology	*Mitral*	*Aortic*
Congenital	stenosis	stenosis (with calcification)
	parachute valve clefts	
Degenerative		
in valve fibroma	mucoid degeneration ('floppy valve')	aortic stenosis
in valve ring	mitral ring calcification	
Mechanical		
dilated ring	stretch lesions	stretch lesions
atrioseptal defect	'Lutembacher syndrome'	
Genetic		
connective tissue disease	floppy valve	stretch lesion
storage diseases	thickening with mucopolysaccharide	thickening in xanthomatosis
Iatrogenic		
surgical		
drugs: methysergide	carcinoid-like thickening	carcinoid-like thickening
Miscellaneous		
carcinoid	fibrous thickening and contractures (left side involvement rare)	
amyloid	nodular thickening affecting any/all valves	
Inflammatory		
virus and unknown:	fibrous scarring and obstruction, contraction	
virus, unknown and thrombus:	rheumatic type of deformity with adherent commisures	

Pericarditis with effusion
Constrictive pericarditis

Causes

Acute idiopathic, or non-specific
Myocardial infarction
- associated with acute myocardial infarction, transient in 20%
- post-myocardial infarction syndrome

Dissecting aortic aneurysm
Connective tissue diseases
- polyarteritis nodosa
- disseminated lupus erythematosus
- giant cell arteritis
- rheumatoid arthritis
- rheumatic fever (in 10% of cases)

Familial Mediterranean fever
Infections
- bacterial, including tuberculosis
- viral, e.g. Type 8 Echo, Coxsackie B
- nocardiosis
- fungal
- histoplasmosis

Malignancy: especially with carcinoma of breast or lung
Trauma
Irradiation
Dissecting aneurysm
Uraemia
Myxoedema
Drugs and toxic actions
- hydrallazine
- procainamide
- practolol
- serum sickness
- methysergide

(Chylopericardium)

Constrictive Pericarditis

Infection

Tuberculous pericarditis
Suppurative pericarditis: acute pericarditis followed by chronic pericarditis
Uraemic pericarditis (uncommon)

Other causes

Sequel to traumatic haemopericardium
Sequel to non-penetrating chest injury
Irradiation of thorax
Connective tissue disorders, e.g. rheumatoid arthritis

Very rare causes

Post-myocardial infarction

Methysergide therapy
Familial Mediterranean fever
Secondary carcinoma invading pericardium
Histoplasmosis
Nocardiosis
Cholesterol pericarditis
? 'Virus infection'

BLOOD PRESSURE

Hypertension

Primary 'Essential' Hypertension: 80% of cases
Secondary (10–30% of cases: renal and blood vessels)
- Renal
  - chronic glomerulonephritis
  - chronic pyelonephritis: unilateral pyelonephritis
  - renal artery stenosis
    - fibromuscular narrowing of artery
    - atheromatous plaques
  - cystic disease of kidney, familial polycystic
  - analgesic nephropathy
  - renal embolism
  - nephrosis
  - acute nephritis
  - Alport's syndrome [R]
  - prostatic obstruction
  - renal transplantation (and renal artery thrombosis following transplantation)
  - haemangiopericytoma (very rare renin-secreting tumour)
  - Diabetic renal damage
- Blood vessels
  - arteriosclerosis
  - coarctation of aorta
- Endocrine
  - phaeochromocytoma
  - Cushing's syndrome
    - idiopathic
    - iatrogenic
  - Conn's syndrome (primary hyperaldosteronism)
  - adrenogenital syndrome
  - steroid contraceptive pills in a few cases
- Pregnancy
  - toxaemia
  - previous hypertension before pregnancy
  - nephritis during pregnancy

Miscellany
- Overtransfusion: iatrogenic, of short duration

Acute intermittent porphyria: in attacks
Acute phase of lead poisoning
Raised intracranial pressure: especially if acute, e.g. subarachnoid haemorrhage
Liquorice derivatives, e.g. carbenoxolone (iatrogenic)
Monoamine oxidase inhibitors followed by cheese
Hypercalcaemia
- hyperparathyroidism
- idiopathic infantile hypercalcaemia
- vitamin D intoxication
- milk-alkali syndrome
- acromegaly

Miscellaneous Causes of Acute Severe Hypertension

Steroid therapy
Burns
Liquorice ingestion
Rapid infusion of methyldopa
Guillain–Barré syndrome
Stevens–Johnson syndrome
Familial dysautonomia

Renovascular Hypertension

Atheromatous disease
Fibromuscular disease
- intimal fibroplasia
- medial fibromuscular dysplasia
- medial hyperplasia
- perimedial fibroplasia
- adventitial fibrosis

Tumour, Trauma, Aneurysm, External pressure } causing renal artery stenosis

Complications of Hypertension

Pulmonary oedema (in hypertensive heart failure)
Hypertensive encephalopathy
Cerebrovascular accident
Renal failure
Malignant or accelerated phase of hypertension
Microangiopathic haemolytic anaemia
Coronary artery disease
Aortic dissection
Fetal death associated with maternal hypertension

Hypertensive Emergencies

(*Indications for Emergency Reduction of Raised Blood Pressure*)

Central nervous system
- intracranial haemorrhage
- subarachnoid haemorrhage
- transient cerebral ischaemic attacks
- thrombotic 'stroke'
- hypertensive encephalopathy

Dissecting or leaking aortic aneurysm
Accelerated or malignant hypertension (associated with hypertension resulting from any cause)
Toxaemia of pregnancy (eclampsia and pre-eclampsia)
- convulsions
- left ventricular failure
- fetal distress

Left ventricular failure with high diastolic blood pressure
Angina
Myocardial infarction
Requirement for emergency surgery
Prolonged epistasis in patient with uncontrolled hypertension
Acute severe hypertensive attacks associated with phaeochromocytoma
Drug action
- overdose with amphetamine etc.
- monoamine oxidase inhibitor with adrenergic substances in the diet, e.g. blue cheese provoking acute severe hypertensive attack
- clonidine withdrawal

Endocrine Disorders associated with Hypertension

Secondary hyperaldosteronism
- Diuretic-induced hyperaldosteronism
- Renal and malignant hypertension
- Renin-secreting tumour [R]
- Oral contraceptives
- Pre-eclampsia

Primary hyperaldosteronism
- Adrenocortical adenoma (Conn's syndrome)
- Adrenocortical macronodular hyperplasia
- Aldosterone-secreting carcinoma

Excess of corticosteroids other than aldosterone
- Deoxycorticosterone excess
  - 17-hydroxylation deficiency
  - 11-hydroxylation deficiency
  - apparently isolated excess of deoxycorticosterone

Corticosterone excess
18-hydroxydeoxycorticosterone excess
ACTH excess: Cushing's syndrome
Liquorice ingestion
Carbenoxolone
Liddle's disease
Low renin 'essential hypertension': occurring in perhaps up to 25% of all cases of 'essential hypertension'
Phaeochromocytoma

Hypotension

Physiological: normal at rest in many people, especially in trained athletes

Pathological

- Acute
  - shock
  - blood loss
  - cardiac tamponade
  - myocardial infarction
  - primary fall in cardiac output
  - ectopic bradycardia
  - postural hypotension
- Chronic
  - hypopituitarism
  - hypoadrenocorticalism

Factors precipitating Postural Hypotension

- Reduction in plasma volume
  - dehydration
  - haemorrhage
- Myocardial insufficiency
  - myocardial infarction
  - dysrhythmias
- Sudden rise in intrathoracic pressure
  - straining at stool
  - bouts of coughing
  - micturition (e.g. after getting up during the night)
- Vasodilatation
  - hot baths
  - during rest following strenuous exercise
  - hot weather
- Decreased muscle movements
  - hemiplegia
  - Parkinsonism
- Sudden change from bending down to the vertical in the elderly

Drugs associated with Postural Hypotension

Hypotensive agents used in the treatment of hypertension
Thiazides
Phenothiazines
Tricyclic antidepressants
Butyrophenones, e.g. haloperidol
Benzodiazepines
Levodopa
Bromocryptine
Barbiturates
Antihistamines
Alcohol

PERIPHERAL CIRCULATORY DISORDERS

Aortic Aneurysm

Atherosclerosis: commonest cause
Post-stenotic dilatation: distal to annular atheroma
Post-trauma
Following bacterial infection: involving ulcerated atheromatous plaque
Syphilitic aortic aneurysm
(The diameter of the normal aorta increases progressively with age)

Ascending aorta
- due to atheroma in over two-thirds of the cases
- due to cystic medial necrosis of aorta in one-fifth of cases
- due to tertiary syphilis in less than one-tenth of cases in the U.K.

Descending aorta
- due to atheroma
- occasionally follows abdominal trauma

Atherosclerosis

Occlusive effects
- Coronary artery disease
  - angina
  - myocardial infarction
  - sudden death
- Cerebral artery disease
  - focal brain damage
  - cerebral insufficiency
- Iliac and femoral arteries
  - intermittent claudication
  - dystrophic changes in the limb
- Intestinal arteries
- Renal arteries

Weakening of artery wall
- aneurysmal formation
- dissection of layers of the aortic wall

Thrombo-embolism initiated on atherosclerotic lesion

Risk factors in atherosclerosis
- Hypertension
- Cigarette smoking
- Raised plasma VLDL and LDL (Very low density and low density lipoproteins)
- Risks inversely proportional to HDL (high density lipoproteins), i.e. HDL are protective

Thrombosis of Superior Sagittal Sinus and Cortical Veins

Local causes
- direct injury
  - fracture of skull
  - surgery
  - after injection into venous sinuses
- spread of infection from local site

General causes
- polycythaemia and increased viscosity of blood
  - dehydration
  - primary and secondary polycythaemia
  - sickle cell disease (HbS)
- thrombocythaemia
- slowed cerebral circulation
- dehydration
- septicaemia
- marasmus

Arteriovenous Fistulas

Congenital
- diffuse
- localized aneurysmal varices
- visceral arteriovenous malformations
  - pulmonary
  - hepatic
  - other sites

Acquired
- trauma
- connective tissue abnormality: Ehlers–Danlos syndrome
- neoplastic invasion
- mycotic aneurysm invading vein

Arterial Embolism

Cardiac conditions associated with embolism
- mitral valve disease with fibrillation
- ischaemic heart disease
  - recent myocardial infarction
  - ventricular aneurysm with thrombosis
  - fibrillation
- atrial fibrillation, e.g. thyrotoxicosis
- bacterial endocarditis
- atrial myxoma [R]

Vascular
- iatrogenic emboli (irrigation of clotted shunt)
- peripheral arterial disease
- paradoxical embolus migrating through patent ductus arteriosus

Pulmonary Embolism Risk Factors

Extensive trauma
Extensive surgery: especially
  hip surgery } especially in the first
  pelvic surgery } three weeks
Splenectomy
Myocardial infarction
Malignancy: especially adenocarcinoma
Previous
  deep vein thrombosis
  pulmonary embolism
Obesity
Elderly
Rare congenital conditions
  antithrombin III deficiency
  vein wall fibrinolytic activating enzyme deficiency
  homocystinuria

Fat Embolism

Fracture of long bones, especially femur, also pelvic fracture
Extensive trauma
Severe burns
Closed cardiac massage, i.e. from rib fractures
Acute pancreatitis

Raynaud's Syndrome

Primary Raynaud's disease: commonly in females, with over-reaction of digital vessels to cold
Secondary Raynaud's syndrome
  systemic diseases affecting smaller blood vessels
    connective tissue disease
      scleroderma
      polyarteritis nodosa
      disseminated lupus erythematosus
      rheumatoid arthritis
    diabetes mellitus
    carcinomatosis
  blood abnormalities
    sickle cell disease (HbS)
    circulating cold agglutinins
    circulating cryoglobulins
    polycythaemia
  arterial disease
    peripheral arteriosclerosis
    thrombo-angiitis obliterans
    arterial embolism
    trauma
      cervical rib pressure
      arterial trauma
      frostbite

vibrating tool damage
arterial spasm due to drugs: ergot

Cerebrovascular Insufficiency

Episodic
carotid artery insufficiency
vertebrobasilar artery insufficiency } possibly caused by
platelet emboli
cholesterol material emboli from atheromatous lesions
vessel spasm

Progressive
subclavian 'steal' syndrome
repeated embolism
progressive thrombosis
cerebral artery haemorrhage

Transient Cerebral Ischaemic Attacks

1. Reduction in cerebral blood flow due to sudden transient reduction in cardiac output from left ventricle
   a. Sudden arrhythmia
   b. Sudden transient hypotension
2. Sudden reduction in cerebral blood flow due to local cerebral vessel spasm associated with hypertension
3. Reduction of blood flow due to compression and temporary occlusion of arteries in the neck following head turning or neck extension in the elderly
4. Carotid artery stenosis
5. Platelet disorders
   a. Formation of platelet aggregations in atheromatous artery, with subsequent embolism into cerebral circulation
   b. Embolism of platelet aggregates formed distal to stenosed artery in neck
   c. Platelet aggregation in arteriosclerotic cerebral artery
6. Haematological abnormality
   a. Polycythaemia – grossly increased haematocrit with corresponding gross increase in whole blood viscosity
   b. Severe anaemia – poor cerebral oxygenation
7. Embolism of degenerated atheromatous plaque material into the smaller cerebral vessels

Arteritis

Infective
Pyogenic
direct spread of infection from

fracture
infected wound
mycotic aneurysm
embolomycotic
erosive
cryptogenic (rare)
Tuberculous arteritis
Syphilitic arteritis
Fungal
Candida arteritis
mycotic aneurysm

Non-infective
Connective tissue diseases
polyarteritis nodosa
disseminated lupus erythematosus
arteritis in rheumatoid arthritis
temporal arteritis (polymyalgia rheumatica)
amyloidosis of arteries
Takayasu's constrictive arteritis
arteritis in tissue transplant rejection syndrome

Acute Limb Ischaemia

Thrombosis in obliterative arterial disease
arteriosclerosis
connective tissue diseases
thrombo-angiitis obliterans
Arterial embolism
Arterial injury, including frostbite
Pathological dissection of artery wall
Raynaud's disease
Raynaud's syndrome
Drug-induced arterial spasms
ergot
periarterial injection of sclerotic solutions
Reduced peripheral blood flow
Severe anaemia or polycythaemia
Haemoglobin S disease
Frostbite

Leg Ischaemia

Acute
Arterial embolism
Arterial thrombosis
Dissecting aneurysm
Ergot poisoning
Trauma
Fractures and soft tissue injuries impeding blood flow
Frostbite

Chronic
  Associated with
    atheromatous disease, chronic obliterative arterial disease
    non-specific arteritis
    diabetes mellitus
    popliteal artery thrombosis
    thrombo-angiitis obliterans (Buerger's disease)
    coronary artery disease: one quarter of patients with intermittent claudication have coronary artery disease
    small artery occlusion
    cerebrovascular disease
    carcinoma of bronchus
    connective tissue disease, rarely
  Causing
    1. Intermittent claudication
    2. Pain at rest
    3. Local gangrene

Digital Ischaemia

Vasospastic ischaemia
  1. Abnormal reactivity locally
    hereditary
    idiopathic Raynaud's disease
  2. Endocrine
    phaeochromocytoma
  3. Hypertension

Organic ischaemia
  Arterial disease
    atherosclerosis
    thrombo-embolism
    cervical rib
    vibrating tool injury
    cold injury
    trauma
    thrombo-angiitis obliterans (Buerger's disease)
    aortic arch syndrome (Takayasu's disease)

Connective tissue disease
  Dermatomyositis
  Systemic scleroderma
    acrosclerosis
    diffuse scleroderma
  Rheumatoid arthritis: sero-positive, skin nodules, and Raynaud's phenomenon
  Disseminated lupus erythematosus
  Acute nodose polyarteritis

Blood disorders
  High titre of cold agglutinins
  Thrombogenic diathesis

High Altitude-induced Disorders

Mountain sickness: including pulmonary oedema and cerebral oedema
Retinal haemorrhages
High altitude proteinuria, associated with acute hypoxia

CENTRAL NERVOUS SYSTEM

Signs and symptoms
- Aphasia
- Mutism, aphasia and alogia
- Neurological syndromes caused by drugs
- Neurological syndromes in renal failure
- Migraine
- Narcolepsy
- Nystagmus
- Lightning pains
- Insensitivity to pain
- Paraesthesia
- Facial paralysis
- Retraction of the head
- Sleep disorders
  - Insomnia
  - Dysomnia
  - Hypersomnia
  - Sleep apnoea syndrome
- Tendon reflexes
- Trismus
- Vertigo
- Vertigo in children

Skull, Cerebrospinal Fluid and Brain
- Fractures of the skull
- Subdural haematoma
- Hydrocephalus
- Intracranial tumours
- Multiple disseminated calcification in brain
- Brain oedema
- Criteria for brain death
- Congenital and infantile hemiplegia
- Cerebral palsy
- Korsakow syndrome
- Transient ischaemic attacks
- Bulbar paralysis
- Higher cerebral function disturbance
- Pseudobulbar palsy
- Microcephaly

Epilepsy
- Epilepsy
  - Varieties
  - Complications
  - Causes
- Status epilepticus
- Temporal lobe epilepsy
- Post-trauma epilepsy
- Drugs known to precipitate epilepsy in susceptible individuals
- Epilepsy presenting in the elderly
- Fits and faints in children

'Attacks' in young children
Infantile spasms, mental subnormality and abnormal EEG
Rare complications of electroconvulsive therapy

Infections of central nervous system
Infections of the nervous system
Recurrent bacterial meningitis
Sterile (aseptic) meningitis
Encephalomyelitis
Viral encephalitis

Spinal cord
Spinal cord disorders
Spinal cord compression
Syringomyelia
Motor neuron disease
Lower motor neuron disease
Haematomyelia

Neuropathy
Peripheral neuropathy
Symmetrical polyneuropathies
Facial neuralgia
Drugs associated with autonomic dysfunction

Eyes and optic nerves
Ptosis
Diplopia
Reflex iridoplegia
Argyll Robertson pupil
Visual field defects
Papilloedema
Optic neuritis
Retrobulbar neuritis
Optic atrophy
Inherited conditions associated with optic atrophy
Optic chiasmal compression

Defects of movement
Tic – habit spasm
Localized involuntary movements
Tremor
Ataxia
Chorea
Hemichorea (hemiballism)
Myotonia
Myoclonus
Torsion dystonia (athetosis)
Involuntary movements caused by drugs
Parkinsonian syndrome

Limbs, gait etc.
Neurotrophic arthropathy – Charcot's joints
Absent knee and ankle jerks with extensor plantar response
Toe gait
Foot drop
Progressive weakening of the legs

Inherited muscular dystrophies
Episodic weakness
Inherited myotonia
Myasthenia

SIGNS AND SYMPTOMS

Aphasia

Posterior aphasia
- Wernicke's aphasia
- Pure word deafness
- Transcortical sensory aphasia
- Conduction aphasia
- Anomic aphasia
- Alexia without agraphia

Anterior aphasia
- Aphemia
- Broca's aphasia
- Transcortical motor aphasia
- Global aphasia

Mutism, Aphasia, Alogia

Lesions of cingulate gyri on both sides
Episodic mutism
- hysteria
- migraine

Electrical stimulation of ventrilateral nucleus, or in the region of the caudate nucleus
'Elective mutism' in children
Drugs
1. Phenothiazine therapy
2. Intracarotid sodium amytal injected into dominant side

Neurological Syndromes caused by Drugs

Peripheral neuropathy
- Nitrofurantoin
- Isoniazid
- Vincristine
- Thalidomide
- Rarely
  - Chloramphenicol
  - Clioquinol

Disulfiram
Gold salts
Phenytoin

Cerebellar disturbance
Carbamazepine
Phenytoin

Extrapyramidal disorders
Haloperidol
Phenothiazines
Tetrabenazine
Reserpine
L-Dopa

Epilepsy
See list

Neurological Syndromes in Renal Failure

Cerebrum
Acute and chronic encephalopathy
Seizures
Psychosis and affective disorders
Amaurosis
Cerebrovascular accident

Basal ganglia
Tremor
Asterixis (abnormal flapping tremor of hands – 'liver flap')
Rigidity
Akinesia
Oculogyria
Trismus
Choreoathetosis
Myoclonus

Brainstem
Cranial neuropathy
Central pontine myelinolysis

Peripheral nerve and muscle
Uraemic polyneuropathy
Restless legs
Myopathy
Muscle cramps

Migraine

Clinical varieties
1. Classical migraine: headache preceded by or accompanied by focal neurological symptoms

2. Common migraine: lacking clear-cut prodromata
3. Ophthalmoplegic migraine: attacks associated with paralysis of one or more oculomotor nerves, lasting for days or weeks after the end of the attack
4. Periodic migrainous neuralgia, cluster headaches, Horton's histamine cephalgia
5. Hemiplegic migraine
6. 'Lower half' migraine: episodic facial pain
7. Facio-plegic migraine: recurrent facial palsy with migraine. Very rare
8. Retinal migraine. Recurrent attacks of retinal ischaemia during attacks of migraine. Rare

Narcolepsy

Narcoleptic syndrome
- narcolepsy alone
  - psychogenic origin
  - myxoedema
  - extreme vigilance (e.g. sentry)
- cataplexy
- sleep paralysis
- hypnogenic hallucinations

Secondary narcolepsy
- encephalitis, including encephalitis lethargica
- cerebral tumours
- head injury
- cerebrovascular disease
- disseminated sclerosis
- cerebellar tumour

Kleine–Levin syndrome [R]
Pickwickian syndrome [R]
South African trypanosomiasis

Nystagmus

Nystagmoid jerks: No pathological significance. Results from following a moving object with the eye too far or too fast

Congenital nystagmus: Usually familial. The eye movements are non-stop and pendular, with the head often wobbling in the opposite direction to stabilize the gaze. The movements are lateral only and never vertical

Spasmus nutans: Occurs in early life. There are fast and variable movements of the eyes with compensatory head nodding. The condition is benign and lasts for a few years.

Distinguish from impaired vision due to –
- congenital macular disease
- congenital cataracts

total colour blindness
albinism
ophthalmia neonatorum

Nystagmus caused by vestibular disease
Nystagmus away from the side of the lesion
Central lesion of vestibular apparatus (often with vertical nystagmus)
multiple sclerosis
cerebral vascular accidents
glioma
syringomyelia
Friedreich's ataxia
Vertical nystagmus: also occurs
distortion of brainstem by extrinsic lesion
phenytoin toxicity

Nystagmus caused by cerebellar lesion
Nystagmus towards the side of the cerebellar lesion
Rarely
barbiturates
glutethimide
anticonvulsants
phenytoin
mysoline
tegretol
alcohol, with Wernicke's encephalopathy
post-head injury
trauma affecting labyrinth
trauma affecting VIIIth nerve
Continuous working in dim light results in 'miner's nystagmus'
'Searching movements' of the eyes occur in people born blind

Classification of types of Nystagmus
Non-voluntary oscillation of the eyes that tend to be rhythmic
vestibular
positional
gaze-paretic nystagmus
rebound nystagmus (associated with cerebellar involvement)
acquired fixation nystagmus
congenital nystagmus
periodic alternating nystagmus
dissociated (disconjugate) nystagmus

Related phenomena
Amblyopic nystagmus
Voluntary nystagmus
Convergence retraction nystagmus
Ocular dysmetria, square waves jerks, ocular flutter, frequently coexist in patient with cerebellar disease

Ocular bobbing, as in massive pontine damage
Ocular myoclonus: rhythmic oscillation of the eyes associated with synchronous oscillation of the palate [R]

Lightning Pains

Tabes dorsalis
Diabetes mellitus
Subacute combined degeneration
Sensory radicular neuropathy (especially alcohol)

Insensitivity to Pain

Congenital
Acquired: lesion in brain especially involving the supramarginal gyrus of the dominant parietal lobe, resulting in pain asymbolia
Associated with –
 Anhidrosis
 Riley–Day syndrome
 Peripheral neuropathy affecting unmyelinated and small myelinated fibres
  Leprosy
  Andrade type of familial amyloidosis
  Associated with carcinomatous neuropathy
  Hereditary and congenital neuropathies –
   not progressive
   progressive
   peripheral nerve axonal degeneration

Paraesthesia

(*Abnormal spontaneous sensations*)
Parietal lobe (cerebral) tumour, especially affecting the postcentral gyrus
Multiple sclerosis: usually in the form of numbness and formication
Migraine: paraesthesiae tend to develop shortly after visual disturbance
Tabes dorsalis: paraesthesia especially affecting the lower limbs
Haematomyelia: numbness and tingling may occur
Compression of spinal cord: symptoms depend on which spinal tracts are compressed
Toxic
1. Alcoholic polyneuritis
2. Neurotoxic poisoning following ingestion of shellfish containing dinoflagellates

Local
1. Cervical rib pressure: pain, numbness, tingling in the affected arm, relieved by raising arm above the head
2. Carpal tunnel syndrome

Facial Paralysis

Supranuclear
- cerebrovascular accident
- cerebral contusion
- abscess
- trauma
- neoplasm
- degenerative cerebral disease

Pontine nuclei
- neoplasm
- multiple sclerosis
- poliomyelitis
- motor neuron disease
- syringobulbia
- pontine infarction
- geniculate herpes

Lower motor neuron
- fracture of skull with associated VIIth nerve damage
- polyneuritis
- parotid tumour
- trauma
- Bell's palsy
- middle ear and mastoid infection
- neoplasm in the cerebropontine angle
- meningovascular syphilis
- herpes zoster (Ramsay Hunt syndrome)
- leprosy
- sarcoidosis
- leukaemic deposits

Muscle disease
- myasthenia gravis
- facioscapulohumeral muscular dystrophy
- dystrophia myotonica

(Congenital bilateral facial paralysis due to absence of the facial nerves (very rare))

Retraction of the Head

Meningism

Meningitis
- Bacterial meningitis
- Virus meningitis
- Spirochaetal and Treponemal meningitis
  - *T. pallidum* (syphilis)
  - *T. recurrentis*
  - *Lept. icterohaemorrhagica*
  - *Lept. canicola*
- Torula histolytica
- Sarcoidosis
- Carcinomatosis

Subarachnoid haemorrhage
- aneurysm
- angioma
- hypertension
- head injury
- cerebral tumour
- associated with generalized purpura

Pressure cone
- intracranial tumour
- intracranial abscess
- subdural haematoma
- extradural haematoma
- cerebral oedema
- hydrocephalus

Severe asphyxia

Intermittent neck retraction
- tetanus
- strychnine poisoning
- rabies
- torsion spasm
- spasmodic torticollis
- spinal and paraspinal disease

Sleep Disorders

Insomnia (Hyposomnia)
- Physiological, in the aged
- Pseudo-insomnia (sleep neurosis)
- Primary idiopathic insomnia
- Secondary insomnia
  - Situation factors
    - discomfort
      - bed
      - noise
      - temperature (ambient)
      - humidity
    - sleeping pill withdrawal, after prolonged use
    - stimulant ingestion, e.g. coffee
  - Physical factors
    - pain while lying prone or supine
    - itching
    - angina decubitus
    - sleep apnoea
    - hypermetabolic state
      - hyperthyroidism
      - hypoglycaemia
    - impending delirium tremens
    - nocturia
    - pregnancy
    - restless legs syndrome

nocturnal cramps or myoclonus
Psychological and psychiatric
tension and anxiety states
depression
acute psychosis
paranoid states

Dysomnia (abnormal sleep pattern)
Excessive bruxism and snoring
Somnambulism
Night terrors

Hypersomnia
Idiopathic
Narcolepsy with/without cataplexy
Daytime sedative or tranquillizer usage

Sleep Apnoea Syndrome

Central apnoea
Obstructive: loud snoring with daytime somnolence
Obesity
Large adenoids and tonsils
Laryngeal stenosis
Failure of the genioglossus muscle to open pharynx in inspiration during sleep

Rare causes
Bulbar poliomyelitis
Bilateral cordotomy
Ondine's curse syndrome
Shy–Drager syndrome
Muscular dystrophy
Pierre Robin syndrome
Bird-like face syndrome

Tendon Reflexes

Exaggerated
Symmetrical
excitement
anxiety
intoxication
Asymmetrical
pyramidal tract damage

Diminished
Transient
shock
haemorrhage
concussion
cerebral
spinal

deep anaesthesia
drugs affecting the central nervous system
severe infections with toxaemia
diabetic ketosis
hyperkalaemia

Persistent
Muscle disease
myotonia dystrophica (in late stages)
non-myotonic dystrophies
dermatomyositis
myotonia congenita
paralytic stage of periodic paralysis
Cerebellum
unilateral effect from an acute cerebellar lesion
Spinal cord disease
compression of cord
advanced motor neuron disease
syringomyelia
haematomyelia
intramedullary tumour
acute poliomyelitis
thrombosis of the anterior spinal artery
Afferent pathway disease
tables dorsalis
polyneuritis
malignancy
toxic
infective
Motor nerve disease
diphtheria
beri-beri
lead poisoning, etc.

Trismus

Local painful lesion in neighbourhood of jaw, e.g. abscess
Mandibular block with local anaesthetic
Encephalitis, e.g. post-vaccinal encephalitis
Strychnine poisoning: complete muscle relaxation between paroxysms
Tetanus
Tetany: only in very severe attacks
Hysteria

Vertigo

Aural vertigo
wax in external acoustic meatus
blockage of Eustachian tube with sudden changes in atmospheric pressure
acute and chronic suppurative otitis media
labyrinthitis
viral infection
bacterial infection – suppurative

otosclerosis
drugs – quinine, salicylate
impairment of blood supply
head injury
herpes zoster of geniculate ganglion
acute non-suppurative labyrinthitis
recurrent aural vertigo (Menière's syndrome) – membranous labyrinth dilated, with destruction of sensory cells in ampullae and cochlea
motion sickness
benign positional vertigo: attacks last a few seconds after sudden head movement or bending down

Eighth cranial nerve
acoustic neuroma
nerve compressed in
abnormal blood vessel
meningitis
meningovascular syphilis

Cerebellar vertigo
lesions especially in flocculonodular lobe
onset of thrombosis of posterior inferior cerebellar artery
primary intracerebellar haemorrhage

Vestibular neuronitis
Increased intracranial pressure, especially due to intracranial tumour
Tumour of fourth ventricle: triad of headache, morning sickness and vertigo
Ocular vertigo
giddiness at height
conversion symptom in hysteria
Vascular or neoplastic lesion of brainstem involving vestibular connexions
Transient ischaemia of brainstem
Multiple sclerosis
Vertigo – an aura in epilepsy: not uncommon in minor epilepsy of temporal lobe origin
Migraine: in attack
Benign paroxysmal positional nystagmus
Epidemic vertigo
Psychogenic
anxiety neurosis
conversion symptom in hysteria
'afraid of heights'
Severe anaemia } giddiness
Severe toxaemia }

Vertigo in Children

Temporal lobe epilepsy
Vestibular neuronitis
Migraine
Psychological causes

Sequelae to
- trauma
- meningitis

Benign paroxysmal vertigo Congenital deafness	No loss of consciousness. Abnormal response to caloric stimulation test

Hypoglycaemia
Cerebral lesions
Multiple sclerosis
Drug action
(Distinguish from an impending vasovagal attack)

SKULL, CEREBROSPINAL FLUID AND BRAIN

Fractures of the Skull

Simple
- Linear
- Depressed
  - dura intact
  - dura torn

Compound
- Linear
  - on vault
  - into ear or sinuses
- Depressed
  - dura intact
  - dura torn

Subdural Haematoma

Trauma to the head
- 'Battered baby' syndrome
- Whiplash injury to neck
- Direct cranial trauma

Intracranial causes
- Ruptured aneurysm
- Cerebral atrophy
- Drainage of hydrocephalus by shunting
- Meningeal metastates

Blood dyscrasias
- Plasma coagulation factor defects
  - primary
  - secondary
    - leukaemia
    - anticoagulant therapy
    - scurvy
    - D.I.C., acute fibrinolysis
- Platelet malfunctions
  - thrombocytopenia

primary
secondary
thrombocytasthenia

Hydrocephalus

1. Obstruction to circulation of cerebrospinal fluid
   Non-communicating
   block at foramen of Monro } due to intracranial tumour or congenital anomaly
   block at aqueduct of Sylvius } due to intracranial tumour or congenital anomaly
   block at foramina of 4th ventricle } due to intracranial tumour or congenital anomaly
   Communicating: interference at basal cisterna
   post-meningitis
   subarachnoid haemorrhage
   trauma

2. Defective absorption of cerebrospinal fluid (via arachnoid villi).
   There is a linear relationship between the rate of absorption of CSF and the intraventricular pressure between 68–250 mm CSF. Below 68 mm CSF there is no absorption
   thrombosis of the sagittal or transverse vein
   Guillain–Barré syndrome
   spinal ependymoma
   reduced numbers of arachnoid granulations

3. Increased production of CSF (rare)
   papilloedema of choroid plexus
   hyperaemia of choroid plexus in acute bacterial meningitis
   cerebral oedema
   (excess or lack of vitamin A ?)

Intracranial Tumours

Intrinsic
glioma
astrocytoma
ependymoma
oligodendroglioma
medulloblastoma

Meninges and cranial nerve sheaths
meningioma
acoustic neuroma

Developmental
haemangioblastoma
craniopharyngioma
epidermoid
dermoid
colloid cyst
chondroma

Pituitary
tumour

Cerebral metastases

Multiple Disseminated Calcification in Brain

Congenital toxoplasmosis
Glioma: calcification occurs in a single area
Cytomegalic inclusion disease occurring in infants and young children
Tuberose sclerosis

Brain Oedema

Vasogenic: increased permeability of brain capillary endothelial cells. Associated with
- Brain tumour
  - abscess
  - haemorrhage
  - infarction
  - contusion
- Lead encephalopathy
- Purulent meningitis

Cytotoxic: all the cellular elements of the brain (neurons, glia, and endothelial cells) may undergo swelling. Associated with
- Acute hypo-osmolality
  - water intoxication
  - acute dilutional hyponatraemia
  - inappropriate secretion of ADH
  - acute sodium depletion
- Severe purulent meningitis
- Cerebral hypoxia with acute cerebral oedema associated with
  - cardiac arrest
  - acute asphyxia

Interstitial: increase in water and sodium contents of the periventricular white matter due to movement of CSF across the ventricular walls. Associated with
- Obstructive hydrocephalus
  1. obstructive lesion in ventricular system (non-communicating hydrocephalus)
  2. obstructive lesion in subarachnoid spaces (communicating hydrocephalus)

Criteria for Brain Death

Unreceptivity and unresponsivity
No movements or breathing
No reflexes

Pupils fixed and dilated, with no response to bright light
No ocular movements in response to head turning, or irrigation of external ears with ice water
No postural activity
Corneal and pharyngeal reflexes absent
Absence of stretch or tendon reflexes

Late electroencephalogram
In the absence of hypothermia (body temperature above 32·2 °C)
In the absence of barbiturates or other cerebral depressants
Following a minimum of not less than 10 minutes of recording time with adequate adjusted apparatus

Congenital and Infantile Hemiplegia

Congenital [R]
- Difficult labour
- Vascular lesion during birth
  - fall in blood pressure
  - compression of artery
  - thrombosis in great cerebral vein
- Congenital – cerebral abnormality
  - porencephaly
  - aplasia of cerebral hemisphere
  - cerebral vascular lesion
  - following fetal encephalitis

Associated with acute infective disorders in childhood

Bacterial	
whooping cough, diphtheria, pneumonia, septicaemia, typhoid, typhus, scarlet fever	leading to cerebral venous thrombosis, meningitis cerebral abscess
Viral	
measles, chickenpox, smallpox, vaccinia	acute haemorrhagic encephalitis

Early childhood: of unknown cause
- ? Encephalitis or encephalopathy
- Haemorrhage
  - angioma
  - aneurysm
  - subdural haematoma

Slow onset: very rare
- Intracranial tumour
- Cerebral tuberculosis
- Diffuse sclerosis

Cerebral Palsy

Congenital diplegia – congenital spastic paralysis: probably the majority result from arrest in development or onset of degeneration in utero. Other possible causes include
- meningeal haemorrhage
- anoxia during labour
- rarely gross maldevelopment of brain

Congenital and infantile hemiplegia, rare: associated with acute infective disorders

Bilateral hemiplegia

Cerebellar diplegia (rare) due to hypoplasia of cerebellum

Minimal cerebral dysfunction: 'clumsy children'

Korsakow Syndrome

Gross defect in memory for recent events, with disorientation for space and time. Gaps in the memory are filled by confabulation

1. Brain damage
   - head injury
   - traumatic encephalopathy, e.g. boxers
   - post-anoxia
   - post-carbon monoxide poisoning
   - intracranial tumour
   - repeated epileptic convulsions
   - electroconvulsive therapy, in some cases
   - post-cingulectomy
2. Infections
   - syphilis
     - general paresis
     - cerebral leptomeningitis
   - acute encephalitis
   - acute post-infective polyneuritis (rare)
3. Deficiency, toxicity
   - chronic alcoholism
   - alcoholic polyneuritis
   - Wernicke's encephalopathy
4. Defective blood supply to brain
   - cerebral arteriosclerosis

Transient Ischaemic Attacks

Hypertensive crises

Hypotensive episodes

Anaemia

Polycythaemia

Episodic cardiac dysrhythmia

Intermittent compression of arteries

Subclavian artery 'steal' syndrome

Emboli
- from heart
- from great vessels

Bulbar Paralysis

Motor neuron disease affecting the medullary nuclei
Bulbar poliomyelitis
Acute post-infective polyneuritis, Guillain–Barré syndrome
Basal meningitis
Diphtheria
Brainstem infarction
Myasthenia gravis. (Bulbar palsy in thyrotoxicosis is almost certainly due to myasthenia gravis affecting the bulbar nuclei in a thyrotoxic patient)
Carcinomatous neuromyopathy
Metachromatic leuco-encephalopathy
Rabies (terminally)
Familial motor neuron disease (very rare)

Pseudobulbar Paralysis
(*a poor term for Spastic dysarthria, usually with dysphagia*)

Upper motor neuron degeneration in motor neuron disease
Gaucher's disease
Vascular lesions involving corticospinal tracts at any point above the medulla, e.g. arteriosclerotic Parkinsonism

Higher Cerebral Function Disturbance

Cerebral dominance
- 99% of right-handed adults: language and related skills lateralized to left hemisphere
- 20–30% of left-handed individuals: language and related skills lateralized to the right hemisphere
- The majority of left-handed adults: language and related skills lateralized to the left hemisphere

Left hemisphere disorders
- Dysphasia
  - Global dysphasia and concurrent impairment of many language functions, with widespread left hemisphere lesion
  - Nominal dysphasia – inability to name objects, but able to describe objects and their uses. Often left temporal lobe lesion
  - Expressive dysphasia
    1. Fluent – circumlocutory speech with a paucity and misuse of nouns. Left posterior temporal and parietal lesions
    2. Non-fluent – short utterances with omission of connecting words. Only key words in sentences. Left frontal lobe lesions
  - Receptive dysphasia – failure to understand spoken language, i.e. individual words, or meaning of words in the context of a sentence. Posterior left hemisphere lesion

Dyslexia – inability to read letters or words, with intact visual functions. Left parieto-occipital lesion if in isolation. Often associated with right homonymous hemianopia

Dysgraphia – either the spelling or the formation of letters is affected. Lesion in left parietal region.

Dyscalculia – loss of ability to carry out numerical calculations. Rare in isolation, but occurs with other dysphasias. Left parietal lesion

Apraxia – defect of movement or action, not paresis or sensory loss. Parietal lobe lesion

Agnosia

1. Failure to recognize objects
2. Failure to recognize colours

These failures are rare in isolation, and occur with other lesions

Short-term memory: short verbal messages can be retained for only 20–30 seconds. Left parietal lesion

Right hemisphere disorders

Visuo-spatial impairment (visuo-spatial agnosia). Failure to appreciate or manipulate spatial relationships between objects. Right posterior parietal lesion

Perceptual difficulties. Inability to recognize common objects photographed from unusual angles. Right parietal lesion

Memory disorders – amnesic syndrome

Bilateral cortical and subcortical damage

1. Left temporal damage – verbal memory affected
2. Right temporal damage – visual memory affected

Disorders of reasoning and problem solving – dementia

Pseudobulbar Palsy

Motor neuron disease
Bulbar poliomyelitis
Brainstem lesion
- infarct
- tumour

Myasthenia gravis
Diphtheria
Basal meningitis
Acute polyneuritis

Microcephaly

Some cases result from disorders at 12–20 weeks' gestation.

At mid-gestation brain cell multiplication ceases, and the cells differentiate into mature neurons

Irradiation of the fetus in-utero

Methyldopa treatment of mother for hypertension in early pregnancy (no effect before 16 weeks or after 20 weeks pregnancy)

- Virus infection in-utero
  - rubella
  - cytomegalovirus
  - other virus infections
- Fetus developing in homozygote phenylketonuric mother without proper control of mother's diet during pregnancy
- Mother treated with high doses of steroids with anti-mitotic properties
- Non-specific, unknown – ?

EPILEPSY

Clinical varieties
- Grand mal
- Focal
- Psychomotor
- Petit mal
- Inhibitory or akinetic
- Myoclonic
- Status epilepticus
  - grand mal
  - focal
  - petit mal
  - myoclonic
- Autonomic
- Reflex

Complications of epilepsy
- Trauma
- Suffocation
- Dehydration
- Electrolyte disturbances
- Uraemia
- Liver damage
- Pneumonitis

Immediate differential diagnosis
- Epilepsy
- Syncope
- Stokes–Adams attack

Causes
- Idiopathic epilepsy
- Post-trauma
  - immediate
  - early
  - late
- Intracranial tumour
  - primary
  - secondary

Cerebrovascular disease
- post-stroke, related to local infarct
- cerebral embolism
- hypertensive disease
- intracranial arteritis
- cortical thrombophlebitis
- general cerebral arteriosclerosis
- ischaemic fits in the very old (falling asleep upright)

Acute infections
- bacterial } especially in young children
- virus }

Extracranial disease – fluid balance disturbance, e.g. water intoxication
- electrolyte disturbance
- endotoxins
- exotoxins
- drugs
  - analeptics
  - withdrawal from barbiturates
    alcohol
    diazepam
- hypoglycaemia
- cerebral hypoxia

Status epilepticus

In an established epileptic
- reduced intake of anticonvulsant
  - reduction in adequate dose
  - lack of supply (e.g. on holiday, etc.)
- drug intoxication
- severe infection
- development of other causes of epilepsy

Epilepsy as presenting feature
- intracranial tumour
- central nervous system infection
- trauma
- intoxicant withdrawal – barbiturates, alcohol, diazepam

Temporal Lobe Epilepsy

Anoxia in early infancy results in sclerosis of medial part of the temporal lobe, including hippocampus (Ammon's horn sclerosis)
Infants
Porencephaly
Small vascular malformations
Traumatic scars in cerebral temporal lobe
Indolent gliomatous tumours
Cortical dysplasia related to tuberose sclerosis

Post-Trauma Epilepsy

Commoner in children than in adults, and especially common in under-5-year-olds

Early: occurring during the first week after injury
- 33% within 1 hour of injury
- 33% during the first day after the first hour
- 33% during the rest of the first week

Late epilepsy occurring after the first week
- Factors increasing risk of late epilepsy
  1. Fit during the first week
  2. Depressed skull fracture
  3. Acute intracranial haematoma
  4. Post-traumatic amnesia lasting more than 24 hours
- Occurrence
  - 50% during the first year
  - 25% delayed until more than 4 years after injury
  - Late epilepsy is focal in 40%
  - Once late epilepsy develops, it persists in 80%

Drugs known to precipitate Epilepsy in Susceptible Individuals

Baclofen
Cholinergic drugs
Cycloserine
Diphenyhydramine (and other antihistamines)
Isoniazid
Monoamine oxidase inhibitors
Niridazole
Phenothiazines
Tricyclic antidepressants
Sudden cessation of prolonged barbiturate therapy
Hexachlorophane

Epilepsy presenting in the Elderly

Intermittent heart block
Drug-induced hypoglycaemia
Uraemia
Cerebral tumour
- secondary (more frequent)
- primary

Cerebrovascular disease
Dementia
Meningitis
- infective
- carcinomatous (uncommon)

Fits and Faints in Children

Behaviour disorders
Syncope

Breath holding attacks
Migraine
Sleep disorders
Epilepsy
Infantile spasms (drop attacks)
Hypoglycaemia
Hypocalcaemia

'Attacks' in Young Children

Epileptic phenomena
- Neonates: fragmented grand mal attacks
  focal or multifocal twitching
- 1–6 months: fragmented grand mal attacks
  infantile spasms
- 6 months–4 years: 'benign febrile' grand mal attacks
  myoclonic epilepsy

Non-epileptic attacks
- Early months–4 years: breath-holding attacks with cyanosis
- 1st year: syncope of infancy: breath-holding with pallor
- 1–8 years: paroxysmal vertigo
- 6 months onwards: infantile masturbation

Infantile Spasms, Mental Subnormality and Abnormal EEG (*West's syndrome*)

Intra-uterine infection
- cytomegalovirus
- toxoplasmosis

Cerebral malformations
- hydronencephaly
- agyria

General and cerebral malformations
- tuberose sclerosis
- Aicard's syndrome
- 'happy puppet' syndrome

Perinatal damage
- hypoxia
- hypoglycaemia
- kernicterus

Inborn errors of metabolism, e.g. phenylketonuria (the commonest in the UK)

Postnatal damage
- meningitis
- encephalitis
- post-immunization

Cause unknown: ? 30% of all cases

Rare Complications of Electroconvulsive Therapy

Status epilepticus
Cerebrovascular accident

Nasal haemorrhage
Subarachnoid haemorrhage
Pulmonary
- prolonged apnoea
- aspiration pneumonia
- pulmonary embolism
- spread or exacerbation of dormant tuberculosis

Cardiac
- arrhythmias
- congestive cardiac failure
- myocardial infarction
- angina

(Unmodified electroconvulsive therapy)
- fractures
  - spinal midthoracic region
  - long bones, with risk of fat embolism

INFECTIONS OF THE CENTRAL NERVOUS SYSTEM

Infections of the Nervous System

Meningitis
- viral
- bacterial
- fungal
- protozoal
- yeasts

Parameningeal infections
- extradural
- subdural
- thrombophlebitic

Cerebral and intraspinous abscess
Encephalitis
Myelitis

Recurrent Bacterial Meningitis

Gross anatomical defects in central nervous system and its coverings
1. Congenital
   - myelomeningocele
   - midline dermal sinuses
     - cranial
     - spinal
2. Acquired
   - skull fracture into paranasal sinus
   - skull fracture into middle ear
   - Spitz–Holter valve

Parameningeal foci of infection
1. Chronic mastoiditis or sinusitis with osteomyelitis
2. Chronic brain abscess

epidural abscess
subdural abscess
4. Spinal
epidural abscess
subdural abscess
Impaired immune states

Sterile (Aseptic) Meningitis

Virus
meningitis } probably the commonest cause
encephalitis } of aseptic meningitis
Fungal meningitis: 'sterile' in the first few days when cultured on routine bacteriological media
Partially treated pyogenic meningitis
Tuberculous meningitis
Cerebral abscess } when there is no direct communication
Subdural empyema } into the cerebrospinal fluid
Eosinophilic meningitis – caused by *Angiostrongylus cantonensis* (rat lung worm)
Carcinomatous meninigitis
Leukaemia infiltration of meninges
Sarcoid infiltration of meninges
Syphilis affecting the central nervous system
Drug reactions, e.g.
PAS
post-myelography
post-spinal anaesthesia
radio-iodinated human serum albumin studies
post-lumbar puncture
Multiple sclerosis
Epidermal cyst rupture, with escape of cholesterol crystals into the cerebrospinal fluid
Uncommon
Mollaret's meningitis. Recurrent sterile meningitis, increased cell count, slight increase in protein ? exists
Behçet's disease
systemic lupus erythematosus
Vogt–Koyanagi–Harada syndrome. Recurrent sterile meningitis uveitis, depigmentation of skin and hair, dysacousis, and deafness

Encephalomyelitis

Post-infection encephalomyelitis
Smallpox vaccination
Measles
Mumps
Rubella
Varicella

Acute encephalomyelitis associated with –
Enterovirus

Echo
Coxsackie
poliomyelitis
Mumps
Herpes simplex
Herpes zoster
Infectious mononucleosis
Influenza
Varicella

Viral encephalomyelitis
Herpes virus simiae (B virus)
Mycoplasma pneumoniae
Cat scratch fever
Rabies
Lymphocytic choriomeningitis
Louping ill

Viral Encephalitis

Conventional, e.g. Coxsackie, herpes simplex, etc.
Temperate, e.g. subacute sclerosing panencephalitis
Slow, e.g. Jakob–Creutzfelt disease, and related conditions including
Kuru – disappears as cannibalism disappears
Scrapie – in sheep and goats
Transmissible mink encephalopathy

SPINAL CORD

Spinal Cord Disorders

Spinal cord compression: *see list on next page*
Development disorders
Spina bifida
Arnold–Chiari syndrome
Syringomyelia: *see* list
Infections
transverse myelitis
poliomyelitis
neurosyphilis
Multiple sclerosis
Motor neuron disease: *see* list
Carcinomatous myelopathy
Vascular lesions
angioma
haematomyelia: *see* list
cord ischaemia
cord infarction
Deficiency diseases
Hereditary disorders
hereditary spastic paraplegia

Friedreich's ataxia
Sanger–Brown ataxia
Marie's ataxia

Spinal Cord Compression

Disease of vertebral column
- Cervical spondylosis with protrusion of disc
- Dorsal (thoracic) disc degeneration
- Primary neoplasm
  - myeloma
  - angioma
  - sarcoma
  - osteoma
- Secondary neoplasm: carcinoma
- Osteitis
  - tuberculosis (Pott's disease)
  - syphilis
  - osteitis deformans (Paget's disease)
  - Staphyloccocal osteitis
- Trauma

Intravertebral (intraspinal) lesions
- Extradural abscess
- Neoplasm
  - extramedullary
  - intramedullary
- Pachymeningitis
  - syphilis
  - tuberculosis
  - pyogenic organisms [R]
- Meningeal infiltration
  - leukaemia deposits
  - reticuloses
- Meningitis circumscripta serosa
- Arachnoiditis
- Parasitic cysts

Syringomyelia

Communicating syringomyelia (syringohydromyelia)
1. With developmental anomalies at the foramen magnum and in the posterior fossa
2. Associated with abnormalities at the base
   - basal arachnoiditis
   - posterior fossa tumour
   - posterior fossa cyst

Syringomyelia as a late sequel to injury, infection, etc.
1. Spinal cord injury
2. Sequel to arachnoiditis confined to the spinal canal
3. Associated with spinal cord tumours
   a. intramedullary
   b. extramedullary

Idiopathic syringomyelia

Motor Neuron Disease

Classical adult motor neuron disease
1. Progressive bulbar palsy
2. Amyotrophic lateral sclerosis (ALS)
3. Progressive muscular atrophy

Inherited disorders similar to adult motor neuron disease –
1. ALS plus Parkinson's disease
2. ALS with dementia

Motor neuron disease with carcinoma

Childhood forms
1. Werdnig–Hoffmann disease
2. Kugelberg–Welander disease

Lower Motor Neuron Disease

Spinal muscular atrophy
- severe spinal muscular atrophy: Werdnig–Hoffmann disease
- intermediate severity spinal muscular atrophy
- mild spinal muscular atrophy: Kugelberg–Welander disease
- progressive bulbar paralysis (Fazio–Londe disease) [R]

Hereditary peripheral neuropathy
- hypertrophic neuropathy: peroneal muscular atrophy (D)
- neuronal type of peroneal muscular atrophy (D)
- hypertrophic neuropathy of infancy: Déjérine–Sottas disease (AR)
- hypertrophic neuropathy in Refsum's disease (AR) [R]
  - due to faulty metabolism in phytanic acid in green leaf foods
- peripheral neuropathy with spastic paraplegia (D)
  - with associated optic atrophy and retinitis pigmentosa (scapuloperoneal muscular atrophy)

Other peripheral neuropathies
- Guillain–Barré syndrome
- poliomyelitis
- relapsing polyneuropathy
- motor neuron disease

Progressive degenerative disorders of the central nervous system
- metachromatic leucodystrophy
- globoid cell leucodystrophy: Krabbe's disease
- neuroaxonal dystrophy

Haematomyelia
(Bleeding within the substance of the spinal cord)

Petechial haemorrhages
- poliomyelitis

toxic states
blood diseases with associated purpura
asphyxia
severe convulsions

Haemorrhages
- injury
- spinal concussions and contusion
- laceration of cord following fracture dislocation
- congenital abnormality
  - intramedullary angioma
  - spontaneous haemorrhage into a syringomyelic cavity
- haemorrhage follows central softening within the spinal cord in the cervical region following previously symptomless cervical spondylosis, often associated with acute flexion or hyperextension of the neck
- ? cause

NEUROPATHY

Peripheral Neuropathy

Genetic
- porphyritic neuropathy
- inherited primary amyloidosis
- peroneal muscular atrophy
- Déjérine–Sottas disease
- Refsum's disease
- hereditary sensory neuropathy
- neuropathy associated with
  - leucodystrophies
  - alpha-lipoprotein deficiency
  - beta-lipoprotein deficiency
  - Chediak–Higashi syndrome

Infections
- Viral: Guillain–Barré syndrome
- Bacterial
  - diphtheria
  - leprosy

Inflammatory and vascular disorders
- sarcoidosis
- polyarteritis nodosa
- Wegener's granulomatosis
- rheumatoid arthritis
- systemic lupus erythematosus
- systemic sclerosis
- vascular lesions in diabetes mellitus

Infiltrative conditions
- amyloid disease

- neoplasms
- xanthomatosis

Mechanical: local pressure

Drugs

- anticonvulsants: phenytoin
- chemotherapy
  - isoniazid
  - nitrofurantoin
  - amphotericin B
  - ethambutol
  - ethionamide
  - sulphonamides
  - clioquinol
- antimitotics
  - nitrogen mustards
  - vinca alkaloids
  - ethoglucid
- sedatives
  - thalidomide
  - glutethimide
- gold
- disulfiram (Antabuse, cronetal)
- others
  - imipramine
  - monoamine oxidase inhibitors
  - hydrallazine
  - stilbamidine

Foods

- alcohol
- cyanogens (cassava)
- lathyrogens

Chemicals

- metals
  - lead
  - arsenic
    - inorganic
    - organic
  - mercury
    - inorganic
    - organic
  - thallium
  - gold
- organic
  - solvents
    - *n*-hexane
    - petrol
    - trichlorethylene
    - carbon tetrachloride
    - carbon disulphide

dimethyl sulphoxide
insecticides
dieldrin
aldrin
2,4 D
DDT
others
trichlocresyl phosphate (TOCP)
acrylamide
diethylthiocarbamate
p-bromophenylacetlyurea

Symmetrical Polyneuropathies

Acute + Subacute
- Predominantly motor
  - Guillain–Barré syndrome
  - porphyria
  - diphtheria
- Mixed motor plus sensory
  - TOCP poisoning
  - acrylamide
  - thallium
  - vincristine
  - uraemia

Chronic
- Predominantly motor
  - lead poisoning
  - peroneal muscular atrophy
- Mixed motor and sensory
  - beri beri
  - alcoholism
  - isoniazid
  - nitrofurantoin
  - arsenic
  - carbon tetrachloride
  - paraproteinaemia
  - hereditary sensory neuropathy
  - systemic lupus erythematosus
  - Sjögren's syndrome
- Relapsing
  - predominantly motor
    - porphyria
    - relapsing Guillain–Barré syndrome
  - mixed motor and sensory
    - Refsum's disease[R]

Facial Neuralgia

Trigeminal neuralgia
Atypical facial neuralgia
Post-herpetic neuralgia

Raeder's neuralgia (paratrigeminal neuralgia)
Costen's syndrome (triggered by dental malocclusion)

Drugs associated with Autonomic Dysfunction
(including urinary retention, dry mouth, blurred vision, paralytic ileus)

Atropine
Hysocine
Amphetamine
Methyldopa
Phenothiazines
- with anticholinergic drugs
- with antidepressants

Phenothiazines or antidepressants
- with alcohol
- with barbiturates
- with narcotics
- with amphetamine

Monoamine oxidase inhibitors: especially with
- ripe cheese
- Chianti wines
- chicken liver
- pickled herring
- amphetamine
- sympathomimetics

Selenium sulphide

EYES AND OPTIC NERVES

Ptosis

Unilateral
- 'Hysterical'
- Voluntary – to suppress diplopia
- Pseudoproptosis
  - thickening of eyelids, e.g. oedema
  - extreme thinning of lids
- Weakness of levator palpebrae superioris
- Neurogenic
  - supranuclear
  - nuclear
  - infranuclear
- Congenital ophthalmoplegia (with superior rectus damage)
- 'Jaw-winking'
- Oculomotor palsy: oculomotor nucleus damage
  - brainstem glioma
  - aneurysm
  - vascular malformations
  - posterior cerebral artery damage
  - compression of cavernous sinus
  - encroachment on the supraorbital fissure

inflammation
neoplasm
retro-orbital mass
Ocular myopathy
Oculo-pharyngeal dystrophy
ophthalmoplegic migraine
diabetes mellitus
myasthenia gravis
slowly progressive hereditary ptosis
hereditary ataxia
tapeto-retinal degeneration
myopathies
Trachoma
Overaction of frontal belly of occipito-frontalis muscle
Paralysis of cervical sympathetic: Horner's syndrome

Diplopia

Nerve nuclei and nerve exit at brainstem
multiple sclerosis
tumours
intrinsic
extrinsic
vascular lesions
Wernicke's encephalopathy

Nerves at skull base
fractures
aneurysms
tumours
malignant infiltration
parasellar lesions
meningitis
bacterial, including tuberculosis
syphilis
carcinomatosis

Third, fourth and sixth nerves in the region of cavernous sinus
aneurysm
carotid-venous fistula
infection
trauma

Third, fourth and sixth nerves in the region of superior orbital fissure
tumour
granuloma
trauma

Third, fourth and sixth nerves in the region of the orbit
tumour
trauma

granuloma
myasthenia gravis
endocrine exophthalmia
orbital myositis
chronic progressive ophthalmoplegia

Cranial nerve damage
1. Third nerve
2. Fourth nerve
3. Sixth nerve
} muscles moving the eyes affected, impairing conjugate vision

Brainstem tumour affecting nuclei of cranial nerves III, IV, or VI
Hereditary ataxias
Multiple sclerosis
Ménière's disease during severe attacks
Migraine: transistory in severe attacks
Ocular myopathy
Exophthalmic ophthalmoplegia
Botulism
Hysteria

Reflex Iridoplegia

Pupil fails to react to light

Lesions of optic nerve
Lesion of optic tract: loss of light reflex in temporal half of ipsilateral and nasal half of contralateral retina
Lesion of upper part of midbrain
Lesions of third cranial nerve
Site of lesion unknown
Alcoholic polyneuritis
Chronic hypertrophic polyneuritis
Diabetes mellitus

Argyll Robertson Pupil

Reflex iridoplegia with small pupil, unaffected by light or shade, but pupils contract fully and completely on convergence, dilating promptly when the effort to converge is relaxed. There is slow and imperfect dilatation with mydriatics

Causes
Congenital neurosyphilis: fixed dilated pupils are more frequently found
Facial hemiatrophy: unilateral AR pupil may occur
General paresis: AR pupils common
Progressive hypertrophic polyneuritis: AR pupils found in a few cases
Peroneal muscular atrophy: AR pupils very rare
Tabes dorsalis: AR pupils common

Visual Field Defects

(generalizations)
Temporal lobe lesion, e.g. tumour: crossed upper quadrantic hemianopia

Occipital lobe lesion, e.g. tumour: crossed homonymous hemianopia

Parietal lesion, e.g. tumour: crossed homonymous defect more likely to affect the lower quadrant

Optic tract lesion: damage to one tract results in crossed homonymous field defect
Causes
1. Pituitary tumour
2. Tumour of base of brain
3. Aneurysm of internal carotid artery
4. Aneurysm of posterior communicating arteries
5. Inflammatory lesions, e.g. basal syphilitic meningitis

Optic chiasma
Pressure from below: upper temporal quadrant defect
Pressure from above: lower temporal quadrant defect
The pressure on the optic chiasma is rarely symmetrical, and the effect is therefore not symmetrical

Optic nerve: the field defect is limited to the eye supplied by the affected nerve
1. Papilloedema – there is enlargement in the size of the blind spot, with deterioration of visual acuity as optic atrophy progresses. Patients are liable to brief attacks of blindness, with ultimately permanent blindness
2. Toxic amblyopia: central scotoma

Pituitary tumour: bitemporal hemianopia is the most frequent lesion, which is usually asymmetrical

Multiple sclerosis: central scotoma frequently found

Tabes dorsalis
Usually peripheral field visual defect progressing to blindness
Less commonly: central scotoma

Migraine: gradually developing hemianopia in attack

Papilloedema

Increased local pressure, or increased intracranial pressure
Intracranial tumour
Cerebral abscess
Carbon dioxide intoxication: marked increase in cerebral oedema
Subarachnoid haemorrhage
Hydrocephalus: some cases develop optic atrophy
Exophthalmic ophthalmoplegia

Hypoparathyroidism
Craniostenosis: some cases develop optic atrophy

Inflammatory disorders
- Inflammation involving
  - optic nerve
  - optic neuritis
- Subdural empyema or effusion
- Meningitis
- Massive increase in cerebrospinal fluid protein content, e.g. Guillain–Barré syndrome

Circulatory disorders
- Cortical thrombophlebitis
- Major intracranial venous sinus thrombosis
- Venous obstruction
  - neoplasm of orbit
  - gumma of orbit
  - thrombosis of central retinal vein
  - cavernous sinus thrombosis (some cases)
  - traumatic arteriovenous aneurysm of internal carotid artery
  - intrathoracic venous obstruction due to
    - neoplasm
    - aortic aneurysm
- Oedema associated with disease of retinal arteries and retina, e.g.
  - malignant hypertension
  - giant cell arteritis
- Severe
  - anaemia
  - polycythaemia
    - primary
    - secondary

Other causes
- Disseminated lupus erythematosus
- Carcinomatous neuropathy
- Reticuloses
- Infective endocarditis
- Multiple sclerosis: slight papilloedema may occur. Optic neuritis frequently

Inherited conditions, in which papilloedema may occur
- Albright's disease
- Apert's syndrome
- Chediak–Higashi syndrome
- Crouzon's craniofacial dysostosis [R]
- Cystic fibrosis
- Hypophosphatasia
- Incontinentia pigmenti
- Neurofibromatosis

Optic Neuritis

Demyelinating disease
- multiple sclerosis
- postinfection encephalomyelitis
- neuromyelitis opticans (Devic's disease)
- diffuse periaxial encephalitis (Schilder's disease)

Systemic infection
- virus
  - poliomyelitis
  - influenza
  - mumps
  - measles
  - chickenpox
  - infectious mononucleosis
- bacterial
  - pneumonia
  - rarely other infections

Nutritional and metabolic
- diabetes mellitus
- pernicious anaemia
- malignancy
- hyperthyroidism

Hereditary atrophy of the optic nerve (Leber's disease)

Local disease affecting optic nerve
- sinusitis
- meningitis
  - purulent
  - tuberculous
  - syphilitic
- orbital inflammation
- intraocular chorioretinitis
- syphilis

Toxic amblyopia
- tobacco
- methanol
- quinine
- arsenic
- salicylate
- lead

Miscellany
- blood dyscrasias
- trauma
- ischaemia

Retrobulbar Neuritis

Demyelinating diseases
- multiple sclerosis: 25–50% of cases
- late neurosyphilis
- toxic amblyopia

Leber's optic atrophy
diabetes mellitus
vitamin deficiency states
(Optic neuritis occurring far enough behind the optic disc for no early optic disc changes to be visible)

Optic Atrophy

Vascular
- central retinal vein occlusion
- retinal artery occlusion
- arteriosclerotic changes affecting the optic nerve
  - faulty blood supply
- sudden severe blood loss

Degeneration
- secondary to retinal disease
  - retinitis
  - choroidoretinitis
- systemic cerebromacular degeneration
- secondary to papilloedema
- secondary to optic neuritis and retrobulbar neuritis
  - tobacco
  - lead (occasional)
  - organic arsenicals
  - methylmercuric iodide
  - methyl alcohol
  - carbon disulphide
  - thallium
  - quinine
  - some insecticides
  - aspidium (*Dryopteris filix-mas*)
- pressure on the optic nerve
  - aneurysm on the anterior part of Circle of Willis
  - bony pressure at the optic foramen
    - osteitis deformans (uncommon)
    - craniostenosis
  - intraorbital tumour
  - intracranial tumour
  - adhesive constricting basal arachnoiditis
- toxic: end-result of toxic amblyopia
- metabolic disorders
  - diabetes mellitus
  - ganglioside storage diseases
- trauma – direct injury to the optic nerve
  - nerve severed
  - nerve avulsed
  - nerve contused
- glaucoma

Deficiency states
- vitamin B_{12} deficiency neuropathy
- other nutritional deficiency neuropathies

Other conditions
- syphilis
  1. congenital neurosyphilis
     a. secondary to choroidoretinitis
     b. secondary to involvement from basal syphilitic meningitis
  2. tabes dorsalis
  3. general paresis
- multiple sclerosis – some degree of optic atrophy may occur

Inherited Conditions associated with Optic Atrophy

Albright's disease
Apert's syndrome
Behr's hereditary optic atrophy (AR)
Charcot–Marie–Tooth disease
Cockayne's syndrome
Cri-du-chat syndrome
Crouzon's craniofacial dysostosis
Juvenile diabetes mellitus with optic atrophy
Friedreich's ataxia (occasional)
Glucose-6-phosphate dehydrogenase deficiency
Homocystinuria
Hyperostosis corticalis generalisata
Hyperostosis frontalis interna
Hypertelorism
Hypophosphatasia
Incontinentia pigmentosa (Bloch–Sulzberger's syndrome)
Krabbe's disease
Leber's optic atrophy (? X-linked)
Menke's disease
Microcephaly
Naegele's syndrome
Necrotizing encephalopathy
Neurofibromatosis
Optic atrophy with demyelinating disease of the central nervous system
Optic atrophy, cataract and neurological disorders
Optico-cochleo-dentate degeneration
Osteopetrosis
Pelizaeus–Merzbacher's disease
Acute intermittent porphyria
Porphyria with conjuctival-scleral necrosis
Progressive muscular atrophy
Rubinstein–Taybi syndrome
Congenital infantile hereditary optic atrophy (AR)
Retinitis pigmentosa – dominant inheritance form
Cerebromacular degeneration – Tay–Sachs disease, amaurotic familial idiocy (AR)
Hereditary ataxias – Sanger–Brown and Marie's ataxia
- Hereditary spastic paraplegia
- Congenital diplegia [R]

Optic Chiasmal Compression

Pituitary tumour: chromophobe adenoma (rarely basophil adenoma)
Craniopharyngioma
Meningioma
Glioma
Chordoma
Epidermoid
Dermoid
Metastatic tumour
Bone tumour
Acromegaly
Arterial aneurysm

DEFECTS OF MOVEMENT

Tic – Habit Spasm

Increasing with excitement and stress, ceasing during sleep
Present in at least 25% of normal children, especially between the ages of 5 and 12 years. Distinguish from rheumatic (Sydenham's) chorea
- Abnormal: Gilles de la Tourette syndrome. Grotesque movements with uncontrolled sounds, and even expletives

Localized Involuntary Movements

Hemifacial spasm
- majority, cause unknown
- minority
  - post-Bell's palsy
  - compression of VIIth nerve
    - Paget's disease
    - acoustic neuroma
    - posterior fossa angioma

Facial myokymia: associated with
- multiple sclerosis
- intrinsic brainstem tumour

Blepharospasm
- unknown cause, occurring in middle or old age
- Parkinson's disease
- torsion dystonia
- neuroleptic drugs

Orofacial spasm
- elderly
- chronic psychiatric disorders
- prolonged neuroleptic drug therapy

Huntington's chorea
torsion dystonia

Palatal myoclonus
vascular lesion or tumour in region of red nucleus, olive or dentate nucleus

Spasmodic torticollis
idiopathic spasmodic torticollis (majority of cases)
trauma or infection of cervical spine
intermittent torticollis in infant, may be in association with hiatus hernia
dystonia musculorum deformans

Writer's cramp
joint disease
carpal tunnel syndrome
spastic hand
ataxic hand
Parkinson's disease
benign essential tremor
torsion dystonia

Tremor

Tremor at rest
Parkinson's disease
Post-encephalitic Parkinsonism
Drug-induced Parkinsonism
Rarely associated with cerebral tumour

Postural tremor
Physiological
Exaggerated physiological tremor
anxiety states
thyrotoxicosis
drugs (e.g. tricyclic antidepressants)
alcohol
heavy metals (e.g. mercury)
Benign essential familial tremor
Structural brain disease
severe cerebellar damage
hepato-lenticular degeneration (Wilson's disease)
neurosyphilis

Intention tremor
Brainstem or cerebellar disease
multiple sclerosis
spinocerebellar degeneration
vascular disease
tumour

Ataxia

Sensory ataxia – incoordination of movement which occurs in a limb or limbs as a result of sensory loss
Cerebellar ataxia – incoordination of movement which occurs in a limb or limbs as a result of loss of normal postural control

Sensory ataxia

1. Polyneuritis
    - diphtheria
    - diabetes mellitus
    - visceral carcinoma
    - polyarteritis nodosa
    - Hodgkin's disease
    - alcoholism
    - arsenical poisoning
    - polyneuritis of Guillain–Barré
    - familial hypertrophic polyneuritis
    - acute porphyria [R]

   Familial ataxias
    - lipid disorders
        - phytanic acid storage disease (Refsum's disease)
        - A-beta-lipoproteinaemia
        - beta-galactosidase deficiency
        - juvenile arylsulphatase A deficiency
    - aminoaciduria
        - Hartnup's disease
        - maple syrup disease
        - gamma-glutamyl-cysteinyl transferase deficiency
    - oxidative metabolism
        - pyruvate dehydrogenase deficiency
        - 'ragged red' neuromuscular disorder
        - Abnormalities of cytochrome-b or NADH oxidation [R]
        - moderate hypoxanthine-guanine phosphoribosyl transferase deficiency
2. Posterior columns of spinal cord
    - tabes dorsalis
    - subacute combined degeneration
    - multiple sclerosis
    - Friedreich's ataxia (generally recessive, rarely dominant)
    - West Africa – dietary cyanide from poorly prepared cassava
3. Cerebellar
    - Midline floculonodular lobe of cerebellum damage results in trunk ataxia
    - Multiple sclerosis
    - Posterior inferior cerebellar artery thrombosis
    - Cerebellar degeneration
        - Schilder's disease
            - cerebromacular degeneration
            - Pelizaus–Merzbacher's disease
            - congenital ataxia

- Hereditary ataxias
  - hereditary spastic paraplegia
  - Sanger–Brown's ataxia
  - Marie's ataxia (? a mixed group which includes Friedreich's ataxia and Sanger–Brown's types)
  - Roussy–Lévy syndrome (hereditary areflexia with amyotrophy)
- Multiple sclerosis
- Head injury, e.g. multiple injury in boxers
- Brain tumour
- Cerebellar abscess
- Encephalomyelitis
- Progressive familial myoclonic epilepsy (AR)
- Hypoglycaemia – especially in childhood
- Uraemia
- Liver disease
- Mercury poisoning
- Pellagra
- Dinoflagellate poisoning (after eating mussels or other contaminated shellfish)
- Virus infection
  - chickenpox
  - other viruses
- Typhus infection: a few cases
- Drugs and chemicals
- 'Hysteria'

Chorea

- Sydenham's chorea
  - Occurring in childhood
  - Chorea gravidarum
- Senile chorea
- Huntington's chorea
- Symptomatic chorea
  - Thyrotoxicosis
  - Systemic lupus erythematosus
  - Polycythaemia rubra vera
  - Idiopathic hypoparathyroidism and osteomalacia
  - Encephalitis lethargica
  - Cirrhosis
  - Drug-induced
    - neuroleptics
    - phenytoin
    - phenothiazines
    - contraceptive pill (may be associated with chorea in women with a history of previous Sydenham's chorea)
    - levodopa

Hemichorea (Hemiballism)

Children with Sydenham's chorea

Capsular hemiplegia
Stereotactic thalamotomy
Elderly hypertensive diabetics, of sudden onset, associated with a vascular lesion in the contralateral subthalamic nucleus
Tumour in region of subthalamic nucleus [R]
Subthalamic nucleus infarction

Myotonia
(*Continuous active muscle contraction persisting after cessation of voluntary effort or stimulation*)

Myotonia congenita
Dystrophia myotonica
Paramyotonia congenita

Myoclonus

Idiopathic epilepsy
Progressive myoclonic epilepsy
- Familial myoclonic epilepsy
- Lafora body disease
- Lipidoses
- Spinocerebellar degeneration

Myoclonus in metabolic disorders, with or without seizures –
- Renal failure
- Hepatic failure
- Respiratory failure
- Alcohol withdrawal
- Drug withdrawal

Myoclonus without seizures, with structural brain disease
- Encephalitis lethargica
- Creuzfeldt–Jakob disease
- Subacute sclerosing leucoencephalitis
- Infantile myoclonic encephalopathy
- Post-cerebral anoxia

Idiopathic benign essential familial myoclonus

Segmental myoclonus
- Subacute myoclonic spinal neuronitis
- Spinal cord tumours
- Spinal cord trauma

Other forms of myoclonus
- Palatal myoclonus
- Hemifacial spasm
- Facial myokymia
- Epilepsia partialis continua

Torsion Dystonia
(*Athetosis*)

Symptomatic

Perinatal trauma
- cerebral anoxia
- kernicterus

Athetoid cerebral palsy
Encephalitis lethargica
Hepatolenticular degeneration (Wilson's disease)
Lesch–Nyhan syndrome
Juvenile Huntington's disease
Hallervorden–Spatz disease
Drug-induced dystonia
- neuroleptics (uncommon complication)
- phenothiazines
- butyrophenones
- diazoxide
- metoclopramide
- levodopa

Idiopathic
- Idiopathic dystonia musculorum deformans: sporadic
- Dystonia musculorum deformans: autosomal recessive
- Dystonia musculorum deformans: autosomal dominant
- Paroxysmal dystonia: paroxysmal choreoathetosis

Unilateral
- Capsular hemiplegia – post-hemiplegic dystonia
- Post-stereotactic thalamotomy

Focal
- Spasmodic torticollis
- Benign hemifacial spasm
- Blepharospasm

Involuntary Movements caused by Drugs

Tremor
- Bronchodilators
- Tricyclics
- Lithium

Pseudo-Parkinsonism
- Reserpine
- Tetrabenazine
- Phenothiazines
- Butyrophenones

Acute dystonia
- Phenothiazines
- Butyrophenones
- Metoclopramide
- Diazoxide

} especially in children and young adults

Akathisia (inability to sit down)
- Phenothiazines
- Butyrophenones

Tardive dyskinesias
Phenothiazines } especially in
Butyrophenones } the elderly

Parkinsonian Syndrome
(*Tremor, rigidity and hypokinesia*)

Idiopathic paralysis agitans: Parkinson's disease
Arteriosclerotic Parkinsonism
Post-encephalitic Parkinsonism
Head injury: 'punch drunk' syndrome in boxers developing after repeated multiple brain injuries
Carbon monoxide poisoning
Manganese poisoning
Hereditary or familial forms: [R]
Drug-induced
- prolonged reserpine therapy
- phenothiazines
- haloperidol
- methyldopa
- tetrabenzene

Parkinsonism with other specific signs and symptoms
- progressive supranuclear palsy
- Shy-Drager syndrome
- olivo-ponto-cerebellar degeneration
- hepatolenticular degeneration
- Huntingdon's chorea: rigid form
- phenylketonuria

Parkinsonism with widespread brain damage
- head injury
- cerebral anoxia
- Alzheimer's disease
- presenile dementia
- cerebrovascular disease
- Creutzfeld-Jakob disease

LIMBS, GAIT ETC.

Neurotrophic Arthropathy (Charcot's Joints)

Tabes dorsalis
Syringomyelia
Diabetes mellitus
Rare causes
- congenital neuropathy
- congenital indifference to pain
- familial dysautonomia (Riley–Day syndrome)
- spinal cord lesions
- leprosy
- yaws
- repeated intra-articular steroid injections

Absent Knee and Ankle Jerks with Extensor Plantar Response

Subacute combined degeneration
Syphilitic taboparesis
Friedreich's ataxia
Motor neuron disease
Diabetic amyotrophy

Toe Gait

Normal in early stages of walking
Muscular dystrophies
- Duchenne type
- mild limb girdle forms

Motor neuropathies: peroneal muscular atrophy
Spastic syndromes
- cerebral diplegia
- spastic paraparesis

Foot Drop

Lateral popliteal nerve palsy
Nerve root lesions
Cerebral infarct
Motor neuron disease
Multiple sclerosis

Progressive Weakening of the Legs

Acute paraplegia
- trauma
- spinal compression, including
  - tumour
  - angioma
  - epidural abscess
  - cord infarction
  - myelitis
    - inflammatory
    - demyelinating
  - acute polyneuritis

Chronic spastic paraplegia
- spinal compression
- multiple sclerosis
- spondylitic myelopathy
- motor neuron disease
- syringomyelia
- prolapsed dorsal discs
- subacute combined degeneration

Unilateral spastic weakness
- lesions affecting spinal cord, connections to the motor cortex, or the motor cortex.

Inherited Muscular Dystrophies

Duchenne type: pelvic girdle severe: (XR)
Becker type: pelvic girdle mild (XR)
Limb girdle: pelvic girdle mild: (AR)
Scapulohumeral: (AR)
Fascioscapulohumeral: (D)
Ocular: oculopharyngeal: (D)

Episodic Weakness

Periodic paralysis
Relapsing polyneuropathy
Dermatomyositis
Polymyositis
Myasthenia gravis
Rhabdomyolysis

Inherited Myotonia

Myotonia congenita: Thomsen's disease: (AD) (AR)
Paramyotonia congenita: Eulenburg's disease
Dystrophia myotonica: Steinert's disease: (AD)
Congenital dystrophia myotonica: (AD)

Myasthenia

Transient neonatal myasthenia: in infant born to myasthenic mother
Congenital or infantile myasthenia in child of non-myasthenic mother [R]
Juvenile myasthenia: no associated thymoma
Adult myasthenia

DERMATOLOGY

Malignancy
- Neoplasms of the skin
- Factors predisposing to squamous cell carcinoma
- Tumours associated with dermatomyositis
- Cutaneous manifestations of malignancy

Skin infections and infestations
- Skin infections
- Skin infestations

Lips, genitalia
- Diseases of the lips
- Genital ulceration

Sweat glands
- Disorders of sweat glands
- Hyperhidrosis

Hair
- Hair loss
- Alopecia
- Hair fall (telogen effluvium)
- Broken hairs (anagen effluvium)
- Diffuse hair thinning
- Non-cicatricial patchy hair loss
- Bald patches
- Hair pigmentation
    - white hair (canities)
    - green hair

Nails
- Disorders of the nails
- Brittle nails
- Shedding of nails
- Nail bed lesions

DISORDERS OF SKIN, CONGENITAL ABNORMALITIES, PIGMENTATION

Disorders of Skin Function

Acne vulgaris. Androgen stimulation of subaceous glands and blockage of pilosebaceous openings with inspissated sebum, keratin and squalenes

Hidradenitis eruptiva

Hyperhidrosis
- Axillary
- Palmar
- Plantar

Miliaria ('Prickly heat')
- Crystalline
- Rubra
- Profunda

Anhidrosis

Disorders of pigmentation
- Albinism (affects 1 in 5000–1 in 25 000)
- Piebaldism
- Vitiligo
- Hyperpigmentation
  - inflammatory
    - sunburn
    - infection
    - drugs
  - inorganic arsenic
  - endocrine, e.g. pregnancy
  - rare incontinentia pigmenti (congenital)

Acne

Mild physiological
Papular-pustular (superficial)
Cystic (acne conglobata)
Juvenile
Premenstrual
'Late onset' – after middle age, especially in males
Acne excorié

External agents
- Drug-induced
  - steroids
  - ACTH
  - phenobarbitone
  - troxidone
  - iodides
  - bromides
  - isoniazid
- Chemicals
  - cutting oils
  - coal tar
  - chlornaphthalene
  - perchlornaphthalene
  - chlordiphenyls
  - chlordiphenyl-oxides
  - chlorbenzole
  - oil acne

Acne necrotica

Differential Diagnosis of Acne

Acne
Rosacea

Perioral dermatitis
Papulo-necrotic tuberculoid
Secondary syphilis
Plane warts
Molluscum contagiosum
Milia
Sarcoid lesions

Congenital and Hereditary Conditions Affecting the Skin

Ectoderm
- Ichthyosis
- Congenital ichthyosoform erythroderma
- Keratosis of palms and hands
- Congenital alopecia
- Albinism
- White forelock
- Pachonychia congenita
- Congenital absence of nails
- Congenital anhydrotic ectodermal defect

Mesoderm
- Epidermolysis bullosa
- Congenital lymphoedema
- Urticaria pigmentosa
- Naevus flammeus
- Simple haemangioma
- Cavernous haemangioma
- Blue naevus

Ectoderm and Mesoderm
- Neurofibromatosis
- Acanthosis nigricans (juvenile)

Ichthyosis

Autosomal dominant conditions
- autosomal dominant ichthyosis
- bullous ichthyosiform erythrodermia
- ichthyosis hystrix

Autosomal recessive conditions
- ichthyosiform erythrodermia
- lamellar ichthyosis
- Refsum's disease
- Sjögren–Larsson's syndrome

Sex-linked recessive condition
- sex-linked ichthyosis

Congenital Skin Anomalies

Birthmarks
- Capillary haemangiomas ('Port wine stains') including Sturge–Weber syndrome

Cavernous haemangioma ('Strawberry mark')
Spider naevi
Hereditary haemorrhagic telangiectasia

Moles
Epidermal naevi
Benign melanoma

Ichthyosis
Ichthyosis vulgaris (dominant inheritance)
Sex-linked ichthyosis (clinically apparent in males)
Bullous ichthyosiform erythroderma
Ichthyosiform erythroderma autosomal recessive inheritance

Infantile eczema: dominant inheritance

Psoriasis: inherited, with onset following 'trigger'

Epidermolysis bullosa
Epidermolysis bullosa simplex
Epidermolysis bullosa dystrophica
Darier's disease: Keratosis follicularis and variant familial benign pemphigus (Hailey–Hailey disease)
Adenoma sebaceum: epiloia, tuberose sclerosis (autosomal inheritance)
Ehlers–Danlos syndrome: cutis hyperelastica
Pseudoxanthoma elasticum (autosomal recessive)
Urticaria pigmentosa (dominant inheritance)
Multiple neurofibromatosis: von Recklinghausen's disease
Hereditary harmorrhagic telangiectasia

Birthmarks

Genetic: These have a higher incidence in pigmented races. Most naevi develop after birth, growing and multiplying during childhood, adolescence, pregnancy, and the climacteric
Mongolian spots
Ashleaf leukoderma in epiloia
Lentigines in Peutz–Jeghers syndrome

Common vascular naevi
Salmon naevi – (found in 40% of neonates)
Strawberry naevi (1% of babies), apparent at birth, maximum size by 1 year, with subsequent spontaneous involution usually complete by puberty
Port wine stain – less than 0·3% present at birth

Uncommon naevi
Naevus sebaceus of Jadassohn: present at birth as a bald patch on scalp becoming warty and darker with age.

Up to 30% develop into neoplastic tumour in middle life

Epidermal naevus: yellow streaks, becoming warty and darker with age, but benign

Genetic or Naevoid Hypermelanosis

Brown
- Neurofibromatosis
- Albright's syndrome
- Freckles
- Multiple lentigines
- Peutz–Jeghers syndrome
- Xeroderma pigmentosa
- Acanthosis nigricans

Grey, slate or blue
- Mongolian blue spot
- Ota's naevus
- Ito's naevus
- Blue naevus

Acquired Hypermelanosis

Brown
- Metabolic
  - liver disease
  - porphyrias
- Endocrine
  - ACTH and MSH producing
  - (pituitary and other tumours)
  - ACTH therapy
  - pregnancy (cloasma)
  - oestrogen therapy
  - Addison's hypoadrenalism
- Chemical
  - arsenic
  - psoralens
- Post-inflammation
  - eczema
  - lichen planus
  - lupus erythematosus
  - amyloidosis
  - scleroderma
- Nutritional
  - malabsorption
  - pellagra
- Tumours
  - melanoma
  - acanthosis nigricans associated with carcinoma
  - adenocarcinoma

Grey, slate, blue
- Metabolic

haemochromatosis
(haemosiderosis)
Chemical
fixed drug eruption
chlorpromazine
Post-inflammation
pinta
ashen dermatosis
Tumours
metastatic melanoma with melanogenuria

Increased Melanin Pigmentation

Focal
- Freckle (ephelis)
- Lentigo: macular increase in pigmentation
  - simple
  - senile
- Peutz–Jeghers syndrome: multiple pigmented macules on face and mucous membranes associated with multiple small intestinal polyps
- Neurofibromatosis: von Recklinghausen's disease
- Albright's syndrome: multiple irregular pigmented macules, precocious puberty, and bone disease
- Leopard syndrome: autosomal dominant, multiple lentigines, ECG abnormalities, ocular hypertelorism, pulmonary stenosis, abnormalities of genitalia, growth retardation, deafness
- Centrofacial lentiginosis: associated with neurological and bony abnormalities
- Melanocytic naevi
  - junctional naevus
  - compound naevus
  - intradermal naevus
  - blue naevus
  - mongolian spot – occurring especially in dark skinned races
  - Ota and Ito naevus
  - halo naevus
  - giant hairy naevus
  - juvenile melanoma (spindle cell naevus)
- Malignant melanoma
- Other conditions
  - poikiloderma: irregular areas of increased and decreased melanin pigmentation: may be associated with
    - dermatomyositis
    - mycosis fungoides
    - progressive systemic sclerosis
    - radiation injury
  - post-inflammatory melanin pigmentation
  - seborrhoeic keratosis (pigmented basal cell papilloma)
  - carcinoid syndrome

incontinentia pigmenti
urticaria pigmentosa
primary biliary cirrhosis
chronic renal disease

General: Physiological: Racial
Endocrine
pregnancy: chloasma uterinum
Addison's disease
pituitary tumours secreting ACTH or MSH
drugs, e.g. chlorpromazine
nutritional deficiencies

Hyperpigmentation Syndromes

Nutritional
Malnutrition and starvation
non-tropical sprue
Whipple's disease
vitamin B_{12} deficiency
folate deficiency

Metabolic
Chronic liver disease: cirrhosis
Hepatolenticular degeneration (Wilson's disease)
Haemochromatosis
Porphyria
porphyria cutanea tarda
porphyria erythropoietica
porphyria variegata

Endocrine (ACTH and melanocyte stimulating hormone)
Addison's disease
Nelson's syndrome
Endocrine and non-endocrine neoplasia

Autoimmune
Addison's disease
Pernicious anaemia
Myxoedema
Graves' disease
Systemic scleroderma
Felty's syndrome

Exogenous agents
Busulphan
Arsenicals
Dibromomannitol
etc.

Loss of Melanin Pigmentation

Albinism: autosomal recessive

Chediak–Higashi syndrome: oculocutaneous albinism with morphological and functional leucoyte defects

Phenylketonuria – tendency to fair skins and blue eyes, with decreased melanin deposition

Vitiligo: macular depigmented areas on the body. Melanocytes replaced by Langerhans' cells. Significant association with
- pernicious anaemia
- Addison's disease
- hyperthyroidism
- diabetes mellitus

Piebaldism
- autosomal dominant. Melanocytes in affected areas contain abnormal melanosomes
- Waardenburg's syndrome – associated with congenital deafness and ocular defects

Tuberous sclerosis: depigmented macular areas contain melanocytes

Leprosy: depigmented skin areas related to hyotrophied nerve trunks

Chemicals
- hydroquinone compounds
- catechols
- 4-isopropylcatechol
- *p*-tertiary phenol

Acquired Hypomelanosis

Endocrine
- Hypopituitarism
- Addison's hypoadrenalism
- Thyroid disease
- Hypoparathyroidism: moniliasis syndrome

Chemical
- Hydroquinone
- Monobenzyl ether of hydroquinone
- Phenolic germicides
- Chloroquine

Nutritional
- Kwashiorkor
- Pernicious anaemia (vitamin B_{12} deficiency)

Post-inflammation
- Eczema
- Psoriasis
- Pityriasis versicolor
- Leprosy

Neoplasm
- Halo naevus (Sutton's neavus: leukoderma acquisitum centrifugum: a white halo appears round naevus and engulfs it)
- Malignant melanoma

Miscellaneous
Vogt–Koyanagi–Harada

Disorders of Pigmentation due to Genetic and/or Naevoid Factors

Vitiligo and naevoid hypomelanosis (1% of population)
Piebaldism: autosomal dominant
Waardenburg's syndrome (congenital deafness plus piebaldism)
Albinism: 1 in 20 000 of population. Autosomal recessive
1. tyrosinase positive
2. tyrosinase negative

Chediak–Higashi syndrome: recessive. Dilution of pigment in skin, eyes, hair
predisposition to infection
abnormal white cells
predisposition to lymphoma
Phenylketonuria: hypomelanosis
Tuberose sclerosis
Naevus depigmentosus

Skin Pigmentation not due to Melanin

Argyria: slaty colour due to prolonged use of silver salts, e.g. for sinusitis. Silver is deposited in areas of skin exposed to sunlight
Ochronosis: homogentisic acid deposited in skin, nails and cartilages
Chrysoderma: due to gold. Lilac-grey to fawn in colour
Carotinaemia: especially in palms and soles of feet. Deposition of carotene occurs following a high carrot diet
Clofazimine (Lamprene): red pigmentation of skin, with blue-black lesions during the treatment of leprosy. The urine is coloured red
Local tattooing
accidental
carbon
asphalt
artistic

Complications of Skin Tattoo

Infective
Hepatitis A
Hepatitis B
Syphilis
Tuberculosis
? Leprosy
(Immediate acute infection at time of tattooing with staphylococci etc. and hence pyogenic local infection)

Reaction to trauma of tattooing

- Psoriasis, Lichen planus — arising in the tattooed area, (Koebner phenomenon)
- Granulomatous reaction ± sarcoid-like illness with uveitis

Allergic reaction to pigments [R]

- Mercury, Cadmium, Cobalt, Chromium — salts in pigments

Skin Problems in Black Subjects
(increased incidence when compared with whites)

Pseudofolliculitis of beard
Keloid
Acne keloid
Dermatitis papulosa nigra
Traumatic marginal alopecia
Perifolliculitis abscedens et suffodiens capitis
Systemic disease associated with depigmentation

Conditions associated with Vitiligo
Loss of melanin pigment following destruction of melanocytes occurs in vitiligo

Hyperthyroidism
Hypothyroidism
Hypoparathyroidism
Pernicious anaemia
Diabetes mellitus
Mucocutaneous candidiasis
Alopecia areata
(Vitiligo is often associated with the presence of thyroid, adrenal, and gastric parietal cell antibodies in the serum

Spider Naevi

Physiological
- a few normal subjects
- early normal pregnancy

Pathological
- cirrhosis of the liver
- rheumatoid arthritis
- thyrotoxicosis

Yellow Pigmentation of Skin

Jaundice
Carotenaemia
- excessive vitamin A or carrot intake
- hypothyroidism
- diabetes mellitus

Clinocrine therapy
- antimalaria
- giardiasis therapy
- (malignancy therapy)

Telangiectasia

Physiological
- Ageing skin: exposure to sun, wind, etc.

Pathological
- Damage
  - prolonged corticosteroid therapy
    - local
    - systemic
  - post-irradiation
- Telangiectasia in skin disease
  - rosacea
  - chronic discoid lupus erythematosus
  - localized scleroderma (morphoea)
  - lichen sclerosus et atrophicus (severe cases)
  - skin tumours
    - keratoacanthoma
    - basal cell carcinoma
    - squamous cell carcinoma
  - necrobiosis lipoidica diabeticorum
  - telangiectasia macularis eruptiva perstans
- Telangiectasis in systemic disease
  - systemic lupus erythematosus
  - progressive systemic sclerosis
  - dermatomyositis
  - biliary cirrhosis with scleroderma
  - sarcoidosis (rarely)
  - lymphomatous infiltration of skin
  - related to local carcinoma
  - poikiloderma (atrophy and pigmentation)
    - congenital
    - endocrine
    - reticulosis
- Iatrogenic telangiectasia
  - drugs
    - corticosteroids
    - hydralazine
    - (mercurial drugs in infants)
- Primary Telangiectasia
  - congenital
    - port-wine stain
    - Sturge–Weber syndrome: facial telangiectasia and leptomeningeal angiomatosis
    - Klippel–Trenaunay syndrome: capillary and sometimes cavernous telangiectatic naevus affecting one or more limbs, with hypertrophy of soft tissues, bones and

arteriovenous communication, usually presenting at birth

hereditary haemorrhagic telangiectasis (Osler–Rendu–Weber disease) (AD) affecting face, lips, tongue, mucous membranes, singly or in combination

ataxia telangiectasia (AR)

poikiloderma congenitale – familial tendency to telangiectasia in girls

angioma serpiginosum [R]. Patches of telangiectasia on various parts of the body

erythrocyanosis puellarum: telangiectasia occurring on the lower legs in young women

poikiloderma atrophicans vasculare (atrophic psoriasis): chronic intractable condition, patches of reticular pigmentation and telangiectasia with atrophy especially in flexures. May progress to reticulosis

SKIN ERUPTIONS

Skin Reaction to Drugs

Exanthema
- toxic exanthema
- erythema multiforme
- toxic epidermal necrolysis (Lyell's disease, 'scalded skin' syndrome)
- erythema nodosa
- fixed drug eruption (occurring at same site each time)
- acute necrotizing angiitis
- polyarteritis nodosa
- drug-induced lupus erythematosus syndrome

Urticaria and angioneurotic oedema
- non-allergic acute urticaria
- allergic acute urticaria
- cutaneous anaphylaxis
  - circulatory collapse
  - pruritus
  - severe widespread urticaria
- serum sickness

Purpura
- macular purpura
- raised purpura
- (purpura can occur with thrombocytopenia, or in its absence)

Eczema (dermatitis)
- generalized eczema, exfoliative dermatitis, and erythroderma
- photodermatitis

Bullous eruptions
- prefuse eruption of subepidermal bullae
- large tense subepidermal bullae

Other forms
- lichen planus-like (lichenoid)
- true acne
- acneiform eruption
- generalized pustular psoriasis [R]
- leukaemoid and lymphoma-like eruptions

Hypersensitivity

Type I	early urticaria
Type II	e.g. purpura
Type III	late urticaria (i.e. about 10 days)
Type IV	sensitization developing during 48 hours after exposure

Erythema Multiforme

Virus infections: commonest cause (one-third of which due to herpes simplex)
Strept. pyogenes, occasional
Mycoplasma pneumoniae, occasional
Drugs
- barbiturates
- sulphonamides

Rarely
- leukaemia
- disseminated lupus erythematosus

Erythema Nodosa

Infections
- Bacterial
  - tuberculosis
  - streptococcal infections
  - leprosy
  - pasteurella infections
  - brucellosis
  - gonorrhoea
- Viral infections, e.g.
  - measles
  - cat scratch fever
  - lymphogranulosa venereum
- Histoplasmosis
- Coccidioidomycosis
- Trichophytosis
- Toxoplasmosis
- Leptospirosis

Sarcoidosis
Drug allergy
- sulphonamide sensitivity
- oral contraceptives

Crohn's disease
Ulcerative colitis

Skin Diseases with associated Eosinophilia

Atopic dermatitis
Dermatitis herpetiformis
Herpes gestationis
Pemphigus
Pemphigoid
Toxic erythema of the newborn
Urticaria

Blushing Erythema of the Face

Rosacea
Menopausal flushing
Perioral dermatitis (especially affecting young females)
Seborrhoeic dermatitis
Contact dermatitis
Chronic discoid lupus erythematosus
Tinea incognito: fungus infection of the skin treated with corticosteroids
- Rare
  - photodermatitis
  - polycythaemia
  - dermatomyositis
  - sarcoidosis
  - erysipelas
  - carcinoid syndrome

Urticaria (Weals)

- Distribution
  - General (*see below*)
  - Local
    - insect bite
    - stinging nettle
    - jelly fish sting
    - factitious urticaria (tache, dermatographia)
    - urticaria pigmentosa (related to hot baths)
    - cholinergic urticaria
    - solar and cold urticaria

- Immunological causes
  - isolated symptom
  - associated with serum sickness
  - associated with generalized anaphylaxis
  - dietary hypersensitivity
    - drugs
      - penicillins
      - sulphonamides
      - barbiturates

salicylates
iodine in contrast media
antisera
indomethacin
tartrazine (food additive)

Non-immunological
Hereditary urticaria and angio-oedema
1. Hereditary angio-oedema: deficiency of alpha-2 globulin inhibiting C1 esterase. Autosomal dominant inheritance. 25% of affected heterozygotes die of respiratory obstruction. Homozygote probably not viable
2. Familial paroxysmal peritonitis (Mediterranean fever)
3. Syndrome of urticaria, perceptive deafness, hyperglobulinaemia and amyloidosis

Idiopathic urticaria
Chemical urticaria
chemicals non-specifically stimulate release of histamine in skin
Physical agent urticaria
mechanical: dermatographia
cold
familial cold urticaria
cryoglobulinaemia
paroxysmal cold haemoglobinuria
heat
solar urticaria
following hot baths
delayed pressure urticaria. Urticaria follows at variable time after prolonged pressure
Cholinergic urticaria
spiced foods, vigorous exercise, hot baths } provoke urticaria

Purpura

Congenital defects in the capillary wall, e.g. Ehlers–Danlos syndrome
Increased vascular permeability, e.g. scurvy
Increased vascular fragility
senile purpura
corticosteroids
infections
drugs
systemic disease
diabetes mellitus
uraemia
liver damage
textile purpura and itching purpura (industrial)
Chronic vascular purpura

gravitational purpura
Schamberg's disease (? nature of the condition)
Purpura due to autoimmune damage to vessel wall
Henoch–Schönlein purpura
allergic vasculitis
Quantitative platelet defect: thrombocytopenia
primary
secondary
Qualitative platelet defects
primary
secondary
Purpura associated with dysproteinaemias, e.g. Waldenström's macroglobulinaemia

Dermatitis

Primary irritant dermatitis
Endogenous eczema
Seborrhoeic dermatitis
inborn tendency
low-grade infection

Contact sensitization dermatitis
(delayed hypersensitivity mediated by sensitized lymphocytes)
Physical agents
Cold
frostbite
chilblains
Raynaud's phenomenon
cold urticaria (rare)
livido reticulare
Heat
erythema ab igne
Light
erythema
freckles
solar keratoses
polymorphous light eruption
xeroderma pigmentosa
Photosensitivity
errors of metabolism, e.g. porphyria
drugs and chemicals
sulphonamides
chlorothiazide
phenothiazines
trimeprazine
tetracyclines
griseofulvin
actinic reticularis
Ionizing radiation

Eczema and Dermatitis

Exogenous
- Primary irritant eczema
- Allergic contact eczema

Endogenous
- Atopic eczema
- Seborrhoeic eczema
- Pompholyx (affecting hands and/or feet)

Other
- Napkin dermatitis in infants
- Pruritus ani
- Stasis eczema, e.g. in association with various veins

Complications of Atopic Eczema

Infection
- Abscess formation
- Erysipelas
- Septicaemia
- Impetiginization
- Superimposed fungus infection

Allergic reactions to immunization and to other foreign proteins
- Generalized vaccinia
- Eczema herpeticum
- Cataract
- Lichenification

Photodermatoses

Idiopathic
- Polymorphic light eruption
- Solar urticaria
- Hutchinson's summer prurigo
- Actinic reticulosis
- Photosensitive eczema
- Hydroa vacciniforme

Drug or chemical induced
- Topical: combination of chemical substance and long-wave ultraviolet rays, e.g. pitch, psoralens (in perfumes and plants)
  - photocontact dermatitis
    - antibacterials
    - essential oils
    - sulphans
    - phenothiazines
- Systemic
  - tetracyclines
  - tolbutamide
  - chlorpropamide

thiazide diuretics
phenothiazines
nalidixic acid
sulphonamides

Metabolic diseases
Porphyria
erythropoietic
protoporphyria
coproporphyria
congenital
erythropoietic porphyria
Hepatic
acute intermittent porphyria
porphyria cutanea tarda
variegate porphyria
hereditary coproporphyria
Pellagra
Xeroderma pigmentosa

Skin lesions aggravated by sunlight
Chronic discoid lupus erythematosus
Pemphigus foliacus
Herpes simplex
Albinism (defective protection)

Dermatoses affecting Skin and Mucous Membranes only

Lichen planus
Pityriasis rosea
Pityriasis lichenoides varioliformis
Necrobiosis lipoidica

Bullous disorders
Dermatitis herpetiformis
Herpes gestationis
Pemphigus vulgaris
Bullous pemphigoid
Erythema multiforme
typical
Stevens–Johnson syndrome

Urticaria
Angioneurotic oedema
Cholinergic urticaria
Factitious urticaria
Papular urticaria
Drug eruptions
Morphoea (localized scleroderma)

Dermatoses of Emotional Origin

Dermatitis artefacts
Trichotillomania

Delusional symptoms referred to skin, with rubbing, etc., of skin
Skin disorders aggravated by self-trauma

Red Scaly Patches on the Skin

- Dermatitis
  - seborrhoeic dermatitis affecting flexor surfaces
  - contact dermatitis
  - organismal dermatitis
- Psoriasis: affecting extensor surfaces especially
- Lichen
  - planus
  - simplex
- Pityriasis
  - rosea
  - tinea versicolor
- Secondary syphilis

Bullae and Blistering Conditions

- Physical
  - Heat
    - burns
    - scalds
  - Cold: frostbite
  - Friction
    - blisters due to ill-fitting shoes, etc.
    - blisters due to manual work
  - Sunlight
    - Severe sunburn due to excessive exposure
    - hydroa aestivale: excessive sensitivity to sunlight

- Toxic
  - Animal
    - bites
    - stings, e.g. jelly fish
  - Vegetable: e.g. poison ivy, nettles, etc.
  - Chemicals
    - occupational dermatitis, etc.
    - mustard gas, etc.

- Drugs
  - Iodides
  - Bromides
  - Quinine
  - Chloral
  - Aconite
  - Barbiturates [R]

- Infections
  - Bullous impetigo
  - Herpes zoster

Herpes gestationis
Gangrene (initial lesions)

Tropho-neuritic conditions
Cerebrovascular accident, and other unconscious patients
Cerebral tumour
Encephalitis
Post-leucotomy
Diabetes mellitus (especially on feet)

Dermatological conditions
Pemphigus
Pemphigoid
Mucous membrane pemphigoid
Bullous erythema multiforme
Toxic epidermal necrolysis
Pompholyx

Acute Dermal Gangrene

(*Meleney's spreading gangrene*)
Associated with a virulent form of coliform infection, with or without *Staph. pyogenes,* with or without anaerobic organisms
This condition may complicate
Diabetes mellitus
Multiple sclerosis
Rheumatoid arthritis
Steroid therapy
Post-surgical treatment of ischiorectal sepsis
Post-groin or genital area surgery

Sclerodermatous Changes in the Skin

Progressive systemic sclerosis
Scleroderma, diffuse
Acrosclerosis
Local changes
Linear scleroderma
Morphoea

Sclerodermatous skin changes
Mixed connective tissue disease
Eosinophilic fasciitis
Associated with
Systemic lupus erythematosus
Dermatomyositis
Scleromyxoedema
Werner's syndrome
Vibration-induced skin changes
Amyloidosis
Buschke's post-infection sclerodema

Scleroderma

Morphoea
- Circumscribed: plaques or bands
- Linear
- Frontoparietal lesions with or without hemiatrophy of face (*en coup de sabre*)
- Generalized

Systemic sclerosis
Scleroderma: associated with other diseases: (pseudo-scleroderma)
Occupational scleroderma

Granuloma of Skin

Local lesion
- Subaceous cyst
- Chalazion
- Chronic skin ulcer

Infection
- Cat scratch fever
- Syphilis
- Leprosy
- Tuberculosis
- Anonymous mycobacterial infection
- Sarcoidosis (? infective in origin)

Physical agents
- Talc
- Silica
- Beryllium
- Zirconium

PRURITUS

Itching

Lowered threshold
- temperature changes } cause itching
- contact }

'Spontaneous' itch

Pruritus associated with Dermatoses

Eczema
Scabies
Pediculosis
Fungal infection
Lichen planus
Dermatitis herpetiformis
Urticaria
Urticaria pigmentosa

Pruritus
- ani
- vulvae

Prickly heat
Asteototic eczema
Pityriasis
Seborrhoeic dermatitis
Psoriasis

Pruritus

Skin diseases
Endogenous
- Diabetes mellitus
- Drug sensitivity
- Hyperthyroidism
- Hypothyroidism
- Internal malignancy
- Liver disease, especially obstructive jaundice, primary biliary cirrhosis
- Lymphoma
- Onchocerciasis
- Polycythaemia vera
- Psychiatric disorders
- Uraemia

Pruritus Ani

- With discharge
  - Male and female
    - Anal
      - Mucoid
        - prolapsing haemorrhoids
        - rectal prolapse
      - Faecal
        - diarrhoea
        - Crohn's disease
        - colitis
        - excess intake of liquid paraffin
      - Inflammation
        - fistula
        - fissure
        - papilloma
        - condyloma
        - carcinoma (anal)
  - Female
    - Urethral
      - incontinence
      - venereal disease
    - Vaginal
      - salpingitis
      - moniliasis
      - trichomonas

No discharge
- Infection
  - Mycotic
    - yeast
    - epidermophyton
    - trichophyton
  - Parasitic
    - threadworm
    - nits from *Pediculosis pubis*
- Non-infection
  - Poor hygiene
  - hyperhidrosis
  - Allergy
    - clothes
    - food etc.
  - Iatrogenic
    - antibiotics
    - creams

Pruritus associated with Internal Disorders

Liver disease
- Primary biliary cirrhosis
- Obstructive jaundice

Endocrine
- Thyroid
  - hyperthyroidism
  - hypothyroidism
- Diabetes mellitus
- Hypoparathyroidism

Renal: chronic renal failure with hyperparathyroidism

Haematological
- Polycythaemia vera
- Chronic lymphatic leukaemia
- Iron deficiency

Lymphoma
- Hodgkin's lymphadenoma
- Mycosis fungoides

Autoimmune
- Sjögren's syndrome
- Systemic lupus erythematosus

Normal pregnancy

Tropical infestation
- Onchocerciasis
- Filariasis

Drugs
- Cocaine
- Opiates
- Chloroquine

Neurology
- Thalamic tumour
- Syphilis affecting central nervous system

MALIGNANCY

Neoplasms of the Skin

Benign
- Seborrhoeic warts
- Senile seborrhoeic adenoma
- Skin tags
- Keloid
- Pyogenic granuloma
- Histiocytoma
- Lipoma
- Kerato-acanthoma

Pre-malignant: factors
- Age
- Skin colour
- Senile or actinic keratoses
- Sunlight intensity
- Tar and mineral oils, etc.
- Inorganic arsenic
- Leucoplakia

Malignant: epidermal
- Rodent ulcer (basal cell epithelioma)*
  - Types
    - ulcer
    - cystic type
    - morphoeic type
    - pigmented
    - superficial
- Squamous epithelioma
- Intra-epithelial epithelioma (Bowen's disease)
- Paget's disease of the nipple
- Malignant melanoma
- Mycosis fungoides
- Secondary tumour deposits in the skin
- Sarcoma
- Hodgkin's disease
- Leukaemic deposits

Factors predisposing to Squamous Cell Carcinoma

Excessive ultraviolet light exposure, e.g. sun
Long-term X-ray exposure
Chemical agents
- machine oil (e.g. mulespinners' carcinoma)
- tar
- pitch
- soot (e.g. chimney sweeps in olden days)
- cigarette smoking (especially with high tar content)
- long-term arsenical therapy (e.g. Fowler's solution – obsolete)

Skin disorders
- senile keratosis
- Bowen's ulcer
- lupus vulgaris

Tumours associated with Dermatomyositis

Incidence in 15–20% of patients (rising to 50% after the age of 50)
- Ovary
- Uterus
- Kidney
- Lung
- Breast
- Stomach
- Gastrointestinal tract
- Leukaemia
- Hodgkin's lymphadenoma
- Carcinoid tumour
- Thymoma

Cutaneous Manifestations of Malignancy

Pruritus
Pallor (due to anaemia)
Erythema } due to polycythaemia
Cyanosis }
Melanosis
Actinoid keratinization
Urticaria
Erythema nodosum
Erythema multiforme
Eczematous dermatitis
Vesicular and bullous eruptions
Purpura
Superficial thrombophlebitis
Acanthosis nigricans
Clubbing digits
Pachydermoperiostosis (usually with carcinoma of lung)
Bowen's disease

SKIN INFECTIONS AND INFESTATIONS

Skin Infections

Bacteria
- *Staph. pyogenes*
- *Strept. pyogenes*
- Gram-negative bacilli attacking moist devitalized skin
- Others
  - Corynebacterium
  - *B. anthracis*

Erysipelothrix
Tuberculosis
Leprosy

Viruses
Warts
Molluscum contagiosum
Cow pox
Orf

Fungi
Ringworm
Microsporum
M. audouini
M. canis
Trichophyton
T. mentagrophytes
T. verrucosum
Epidermophyton
Yeasts
Pityrosporon ovale – pityriasis versicolor
Candida – candidiasis

Protozoa
Cutaneous leishmaniasis

Deep or systemic mycoses
Histoplasmosis
Coccidioidomycosis (New World)
Blastomycosis (New World)
Rhinosporidiosis (India)
Mycetoma
Chromoblastomycosis (Central America and Australia)
Phycomycosis (Central Africa and Indonesia)

Actinomycosis, Nocardiosis, Torulosis, Sporotrichosis } can affect skin

Skin Infestations

Scabies: *Sarcoptes scabei*
typical eruption
non-specific, e.g. Norwegian scabies
Flea infestation
Bed bugs
Lice
Sand fly infestation
Pediculosis
P. capitis (scalp and hair)
P. pubis (body hair)
P. corporis (infesting clothing)
Ticks (Ixodidae)

Mites (Acarina)
- Demodex folliculorum (hair follicles and sebaceous glands)
- Grain mites (Pyemotes ventricosus)
- Food mites
  - Acarus siro (grain amd cheese)
  - Tyroglyphus longior (cheese)
  - Tyroglyphus castellani (copra and cheese)
  - Glycyphagus domesticans (dried fruit)
- Rodent and bird mites
  - Ornithonyssus bacoti (bats)
  - Allodermanyssus sanguinis (house mouse)
  - Dermanyssus gallinae (hen houses)
- Harvest mites
- Cheyletiella parasitovorax: on cats and dogs
- House dust mites (Dermatophagoides pteronyssinus in beds, upholstery, dust on floors)

Insects causing isolated local lesions: bees, wasps, hornets, ants, mosquitoes, gnats, midges, horse flies, etc.

LIPS, GENITALIA

Diseases of Lips

Dermatitis–eczema
- Contact cheilitis
- Seborrhoeic dermatitis
- Atopic dermatitis
- Perioral dermatitis
- Actinic cheilitis

Infections
- Herpes simplex
- Warts
- Coccal infections
  - syphilis
  - tuberculosis
  - leprosy
- Candidiasis

Granulomas
- Boeck's sarcoid
- Crohn's disease

Aphthous

Erythema multiforme

Angio-oedema

Malformations
- Cavernous haemangioma
- Granuloma pyogenicum
- Keratoacanthoma (*Molluscum sebaceum*)

Tumours
- Squamous cell carcinoma
- Moles

Deficiency disease

Vitamin deficiency
Mineral deficiency

Genital ulceration

Syphilis
- Primary chancre
- Secondary papules ulcerating

Bacterial infection
- Folliculitis
- Furunculosis
- Gonorrhoea (very rarely ulcerative small postules)

Yeast infection: *Candida albicans*
Protozoa: granuloma inguinale (Donovania granulomatosis)
Parasites: scabies: shallow ulcers following scratching
Chancroid
Virus infection: herpes simplex
Erosive balanitis (males)
Trauma
Torn fraenum in men
Paraphimosis
Local caustics (in females)
Drug eruptions

Less common
- Carcinoma
- Circinate balanitis of Reiter's disease (males)
- Erosive balanitis (males)
- Trauma
- Behçet's syndrome
- Sutton's ulcer affecting the vulva } confined to the female
- Acute vulval ulceration of Lipschütz } confined to the female
- Chancroid
- Ecthyma
- Gonorrhoea – rarely small ulcerative pustules
- Pemphigus vulgaris
- Pemphigus vegetans
- Stevens–Johnson syndrome

SWEAT GLANDS

Disorders of Sweat Glands

Excessive sweating: hyperidrosis
Reduced sweating: hypoidrosis, which can lead to miliaria rubra (prickly heat)
Anidrosis: lack of sweating
Dysidrosis: coloured sweat
Bromodrosis: sweat with unpleasant small (especially of axilla and feet)
Lyell–Ritter's disease: toxic epidermal necrolysis in children

Hyperhidrosis

Physiological
- Anxiety
- Heat

Pathological
- General
  - fever
  - thyrotoxicosis
  - pathological anxiety state
- Abnormality of autonomic nervous system
  - cord compression
  - stroke
  - von Frey syndrome
  - diabetic facial sweating
- Abnormality of sweat glands
  - axillary hyperhidrosis, palmar hyperhidrosis, plantar hyperhidrosis } especially in females
  - gustatory hyperhidrosis: occurring in both sexes

HAIR

Hair Loss

Examination of hair roots

1. Telogen root: root produced at the end of growth period. Most normal shed hairs are telogen hairs
2. Anagen root: actively growing flask-shaped, hyperpigmented proximally. 80% of normal hair is in the anagen phase
3. Tapered root: artefact produced by plucking or overvigorous brushing or combing.
4. Period of regression: catagen: a very low per cent of normal hair

Classification of loss
- Increased rate of hair shedding
  - loss of telogen hairs
  - loss of broken hairs
  - loss of whole anagen hairs
- Diffuse hair thinning
  - decrease in hair shaft diameter in a proportion of hairs
- Patchy alopecia
  - non-cicatricial
    - loss of telogen hairs
    - loss of broken hairs
    - loss of whole anagen hairs
    - decrease of hair shaft diameter
  - cicatricial

Failure to grow long hair
- loss of telogen hairs
- loss of broken hairs

Alopecia

Congenital

Acquired
- Seborrhoea capitis
- Ringworm
- Post-febrile alopecia
- Post-puerperal alopecia
- Endocrine disorders
  - hypothyroidism
  - myxoedema
- Diffuse alopecia in women
- Mechanical
- Post-drugs and poisons
- Alopecia areata
- Cicatricial alopecia

Hair Fall (Telogen Effluvium)

Systemic disease
- Following febrile illness
- Following starvation, or severe dieting
- Endocrine
  - thyroid disease
  - postpartum (in the months after delivery)
- Malignancy: widespread disease

Drugs
- May occur with antithyroid drugs
- ? After discontinuing oestrogens
- Long-term heparin therapy

Broken Hairs (Anagen Effluvium)

Disease of the hair: alopecia areata
Systemic disease: systemic lupus erythematosus
Drugs: cytotoxic drugs
- methotrexate
- azathioprine

Diffuse Hair Thinning

Hair follicle disease
- Genetic
  - male pattern: early onset (autosomal dominant)
  - male pattern: late onset (? autosomal dominant)
  - female pattern: ? inheritance pattern

Systemic disease
- iron deficiency
- thyroid disease
- hyperandrogen conditions

Non-Cicatricial Patchy Hair Loss

Loss of telogen hairs: alopecia areata
Loss of broken hairs
- alopecia areata
- tinea capitis
- mechanical trauma

Loss of anagen hairs: tinea amiantacea
Decrease in hair diameter: prolonged traction

Bald Patches

Infections
- Bacterial
  - Boils
  - Impetigo
  - Infected eczema
- Fungal
  - Tinea capitis

Acute psoriasis

Discoid lupus erythematosus

Alopecia areata associated with –
- Autoimmune thyroid disease
- Other endocrine diseases
- ? Family history
- 'Idiopathic'
- Emotional stress

Hair pulling
- Children
- Adult neurosis

HAIR PIGMENTATION

White Hair (Canities)

Physiological: after 40 years of age, variable

Pathological
- endocrine
  - hyperthyroidism
  - hypopituitarism
- partial, or general, after recovery from alopecia areata
- after 'psychological shock or stress'

Green Hair
(Deliberate use of green hair dye)

Copper workers
Excess copper in washing or bath water
Brass workers
Mercury workers
Phenylketonuria: } green hair has been reported
Chlorinated swimming baths when copper-based algicides are used

NAILS

Disorders of the Nails

Congenital
- absence
- irregular growth

Nail disease
- paronychia
- warts
- fungus infections
- subungual exostosis
- glomus tumour
- melanotic whitlow

Nails involved with skin disease
- psoriasis
- dermatitis
- lichen planus
- epidermolysis bullosa

Oncholysis: separation of nail plate from underlying bed with increased distal separation
- 10% of thyrotoxic patients (usually beginning with fourth finger)
- trauma
- arthritis
- hypothyroidism

Involvement with systemic disease
- Beau's lines: any serious illness
- clubbing: (from many causes)
- koilonychia: hypochromic anaemia
- connective tissue disease: telangiectasia and interference with growth if associated with Raynaud's phenomenon

Pigmentation of nails
- Mees' lines in arsenic poisoning
- white parallel bands in hypoalbuminaemia
- white nails associated with chronic liver diseases
- green nails: pseudomonas infection under nail

yellow nails
- associated with lymphoedema
- rarely with pleural effusion
- very slow nail growth
- yellow nails of lower extremities in diabetes mellitus

blue lanulae: hepatolenticular degeneration
longitudinal bands: Cushing's syndrome
broad white parallel bands and solid proximal pigmentation during chemotherapy for cancer

Nail anomalies
- leuconychia – white spots on nails commonly found, probably results of trauma
- splitting of nail edges – common in women, and may be the result of alkaline household cleansing agents and nail varnish solvents
- onychogryphosis: large horn-like nails, especially on toes, the result of trauma and failure to cut nails
- ingrowing toenails: result of tight footwear
- nail ridging: result of trauma
- racket nails
- periodic shedding

Drug effects on nails
- Pigmentation
  - blue-black
    - phenolphthalein
    - chloroquine
  - blue: mepacrine
  - yellow: tetracycline
- Temporary loss
  - cloxacillin
  - cephaloridine

Brittle Nails

Congenital

Acquired
- detergents
- nail polish
- nail polish remover
- myxoedema

Physiological: old age

Shedding of Nails

Severe infectious fevers
Alopecia areata (some cases)

Nail Bed Lesions

Haematoma
Malignant melanoma
Exostosis
Glomus tumour

EAR, NOSE AND THROAT

MOUTH

Oral Pigmentation

White

- Moniliasis: pearly white
- Lichen planus: pearly white

Red
- Pernicious anaemia tongue: red and smooth
- Vitamin B deficiency: magenta tongue
- Polycythaemia: blue-red

Yellow
- Herpangina: yellow grey
- Syphilitic rhagades: golden
- Cadmium poisoning: golden gingivitis

Black
- Addison's disease: black patches
- Peutz–Jeghers' syndrome: black
- Bismuth, Mercury, Lead } poisoning: blue–black gums

Halitosis

Diet
Smoker's breath
Faulty oral hygiene
Continued mouth breathing
Acute ulcerative gingivitis
Chronic periodontitis
Infected tooth socket
Pericoronitis
Descending pharyngeal exudate from infected sinus
Tonsillitis
Bronchiectasis
Lung abscess
Rare
- pharyngeal pouch
- oesophageal diverticula

Gum Hyperplasia

Physiological
- In mouth breathers during childhood
- Pregnancy

Pathological
- Long-term therapy with phenytoin (anticonvulsant)
- Chronic infection of gums
- Ill-fitting dentures
- Vitamin C deficiency
- Acute myeloblastic leukaemia

Bleeding Gums

Bleeding gums in systemic disease
- Scurvy
- Associated with purpura
  - any thrombocytopenia, platelet dysfunction } including acute leukaemia

Bleeding diathesis associated with plasma coagulation factor deficiencies

Bleeding gums due to local conditions
- Injury
- Pyorrhoea alveolaris
- Receding gums
- Local lesion
  - papilloma
  - epulis
  - epithelioma
  - stomatitis
  - etc.

Bilateral Parotid Gland Enlargement

Mumps
Infectious mononucleosis
Mickulicz's disease
Sarcoidosis
Sjögren's syndrome
Chronic pancreatitis
Cirrhosis

NOSE

Nasal Stuffiness

Adenoidal hyperplasia (children 2–7 years)
Nasal polyps (adults)
Nasal allergy/allergic rhinitis. Seasonal or perennial
Vasomotor rhinitis. Reaction to stimuli, including:
- Climatic
- Hormonal
- Psychomotor
- Drugs
- Tobacco
- Alcohol

Rare causes
- Atrophic rhinitis (ozaena)
- Sarcoid
- Lupus vulgaris
- Malignant granuloma
- Wegener's granulomatosis
- Tumours arising in
  - nasal passages
  - postnasal space
  - antro-ethmoidal region

Nasal Catarrh

Acute coryza

Seasonal allergic rhinitis ('hay fever')
Non-seasonal allergic rhinitis, e.g. house dust mite
Vasomotor rhinitis
Iatrogenic rhinitis: 'rebound' congestion following decongestant drops or sprays
Rhinitis: due to occupational causes
- welders' hot metal fumes
- farmer's nose
- office workers } dusts and epithelial
- 'pop' singers } cells and human hair

Nasal polyps: frequently associated with
- 'hay fever'
- asthma
- occasional hypersensitivity to aspirin

Acute Rhinitis

Virus infection
Bacterial infection
Allergy
Local irritants
Trauma
Drugs
- iodides
- rarely: mercury, arsenic, antimony

Chronic Rhinitis

Simple
Hypertrophic
Polypoid
Sicca
Atrophic
Caseous
Malignant granuloma
Gangrinosa

Bacterial
- Diphtheria
- Tuberculosis
- Leprosy
- Scleroma
- Glanders
- Rhinosporidiosis

Treponemal
- Syphilis
- Yaws

Protozoal: leishmaniasis
Fungus
- Moniliasis
- Histoplasmosis
- Sporotrichosis

Mycoses
- actinomycosis
- blastomycosis
- aspergillosis

Uncertain origin: Boeck's sarcoid

Nasal Collapse

Infection
- Syphilis
  - congenital
  - tertiary
- Yaws
- Leprosy
- Cutaneous leishmaniasis
- Blastomycosis
- Phycomycosis

Vasculitis (collagen disorders)
- Wegener's granuloma } Rare causes
- Lethal midline granuloma } Rare causes
- Polyarteritis nodosa } Rare causes
- Systemic lupus erythematosus
- Rheumatoid arthritis
- Scleroderma
- Psoriatic arthritis

Malignancy: carcinoma of the nose and nasopharynx

Perforation of Nasal Septum

Trauma

Infection
- staphylococcal
- syphilis
- tuberculosis

Epistaxis

Physiological
- Vicarious menstruation. Increased incidence of epistaxis during menstruation
- Excessive vigorous nose blowing

Pathological
- Local
  - Trauma
  - Dilatations and tortuosity of nasal veins
  - Local inflammation
    - virus infection
    - bacterial infection
  - Alterations in atmospheric pressure
    - high altitude

caisson disease
Foreign bodies
Malignant growth
Congestion and local vasomotor changes, e.g. allergy
General
Hypertension
In older patients, much more common than younger
Uraemia and chronic nephritis
Mitral valve stenosis
Cirrhosis
Aortic stenosis
Plasma clotting defects
Congenital plasma defect
haemophilia
von Willebrand's disease
Christmas disease
Acquired: overdose with heparin, oral anticoagulants, streptokinase
Platelet disorders
Thrombocytopenia
Thrombocytasthenia
Vessel abnormality: hereditary haemorrhagic telangiectasia, with lesions in the nose

THROAT

Membrane in Throat

Moniliasis
Infectious mononucleosis
Diphtheria
Vincent's angina
Acute leukaemia
Agranulocytosis
(Haemolytic streptococcal infection: follicular patches)

Trachea: Upper Respiratory Infection

Pharyngitis, Tonsillitis, Acute laryngitis } virus and/or bacterial infection
Virus infection
'Common cold'
Infectious mononucleosis
Herpangina (Type A Coxsackie virus)
Herpes simplex
Bacterial infection
Diphtheria
Streptococcal pharyngitis
Predisposition: agranulocytosis

Larynx: Vocal Cord Paralysis

Thyroid
  enlargement
  damage during thyroid surgery
Trauma
Deep cervical lymph glands
  enlarged
  neoplasm
Mediastinal lymph nodes
  enlarged
  neoplasm
Extension from carcinoma of oesophagus
Pressure from aortic aneurysm
Pressure from left atrial hypertrophy
Neurological PICA syndrome
  syringobulbia
  motor neuron disease
  poliomyelitis
  tumours

EAR

Tinnitus

External ear
  foreign body
  wax
Middle ear
  otitis
    acute
    chronic
  Eustachian catarrh
  otosclerosis
  spasm of stapedius associated with hemifacial spasm
Internal ear
  labyrinthitis
  Menière's disease
  drugs
Auditory nerve
  neuronitis
  streptomycin and other vestibular toxins
  Paget's disease
  (rarely tumour)
Pons (tegmentum)
  vascular lesion
  neoplasm
Cerebrum
  temporal lobe tumour
  temporal lobe epilepsy (before attacks)
Carotico – cavernous fistula
Congenital intracranial aneurysm
Arterial angioma
} sound conducted to the ear

Aortic incompetence
Drugs
- quinine
- salicylate
- amyl nitrite
- streptomycin (tinnitus precedes deafness)

Earache

Auricle
- Injury
  - trauma
  - infection
- Malignancy
  - rodent ulcer
  - epithelioma

Meatus
- Infection
- Hard wax
- Foreign body
- Trauma
- Malignancy

Middle ear
- Otitis media
- Mastoiditis
- Malignancy

Referred pain
- From lesions outside ear
  - unerupted lower molars
  - acute tonsillitis
  - pharyngeal and retropharyngeal lesions
  - epithelioma of tongue
- From nervous pain
  - neuralgia
  - herpes zoster
  - glossopharyngeal neuralgia

Non-Suppurative Otitis Media, 'Glue Ear', Mucinous or Serous Otitis Media

Due to dysfunction of Eustachian tubes, associated with

Deficient palatal musculature in cleft palate Enlarged adenoids Chronic sinusitis Allergic rhinitis	aggravated by upper respiratory tract infections

Long-term sequelae
- Adhesive otitis media
- Thinning of the drum head
- Development of tympanic membrane pouches
- Cholesteatoma
- Atrophy of the ossicles

Chalk patches
Prolonged malfunction of the Eustachian tubes

Deafness

Mechanisms

Conductive deafness
- Deafness following any affection of the conducting apparatus
  - external auditory canal
    - wax in external auditory canal
    - foreign body
    - inflammation of external auditory canal
    - atresia of the canal
    - new growth of the canal (very rare)
  - middle ear cleft
    - middle ear injury
    - acute inflammation with occlusion of Eustachian tube
    - chronic inflammation
      - glue ear
      - suppurative otitis media
      - perforation of drum
      - cholesteatoma
  - labyrinthine windows
    - new growth
    - otosclerosis

Sensorineural deafness
- Deafness following affection of the perceiving apparatus
  - cochlear apparatus (sensory)
  - auditory nerve (neural)
  - central area (brain)

Mixed deafness
- Conductive and perceptive deafness in one and the same ear

Lesions

Developmental receptor aphasia: hearing normal, but spoken language not understood. 5 males: 1 female

Nerve deafness
- terminals of cochlear part of VIIIth nerve damaged
  - low grade infection of the middle ear
  - acute labyrinthitis
- internal ear
  - congenital syphilis
  - congenital deaf mutism
- vestibulocochlear nerve damage
  - fracture of skull

intratemporal epidermoid
bony deformity in osteitis deformans
acoustic neuroma
meningovascular syphilis
avitaminosis
polyneuritis cranialis
geniculate zoster
complication of mumps
Refsum's disease

Brainstem damage [R]
head injury
multiple sclerosis

Central deafness
birth injury, anoxia at birth, kernicterus

Menière's syndrome
Hysteria

Acute Sensorineural Deafness

Central
Encephalitis
Meningomyelitis
Pontine glioma
Concussion
Psychogenic, of sudden onset

Cochlear
Viral
herpes zoster, measles, mumps
Vascular lesions
Suppurative labyrinthitis
Cochlear otosclerosis
Tumours
Autoimmune disease
Ototoxic drugs, e.g. gentamycin, streptomycin
Menière's disease
Late syphilis

Retrocochlear
Multiple sclerosis
Acoustic neuroma
Meningitis
leptomeningitis
tuberculous meningitis
syphilitic meningitis
Arachnoiditis
Angle meningioma

Results of trauma
Concussion

Labyrinthine window rupture
Stapes fracture
Fractured otic capsule
Decompression deafness
Blast sensory loss
Persistent high-pitched noise

Idiopathic (up to a quarter of all cases)
Presbyacusis: senile deafness

Drug-induced Deafness

Antibiotics
Aminoglycosides
streptomycin: vestibular, labyrinthine and cochlear damage
gentamycin, kanamycin, neomycin, tobramycin, framycetin, bleomycin, vancomycin, ristocetin, viomycin, capreomycin, paromycin: cochlear damage
Chloramphenicol: topical application can cause damage to hair cells and supporting cells of organ of Corti
Ampicillin: rare reversible deafness
Erythromycin: deafness may follow high intravenous dosage
Polymixin F, Actinomycin C, Actinomycin D: high plasma levels may be associated with deafness
Co-trimoxazole: slight reversible deafness
Rifampicin: rare transient deafness

Diuretics
Ethacrynic acid in high dosage

Anti-inflammatory
Aspirin: retrocochlear rapidly reversible deafness: high-pitched whistle heard by patient
(Isolated cases reported after indomethacin, ibuprofen, phenylbutazone)

Antimalarial
Quinine: reversible deafness following prolonged treatment
Chloroquine

Mustine: severe irreversible deafness

Polybrene: severe irreversible deafness

Thalidomide: Bilateral congenital labyrinthine defects with meatal atresia

Topical applications
- Chloramphenicol: topical applications can cause damage to hair cells and supporting cells of organ of Corti
- Chlorhexidine: 0·5% in 70% alcohol: entry into the middle ear results in total and irreversible deafness
- Formaldehyde: severe middle ear damage
- Lignocaine: irreversible fall in endocochlear potentials
- Cocaine, phenol and thymol solution to tympanic membrane results in sudden deafness

Drugs associated with Auditory Vestibular System Disorders
- Salicylates, when the plasma level exceeds 40 mg/100ml
- Streptomycin and dihydrostreptomycin
- Aminoglycoside antibiotics, e.g. kanamycin sulphate
- Quinine
- Quinidine
- Sodium nitroprusside
- Nitrogen mustard

Genetic Hearing Loss

Congenital and early-onset hereditary hearing loss accounts for up to 50% of all those born deaf. The major cause late-onset hearing loss is genetic in origin. Inheritance may be (1) Autosomal dominant, (2) Autosomal recessive, (3) X-linked, and with variable penetrance and variable expression

Genetic Hearing Loss with no associated Abnormalities
- Dominant congenital severe sensorineural deafness (many D)
- Dominant progressive early-onset sensorineural deafness (D)
- Dominant unilateral sensorineural deafness (AD)
- Dominant low-frequency sensorineural hearing loss (AD)
- Dominant mid-frequency sensorineural hearing loss (AD)
- Dominant high-frequency sensorineural deafness (AD)
- Otosclerosis (dominant with variable penetrance)
- Recessive congenital sensorineural deafness (AR)
- Recessive congenital moderate sensorineural hearing loss (AR)
- Recessive early onset sensorineural deafness (AR)
- X-linked congenital sensorineural deafness (XR)
- X-linked early onset sensorineural deafness (XR)
- X- linked moderate sensorineural deafness (XR)
- X-linked hearing loss with congenital fixation of the stapedal footplates (XR)
- Hereditary Menière's syndrome (?AD)

Absence of external auditory canal and conduction deafness (AD)

Genetic Hearing Loss with External Ear Abnormalities

Otofaciocervical syndrome (AD)
Ear malformation, cervical fistula or nodules, with mixed hearing loss (AD)
Pre-auricular pits, branchial fistulas and sensorineural hearing loss (?AD)
Thickened ear lobes and incudostapedial abnormalities (D)
Lop-ears, imperforate anus, triphalangeal thumbs and sensorineural deafness (AD)
Cup-shaped ears, mixed hearing loss and lacrimo-auriculo-dento-digital syndrome (AD)
Malformed low-set ears and conduction hearing loss (AR)
Microtia, meatal atresia and conducting hearing loss (AR)
Microtia, hypertelorism, facial clefting and conduction hearing loss (AR)
Lop-ears, micrognathia and conduction hearing loss

Genetic Hearing Loss with associated Eye Disease

Retinitis pigmentosa and congenital sensorineural deafness (Usher's syndrome)
Retinal degeneration, diabetes mellitus, obesity and sensorineural hearing loss
Retinitis pigmentosa, nystagmus, hemiplegic migraine and sensorineural deafness (?AD)
Retinitis pigmentosa, progressive quadriplegia, mental handicap and sensorineural deafness (AD?)
Cockayne's syndrome (AR)
Refsum's disease (AR)
Inverse retinitis pigmentosa, hypogonadism, and sensorineural deafness (AR)
Retinal changes, muscular wasting, mental retardation and deafness (AR)
Cryptophthalmic syndrome with mixed deafness (AR)
Myopia, cataract, saddle nose and sensorineural deafness (Marshall syndrome) (D)
Myopia, blue sclerae, marfanoid habitus and sensorineural deafness syndrome (D)
Myopia, peripheral neuropathy, skeletal abnormalities and sensorineural deafness (AD)
Optic atrophy, polyneuropathy and sensorineural deafness. (Rosenberg–Chutorian syndrome) (2 types:– X-linked R or AR)
Optic atrophy, juvenile diabetes, and sensorineural hearing loss (AR)
Progressive optic atrophy and congenital sensorineural deafness (AD)
Optic atrophy, ataxia and progressive sensorineural hearing loss (AD)
Optico-cochleo-dentate degeneration (AR)

Iris dysplasia, ocular hypertelorism, psychomotor retardation and sensorineural deafness (D)
Congenital corneal dystrophy and progressive sensorineural hearing loss (Harboyan syndrome) (AR)
Familial corneal degeneration, abnormal calcium metabolism and hearing loss
Norrie syndrome (oculo-acoustico-cerebral degeneration) (XR)
Keratoconus, blue sclerae, loose ligaments and conduction deafness (AR)
Progressive external ophthalmoplegia, retinitis pigmentosa degeneration, cardiac conduction defects and mixed hearing loss

Genetic Hearing Loss associated with Musculoskeletal Disease

Otopalatodigital syndrome (XR)
Orofaciodigital II syndrome (Mohr syndrome) (AR)
Dysplasia of the capital femoral epiphyses, severe myopia and sensorineural deafness (AR)
Absence of tibia and congenital deafness (AR)
Broad terminal phalanges, abnormal facies and sensorineural deafness (AR or XR)
Dominant craniometaphysial dysplasia (AD)
Recessive craniometaphysial dysplasia (AR)
Craniodiaphysial dysplasia (AR)
Frontometaphysial dysplasia AD)
Recessive osteopetrosis (Albers–Schönberg disease) (AR)
Dominant symphalangism and conduction deafness (AD)
Multiple synostoses and conduction deafness (symphalangism–brachydactyly syndrome) (AD)
Paget's disease of the bone (osteitis deformans) (? inheritance)
Hyperostosis corticalis generalisata (van Buchem's disease) (AR)
Sclerosteosis (AR)
Ectrodactyly, ectodermal dysplasia, clefting and mixed hearing loss
Bone dysplasias and sensorineural deafness (AR)
Metaphysial dysostosis, mental retardation, and conduction deafness (AR)
Kniest syndrome (AD)
Arthrogrypotic hand anomaly and sensorineural deafness (AD)
Klippel–Feil anomalies, abducens paralysis with retracted bulb, and sensorineural or conduction deafness (cervico-oculoacoustic dysplasia – Wildervanck syndrome – ? multifactorial)
Craniofacial dysostosis (Crouzon's syndrome) (AD)
Acrocephalo-syndactyly Type 1 (Apert's syndrome) (?AD)
Hereditary hyperphosphatasaemia (AR)
Hereditary artho-ophthalmopathy (Stickler syndrome) (AD)
Osteogenesis imperfecta (AD)

Spondylo-epiphysial dysplasia congenita with sensorineural deafness (AD)
Joint fusions, mitral insufficiency and conduction hearing loss (AD)
Mandibulofacial dysostosis (Treacher–Collins or Franceschetti–Klein syndrome) (AD)

Hereditary Hearing Loss with Integumentary System Disease

Waardenburg's syndrome (AD)
Dominant lentigines and deafness (Leopard syndrome) (AD)
Recessive albinism and congenital deafness (?AR)
Recessive vitiligo, congenital deafness, muscle wasting and achalasia (AR)
Hereditary piebaldness and congenital deafness (?AR)
Sex-linked pigmentary abnormalities and congenital deafness (X-linked)
Recessive ectopic dermatitis and neural hearing loss
Dominant keratopachydermia, digital constrictions and deafness (?AD)
Dominant knuckle pads, leuconychia and mixed hearing loss (AD)
Dominant onychodystrophy, coniform teeth and hearing loss (AD)
Dominant onychodystrophy and congenital deafness (D ? X-linked)
Recessive onychodystrophy, digital abnormalities and deafness (AR)
Familial pili torti and hearing loss (?AR)
Dominant piebald trait, ataxia, and sensorineural hearing loss (AD)
Anhidrosis and progressive sensorineural hearing loss (AD)
Generalized alopecia, hypogonadism and sensorineural deafness (R ? X-linked)
Scanty hair, camptodactyly and sensorineural hearing loss (AR)
Atopic dermatitis and sensorineural hearing loss (AR)

Genetic Hearing Loss with Renal Damage

Nephritis with sensorineural deafness (Alport syndrome)
Severe hypertension, renal failure, abnormal steroidogenesis, hypogenitalism and sensorineural deafness (AR)
Charcot–Marie–Tooth syndrome: nephritis and sensorineural deafness
Macrothrombocytopathia, nephritis and sensorineural deafness (AD)
Infantile renal tubular acidosis and congenital sensorineural deafness (AR)
Adolescent or young adult renal tubular acidosis with slowly progressive sensorineural deafness (AR)
Renal disease, hyperprolinuria, ichthyosis and sensorineural deafness (AD)

Nephritis, urticaria, amyloidosis and sensorineural deafness (Muckle–Wells syndrome) (AD)
Renal, genital and middle ear anomalies (AR)
Renal disease, digital anomalies, and conduction hearing loss (AR or XR)

Genetic Hearing Loss with Nervous System Disease
Ataxia, pes cavus and sensorineural deafness of adult onset (AR)
Ataxia, hypogonadism, mental retardation and sensorineural deafness (Richards–Rundle syndrome) (?AR)
Ataxia, oligophrenia, myocardial sclerosis and sensorineural deafness (?AR)
Ataxia, mental retardation and sensorineural hearing loss (? AR or sex X-linked)
Ataxia, hypotonia, depressed deep tendon reflexes and progressive sensorineural deafness (AR)
Ataxia, cataract, psychosis and/or dementia and sensorineural deafness (AD)
Photomyoclonus, diabetes mellitus, nephropathy and sensorineural deafness (AD)
Myoclonic epilepsy, ataxia and sensorineural deafness (AD)
Myoclonic epilepsy and congenital sensorineural deafness (AD)
Acoustic neuromas and neural deafness (AD)
Sensory radicular neuropathy and progressive sensorineural deafness (AD)
Progressive sensory neuropathy, absent gastric motility, small bowel diverticulitis and profound childhood sensorineural deafness (AR)
Bulbopontine paralysis with progressive sensorineural hearing loss (AR)

Genetic Hearing Loss with Metabolic and other Abnormalities
Goitre and profound congenital sensorineural deafness (Pendred syndrome) (AR)
Goitre, elevated protein-bound iodine, stippled epiphyses and congenital sensorineural deafness (AR)
Aplasia of nasal alae, hypothyroidism, growth retardation, malabsorption, absent permanent teeth and sensorineural deafness occurring in females only
Prenatal dwarfism, elevated growth hormone levels, mental retardation and congenital deafness (AR)
Hypothalamohypophysial dwarfism and sensorineural deafness (AR)
Mucopolysaccharidosis
Type I: Scheie (AR)
Type II: Hunter: (X-linked recessive)
Type III: Sanfilippo: (AR)
Type IV: Morquio (AR)
Type VI: Maroteaux–Lamy (AR)
Mannosidosis (AR) [R]

Skeletal dysplasia, mental retardation, skin granulomas and profound congenital sensorineural deafness (AR)

Storage diseases
- Tay–Sachs disease
- Gm_1-gangliosidosis Type 1
- Beta-galactosidase deficiency
- Metachromatic leucodystrophy
- Fabry disease (many cases)

Chronic lactic acidaemia, metabolic myopathy, growth retardation and sensorineural deafness (AR)

Hyperprolinaemia and hyperprolinuria (iminoglycinaemia) with sensorineural deafness (AR)

Lesch–Nyhan syndrome

Chromosomal abnormalities
- Turner syndrome (XO): many deaf cases
- XX gonadal dysgenesis with congenital sensorineural deafness
- Trisomy 21 with mixed deafness
- Trisomy 13 with mixed deafness
- Trisomy 18 with mixed deafness
- Chromosome 18 long arm deletion syndrome

Haematological disorder
- Sickle cell disease: moderate bilateral hearing loss develops in the higher frequencies

ENDOCRINE DISORDERS

General

Major endocrine syndromes
Galactorrhoea with hyperprolactinaemia
Gynaecomastia
Endocrine disorders associated with diarrhoea
Hyperthermia associated with endocrine disorders

Adrenal

Congenital adrenal hyperplasia
Adrenocortical excess
Cushing's syndrome
Adrenocortical insufficiency
Conditions associated with hypoadrenocorticalism
Aldosteronism
Phaeochromocytoma

Diabetes mellitus

High incidence of diabetes mellitus
Genetic syndromes associated with diabetes mellitus
Insulin resistance in diabetes mellitus
Insulin resistance and insulin receptor involvement
Resistance to the action of insulin
Indication for glucose tolerance test in pregnancy
Diabetes mellitus secondary to chemical agents

Parathyroid

Hypoparathyroidism
Hyperparathyroidism
Pluriglandular syndrome

Pituitary

Pituitary tumours
Hypopituitarism
Pituitary dwarfism
Coma in hypopituitarism
Diabetes insipidus
Inappropriate ADH secretion

General sex disorders

Delayed puberty
Precocious puberty
Precocious pseudopuberty
Sexual ateliotic dwarfism

Female sex disorders

Precocious puberty in the female
Heavy periods
Climacteric syndrome
Hyperfunction of the ovary
Dysfunction of the ovary
Hypofunction of the ovary
Oral contraceptives
Amenorrhoea and oligomenorrhoea
Infertility in the female
Female hirsutism
Factors predisposing to pre-eclampsia and eclampsia

ENDOCRINE DISORDERS: GENERAL

Major Endocrine Syndromes
(*signs and symptoms suggesting endocrine disorder*)

Weakness and increasing fatiguability
Hirsutism
Impotence and decreased libido
Menstrual irregularities
Gynaecomastia and galactorrhoea
Obesity
Hypertension
Polyuria and polydipsia
Growth abnormalities
Skin changes
Arthropathy
Tetany and convulsive seizures
Oedema
Psychological abnormalities

Galactorrhoea with Hyperprolactinaemia

Centrally-acting drugs
- Phenothiazines
- Oral contraceptives
- Reserpine
- Methyldopa
- Haloperidol
- Tricyclic antidepressants
- Some antihistamines

Hypothalamic and pituitary stalk lesions
- Tumour
- Meningitis
- Granuloma

Pituitary tumour
- Acromegaly
- Cushing's diseases
- Otherwise non-functioning tumour

Ectopic prolactin production: tumour, especially carcinoma of lung

Primary hypothyroidism [R]

Chest wall injury
- Surgery
- Trauma
- Herpes zoster

Gynaecomastia

Physiological
- Neonatal
- Puberty
- Involutional

Pharmacological
- steroids
  - oestrogens
  - androgens
  - anabolic steroids
  - adrenocorticosteroids
  - progestogens
- digitalis
- spironolactone
- griseofulvin
- phenothiazines
- reserpine
- tricyclic tranquillizers
- methyldopa
- diethylpropion
- amphetamines
- radioactive iodine
- possibly antituberculous drugs

Pathological
- Endocrine
  - testis
    - prepubertal testicular failure, e.g. Klinefelter's syndrome
    - tumour
    - teratoma
      - chorionepithelioma
      - seminoma
      - interstitial cell tumour
      - Sertoli cell tumour

true hermaphroditism
thyroid: hyperthyroidism
adrenal
adrenocortical tumour
Addison's disease
hypothalamic disease
pituitary disease
acromegaly
chromophobe adenoma
Metabolic
chronic liver disease
chronic renal failure
Albright's syndrome
Reifenstein's syndrome
refeeding
after starvation
after severe illness
carcinoma
of lung
of other sites
exfoliative dermatitis
Central nervous system
traumatic paraplegia
Friedreich's ataxia
syringomyelia
myotonica congenita

Endocrine Disorders associated with Diarrhoea

Thyroid
thyrotoxicosis
medullary carcinoma of the thyroid
Zollinger–Ellison syndrome
VIPOMA: Pancreatic cholera, WDHA syndrome
Carcinoid syndrome
(Hypoadrenal crisis may present with diarrhoea)

Hyperthermia associated with Endocrine Disorders

Thyroid
'masked' thyrotoxicosis
tri-iodothyronine (T_3) thyrotoxicosis
subacute thyroiditis
Adrenal
primary adrenal insufficiency
secondary adrenal insufficiency
phaeochromocytoma

ADRENAL

Congenital Adrenal Hyperplasia

The most frequently found varieties are:

20–22 desmolase deficiency
3-beta-hydroxysteroid dehydrogenase deficiency
21-hydroxylase deficiency
11-hydroxylase deficiency

Suspect the possibility of this diagnosis in a vomiting newborn baby with low plasma sodium and raised plasma potassium levels, especially if the genitalia are ambiguous

Adrenocortical Excess

Cushing's syndrome: glucocorticoid excess
Conn's syndrome: aldosterone excess
Adrenal virilism: androgen excess
Congenital adrenal enzyme defects
Congenital adrenal hyperplasia

Cushing's Syndrome

Adrenal hyperplasia
- secondary to pituitary-hypothalamic dysfunction
- secondary to ACTH-producing tumour
  - pituitary tumour
  - non-endocrine tumour, e.g. bronchogenic carcinoma

Adrenal nodular hyperplasia*
Adrenal neoplasm
- adenoma*
- carcinoma*

Iatrogenic
- prolonged high doses of glucocorticoid steroids*
- prolonged use of high doses of ACTH

*ACTH independent – blood ACTH undetectable

Adrenocortical Insufficiency

Primary adrenal destruction
- autoimmune adrenalitis
- tuberculous destruction
- rare
  - infarction of adrenal gland
  - haemorrhage into adrenal
  - destruction by secondary metastases
  - sarcoidosis
  - histoplasmosis
  - amyloidosis

Secondary adrenal atrophy: following ACTH deficiency

Conditions associated with Hypoadrenocorticalism

Thyroid disease
Diabetes mellitus
Addisonian pernicious anaemia

Hypoparathyroidism
Vitiligo
Premature menopause

Aldosteronism

Primary hyperaldosteronism: aldosterone-producing adenoma

Secondary aldosteronism
- Physiological
  - pregnancy
  - sodium depletion
- Pathological
  - With hypertension
    - accelerated hypertension
    - renovascular hypertension in malignant phase
    - hypertension associated with oral contraceptives
    - 17-hydroxylase deficiency
    - juxtaglomerular cell tumour
    - thiazide-induced aldosteronism
  - Without hypertension
    - associated with oedema
      - nephrosis
      - cirrhosis with ascites
      - congestive cardiac failure
      - cyclic oedema
    - juxtaglomerular hyperplasia (Bartter's syndrome)
    - sodium-losing renal disease
  - Idiopathic aldosteronism
    - adenomatous hyperplasia
    - glucocorticoid-responsive aldosteronism
  - Tertiary aldosteronism: secondary aldosteronism developing autonomous control of function

Phaeochromocytoma

Tumour sites
- thoracic sympathetic chain
- spleen
- adrenal medulla
- renal capsule
- renal hilum
- coeliac ganglion
- paraganglion of Kohn
- organ of Zuckerkandl
- para-ureteric
- bladder wall

DIABETES MELLITUS

Potential
- Identical twin of a known diabetic

Both parents known diabetics
One parent and first degree relative of other parent known diabetic
Large babies, exceeding 10 lb at birth
History of recurrent stillbirths or intra-uterine death especially with islet cell hypertrophy at fetal postmortem, before live birth
Hydramnios

Latent

Diabetes mellitus develops under stress but glucose tolerance test normal at time of examination } pregnancy, obesity, trauma, surgery, steroid therapy
Normal glucose tolerance test, but abnormal cortisone-stressed glucose tolerance test

Asymptomatic (chemical)
Abnormal glucose tolerance test, but no sign of symptoms

Clinical diabetes mellitus
Clinical manifestations with abnormal glucose tolerance test
1. Primary
    a. Type 1: Juvenile onset, or insulin dependent
    b. Type 2: Maturity onset, non-insulin dependent
2. Secondary
    a. Pancreatic disease
    b. Liver disease
    c. Hormone-induced
        endogenous
        exogenous
    d. Obesity
    e. Drugs

High Incidence of Diabetes Mellitus

Mechanisms underlying development of diabetes mellitus
Defective beta cell mechanism
Impaired beta cell receptor site
Virus damage to beta cells in pancreas
Impairment of immunity system leading to beta cell damage
Hormonal imbalance
Destruction of beta cells

Conditions associated with a high incidence of diabetes mellitus
Obesity
Hyperlipidaemia
Widespread atherosclerosis
Chronic liver disease
Gout

Autoimmune disease
- Pernicious anaemia
- Addison's disease
- Vitiligo
- Alopecia
- Hypogonadism
- Thyroid disorders

Pancreatic disease
- Acute, relapsing and chronic pancreatitis
- Haemochromatosis
- Pancreatectomy

Endocrine
- Cushing's syndrome
- Acromegaly
- Hyperthyroidism

Genetic syndromes associated with Diabetes Mellitus

Klinefelter syndrome
Down's syndrome
Turner's syndrome
Werner's syndrome
Schmidt's syndrome
Prader–Willi syndrome
Laurence–Moon–Biedl syndrome
Alström syndrome
Cockayne syndrome
Hereditary relapsing pancreatitis
Cystic fibrosis
Ataxic telangiectasia
Friedreich's ataxia
Huntington's chorea
Muscular dystrophy
Dystrophia myotonica
Optic atrophy and diabetes insipidus
Retinitis pigmentosa
Glucose-6-phosphate dehydrogenase deficiency
Glycogen storage diseases
Haemochromatosis
Hyperlipidaemia Types IIb, III, IV and V
Ateliotic dwarfism
Lipodystrophies
Acute intermittent porphyria

Insulin Resistance in Diabetes Mellitus

Defective absorption of insulin from the subcutaneous tissues
Resistance to insulin infused intravenously

1. High concentration of insulin antibodies
2. Presence of antibodies to insulin receptors
3. Insulin resistance due to subnormal insulin receptors

Insulin Resistance and Insulin Receptor Involvement

Obesity
Diabetes mellitus
Uraemia
Ataxia telangiectasia
Diabetes mellitus with scleroderma: antireceptor antibodies
Congenital generalized lipodystrophy
Acanthrosis nigricans Type A
Acanthrosis nigricans Type B (antireceptor antibodies)

Resistance to the Action of Insulin

Endocrine
- Pregnancy
- Oral contraceptives
- Cushing's syndrome
- Acromegaly
- Hyperthyroidism
- Pancreatic alpha-cell tumour
- Insulin antibodies
- Phaeochromocytoma

Muscle disease
- Myotonic dystrophy
- Malignant cachexia

Metabolic: intercurrent infection

Indications for Glucose Tolerance Test in Pregnancy

First degree family history of diabetes mellitus
Second fasting glycosuria specimen during pregnancy
Previous infant's birth-weight exceeding 4·5 kg
Previous unexplained perinatal deaths
Maternal obesity (more than 20% above ideal body weight)
Acute hydramnios
Previous gestational diabetes

DIABETES MELLITUS SECONDARY TO CHEMICAL AGENTS

(*often with regression of diabetes after cessation of administration of the agent concerned*)

Direct beta-cell cytotoxic agents
- Alloxan
- Streptomycin

Inhibition of insulin synthesis
- Some antimitotics
- Some immunosuppressors
- Alpha-adrenergic agents
- Beta-blockers
- Somatostatin

Thiazide diuretics
Dioxide
Phenytoin

Blockade of glucose stimulation
Mannose heptulose

Gluconeogenesis, lipolysis, and possible tissue resistance to insulin
Corticosteroids
ACTH
Growth hormone
Oestrogen/progesterone contraceptive pill

PARATHYROID

Hypoparathyroidism

Uncommon
Surgical damage either to the parathyroid glands or to their blood supply in the neck. Onset 6 hours–3 days after operation of thyroidectomy. Recovery in 2 weeks

Rare
Parathyroid damage by ^{131}I during treatment of hyperthyroidism
Autoimmune hypoparathyroidism. Autosomal recessive. Hypoparathyroidism with other endocrinological abnormalities
Congenital hypoparathyroidism
sporadic
X-linked recessive
autosomal dominant
Transient neonatal hypoparathyroidism
infant born to hypoparathyroid mother
prematurity
dysmaturity
cerebral injury
hypoglycaemia
maternal diabetes mellitus
introduction of cow's milk
Di-George syndrome: absent thymus, susceptibility to infection
Primary hypomagnesaemia: X-linked recessive
Metastatic neoplasia affecting all four glands
Haemochromatosis
Idiopathic

Hyperparathyroidism

Parathyroid adenoma

single 85%
multiple 3%
Parathyroid hyperplasia
chief cell hyperplasia 6%
water-clear cell hyperplasia 0·6%
Parathyroid carcinoma: about 3%

Pluriglandular Syndrome

Parathyroid tumour associated with
pituitary adenoma
pancreatic adenoma
Parathyroid tumour associated with
phaeochromocytoma
medullary thyroid carcinoma
rarely Cushing's syndrome

PITUITARY

Pituitary Tumours
(*10% of all intracranial tumours*)

Anterior lobe
Chromophobe – rare in childhood, equal sex incidence
Eosinophilic adenoma
Basophilic adenoma

Posterior lobe (primary tumour rare)
Astrocytoma
Ganglioneuroma
Tumours of cells resembling pituicytes

Epithelial remnants of craniopharyngeal duct
Craniopharyngioma: commonest pituitary tumour in childhood

Tumours affecting the pituitary–hypothalamic region
Tumours of optic chiasma
Tumours of hypothalamus
Tumours of third ventricle
Midbrain tumours
Pineal tumours
Sphenoidal ridge meningioma

Secondary carcinoma from breast, lung or other sites } may involve pituitary
Reticuloses } may involve pituitary

Infiltrations and granuloma
Sarcoidosis
Histiocytosis
Haemochromatosis

Infections
- Tuberculosis
- Pyogenic abscess
- Syphilis

Hypopituitarism

Tumours
- Pituitary
  - chromophobe
  - eosinophil
  - basophil
  - secondary
    - metastatic tumour
    - leukaemia
    - lymphoma
- In region of hypothalamus and pituitary stalk
  - craniopharyngioma
  - meningioma
  - pinealoma
  - secondary carcinoma (especially from breast)
  - hypothalamic and chiasmal gliomas
  - hamartoma

Granulomas
- sarcoidosis
- tuberculosis
- histiocytosis X (Hand–Schüller–Christian)
- Syphilis

Infarction
- postpartum necrosis (Sheehan's syndrome)
- pituitary apoplexy
  - haemorrhage
  - thrombosis
- pituitary tumour infarction
- aneurysm

Idiopathic
- isolated deficiency of hypothalamic hormone } unknown cause
- insensitivity to growth hormone releasing hormone } unknown cause

Acquired and developmental
- vascular malformations of the hypothalamus
- trauma
  - with or without skull fracture
  - surgery
  - irradiation
- with congenital rubella
- with cerebellar ataxia and retinitis pigmentosa
- with anosmia (Kallman's syndrome)
- emotional deprivation

Pituitary Dwarfism

Congenital hypopituitary dwarfism

Pigmy is probably subresponsive to normal human growth hormone, i.e. a tissue defect

Acquired hypopituitary dwarfism
- Pituitary
  - adenoma
    - chromophobe
    - eosinophilic
  - craniopharyngioma
- Malignancy
  - glioma of optic chiasma
  - meningioma
- Infections
  - tuberculous basal meningitis
  - syphilis
  - encephalitis
- Granulomatous disease
  - sarcoidosis
  - multiglandular syndrome
  - Hand–Schüller–Christian disease
  - eosinophilic granuloma
- Vascular disease
  - severe haemorrhage with hypotension
  - diabetes mellitus
  - cranial arteritis
  - vascular malformations
- Iatrogenic
  - post-surgery
  - radiotherapy
- Trauma: head injury
- Secondary to hypothalamic disease
  - craniopharyngioma associated with diabetes insipidus
- Nutrition: secondary to
  - severe malnutrition
  - starvation
  - malabsorption syndrome

Coma in Hypopituitarism

Following surgery to the gland area
Pituitary apoplexy
Infections
Hypoglycaemia
Hypersensitivity to drugs and anaesthetics
Sodium depletion
Water retention
Cerebral anoxia
Hypothermia

Diabetes Insipidus

Tumours in the region of pituitary gland and hypothalamus
- secondary carcinoma
- primary

craniopharyngioma
large adenoma
chromophobic
eosinophilic
basophilic
glioma
meningioma near hypothalamus
Surgical or irradiation damage to pituitary
Head injury, with or without skull fracture
Infective or granulomatous lesions
encephalitis
basal meningitis (syphilis, tuberculosis)
sarcoidosis
histiocytosis-X (Hand–Schüller–Christian disease)
Vascular lesions e.g. arteriovenous malformations or fistulas
Idiopathic: may have familial incidence
dominant
recessive
(*see* other causes of Polyuria – Renal p. 417)

Inappropriate ADH Secretion
(*results in hyponatraemia and haemodilution with a urine hyperosmotic relative to the plasma*)

Malignancy
oat cell carcinoma of lung
carcinoma of pancreas
lymphosarcoma
reticulum cell sarcoma
Hodgkin's disease
thymoma
Non-malignant pulmonary disease
pneumonia
lung abscess
tuberculosis
Central nervous system
fracture of skull with damage to posterior pituitary or hypothalamus or pituitary stalk
subdural haematoma
subarachnoid haemorrhage
cerebral vascular thrombosis
cerebral atrophy
acute encephalitis
meningitis
purulent
tuberculous
Guillain–Barré syndrome
systemic lupus erythematosus
acute intermittent porphyria
stress, including pain
Miscellaneous
hypothyroidism
positive pressure respiration

Drugs
- chlorpropamide
- thiazide diuretics
- tricyclic antidepressants
- narcotics
- barbiturates
- general anaesthesia
- oxytocin
- vincristine
- cyclophosphamide

GENERAL SEX DISORDERS

Delayed Puberty

Constitutional

Hypothalamic disorders
- Deficiency of gonadotrophin-releasing hormone
    1. Congenital
        - Familial
        - Sporadic
        - Prader–Willi syndrome
        - Laurence–Moon–Biedl syndrome
        - Kallman's syndrome
    2. Acquired
        - Infections
            - viral encephalitis
            - sarcoidosis
            - tuberculosis
        - Neoplasm
            - craniopharyngioma
            - primary hypothalamic tumour
            - histiocytosis
            - pinealoma

Pituitary disorders
- Gonadotrophin deficiency
    1. Congenital
    2. Acquired
        - infections
        - neoplasms
        - trauma

Gonadal disorders
1. Congenital
    - chromosomal
        - Turner's syndrome
        - Klinefelter's syndrome
    - gonadal agenesis
    - myotonia dystrophica
2. Infections
3. Trauma
    - injury

irradiation
Chronic systemic disease
including
cardiac
renal
pulmonary
gastrointestinal
endocrine
haematological
connective tissue disease
hepatic
malnutrition

Precocious Puberty

Constitutional
Gonadotrophins in excess of the patient's age
Midbrain lesion

Precocious Pseudopuberty

Premature secondary sexual characteristics develop without gonadal maturation, and without achieving active sexual maturity or capacity to procreate
adrenal – congenital adrenal hyperplasia
gonadal

Sexual Ateliotic Dwarfism

Group I – Dwarfism associated with monotrophic human growth hormone (HGH) deficiency, with insulin hypersensitivity and low insulin levels

Group II – Dwarfism associated with monotrophic HGH deficiency. Normal sensitivity to insulin and hyperinsulinism.

Group III – Dwarfism with normal or high peripheral levels of immunoreactive HGH, but clinically HGH deficiency (i.e. biologically inactive HGH). Sulphation factor after exogenous HGH low

Group IV – Dwarfism with normal peripheral levels of immunoreactive HGH, with a metabolic profile consistent with HGH deficiency. Sulphation factor after exogenous HGH normal

FEMALE SEX DISORDERS

Precocious Puberty in the Female

Constitutional
inherited familial

developmental
Central nervous system disorders
hypothalamic tumour
pituitary tumour
pineal tumour
infections
trauma
McCune–Albright syndrome
Ovarian tumours
Adrenal disorders
Gonadotrophin-producing tumours
Exogenous causes
oestrogens
gonadotrophins

Heavy Periods

Dysfunctional uterine bleeding
Carcinoma of uterus
Carcinoma of cervix
Cervical polyp
Cervical erosion
Adenomyoma
Endometriosis

Climacteric Syndrome

Vasomotor
hot flushes
night sweats
palpitations
angina
Other symptoms
fatigue
insomnia
headaches
depression
dizziness
anxiety
forgetfulness
pruritus
Genito-urinary
pruritus
dyspareunia
urinary urgency
urinary stress incontinence
decreased libido

Hyperfunction of the Ovary

Primary
feminizing tumour
masculinizing tumour

Secondary
- general – true precocious puberty
- constitutional
  - persistent follicular cyst
  - corpus luteum cyst
  - Stein–Leventhal syndrome and hyperthecosis

Dysfunction of the Ovary

Dysfunction
- chlorioncarcinoma
- Struma ovarii
- carcinoid tumour

Hypofunction of the Ovary

Primary: gonadal dysgenesis
- Turner's syndrome
- menopause
  - normal
  - premature

Secondary
- hypothalamic disorder
- hypopituitarism
- constitutional and metabolic disorders
- anovulatory bleeding
- inadequate luteal phase
- iatrogenic
  - ovariectomy
  - pelvic irradiation
  - cytotoxic drugs
- Addison's disease

Oral Contraceptives

Possible side-effects
- circulatory
  - thrombo-embolism
  - cerebral thrombosis
  - myocardial infarction
  - hypertension
- metabolic
  - jaundice
  - hyperlipidaemia
  - glucose intolerance
- gynaecological
  - 'post pill' amenorrhoea
  - 'breakthrough' bleeding
  - chloasma
  - breast tenderness
- other
  - depression

- headache
- weight gain

Absolute contra-indications to use
- thrombo-embolism
- arterial disease
- diabetes mellitus
- hyperlipidaemia
- liver disease
- carcinoma of breast
- carcinoma of uterus
- migraine
- pregnancy

Relative contra-indications
- oligomenorrhoea or amenorrhoea
- depression
- hypertension
- epilepsy

Amenorrhoea and Oligomenorrhoea

Physiological
- pre-reproductive
- reproductive age group
  - pregnancy
  - lactation
- post-reproduction period

Pathological
- Hypothalamus
  - injury
  - tumours
  - encephalitis
  - idiopathic: functional
    - 'stress'
    - anorexia nervosa
    - starvation
  - drugs
    - phenothiazines
    - contraceptive pill
- Pituitary
  - panhypopituitarism
    - postpartum necrosis (Sheehan's syndrome)
    - tumour
    - surgical hypophysectomy
    - tuberculosis
    - sarcoid
    - cavernous sinus thrombosis
  - isolated gonadotrophin deficiency
- Gonadal
  - ovarian dysgenesis
  - premature ovarian failure

ovarian tumours
Uterine and vaginal abnormalities
Amenorrhoea–galactorrhoea syndromes

Infertility in the Female

Fertility depends on
Production of ova
Fertilization of ova
Tubal transport of ova
Uterine entry of ova
Development implantation
Maintenance of fertilized ovum

Relative infertility
Uterine abnormality, e.g. bicornuate or subseptate uterus
Incompetent cervix
Deficient corpus luteum

Absolute infertility
Tubal blockage
Abnormalities of menstruation
anovulatory menstruation
specific endocrine disorders
hyperprolactinaemia
thyroid disorders
disorders of hypothalamic–pituitary–ovarian control
impaired follicular phase – relieved by clomiphene
impaired midcycle LH secretion – relieved by midcycle HCG
both – relieved by clomiphene plus midcycle HCG
amenorrhoea
primary ovarian failure
pituitary failure
hypopituitary failure
hyperprolactinaemia
thyroid disorders
disorders of pituitary–ovarian–hypothalamic control
Stein–Leventhal polycystic ovary syndrome
Genetic, e.g. Turner's syndrome

Female Hirsutism

Heredity
Familial hypertrichosis
Racial
Hair follicles increased sensitivity to normal endogenous androgens
Male hermaphrodite raised as female
Precocious puberty

Idiopathic

Physiological
- Pregnancy
- Menopause

Drugs
- Androgens*
- Anabolic steroids*
- Corticosteroids
- Phenytoin
- Dilantin
- Some synthetic progestins
- ACTH

Pituitary
- Acromegaly
- Achard–Thiers syndrome (bearded diabetic)

Adrenal cortex
- Cushing's syndrome*
- Virilizing adrenal tumours*
  - adenoma
  - carcinoma
- Mild adrenal dysfunction
- Congenital adrenal hyperplasia*
  - adrenogenital form
  - hypertensive form
  - delayed onset form

Ovaries
- Stein–Leventhal syndrome
- Polycystic ovaries*
- Hilus cell hyperplasia
- Hyperthecosis syndrome
- Virilizing tumours
  - hilar cell adenoma
  - luteoma
  - arrhenoblastoma
  - adrenal rest tumour
- (N.B. adrenal feminization from tumour very rare indeed)

Sexual abnormality
- Gonadal dysgenesis with androgenic manifestations
- Intersex states

Thyroid
- Juvenile hypothyroidism

Cerebral and hypothalamus
- Encephalitis
- Multiple sclerosis
- Hyperostosis frontalis interna

*Can also cause virilism

Miscellaneous
- Anorexia nervosa
- some stress situations
- porphyria

Factors predisposing to Pre-eclampsia and Eclampsia

Associated with hypertension
- Chronic hypertension
- Chronic hypertension in chronic renal disease
- Previous pre-eclampsia
- Family history
  - hypertensive disease
  - pre-eclampsia

Associated with excessive amounts of chorionic tissue
- Multiple pregnancy
- Hydatidiform mole
- Poorly controlled diabetes mellitus
- Severe fetal haemolytic disease

MALE SEX DISORDERS

Testicular Failure

Secondary
- isolated gonadotrophin deficiency
- isolated ICSH deficiency (fertile eunuch)
- multiple pituitary deficiency
  - idiopathic prepuberty
  - secondary to lesions of neurohypophysis
  - congenital: Laurence–Moon–Biedl syndrome

Hypergonadism

Primary: functioning interstitial cell tumour

Secondary
- familial
- tumour in the region of third ventricle
  - pinealoma
  - astrocytoma
  - hamartoma
  - teratoma
  - craniopharyngioma

Neoplasm of the Testis

Seminoma: germinoma
Teratocarcinoma

Embryonal carcinoma
- chorionepithelioma
- various

Teratoma
Interstitial cell tumour
Fibroma
Lipoma
Adenoma
Myxoma
Unclassified

Male Pseudohermaphroditism

Disorders of testicular differentiation: chromosome or gene deletion involving Y-chromosome

Disorders of testicular function
- gonadotrophin unresponsiveness
- abnormalities of Müllerian inhibiting factor synthesis or action
- testosterone biosynthesis deficiencies
- cholesterol 20-alpha, 22-hydroxylase, and/or 20, 22 desmolase deficiency
- 17-alpha-hydroxylase deficiency
- 17, 20-desmolase deficiency
- 3-beta-ol, dehydrogenase: Δ 5-isomerase deficiency
- 17-beta-hydroxysteroid dehydrogenase deficiency

Disorders of functions at the androgen-dependent target areas
- androgen receptor defects
- enzyme deficiences in testosterone metabolism
- 5-alpha-reductase deficiency

Male Hypogonadism

Abnormalities in hypothalamic–pituitary function
- Panhypopituitarism
- LH-FSH deficiency (Kallmann's syndrome)
- Isolated FSH deficiency
- Prader–Willi syndrome
- Laurence–Moon–Biedl syndrome
- Cerebellar ataxia

Primary gonadal abnormality
- Chromosomal abnormality
  - Klinefelter syndrome: XXY or XXYY
  - XX males: sex reversal syndrome)
- Reifenstein's male pseudo hermaphroditism (X-linked recessive)
- True hermaphroditism
- Streak gonads with XY karyotype
- Anorchia
- Testicular agenesis (the vanishing Testes syndrome)

Noonan's syndrome
Sertoli cell only syndrome
Adult seminiferous tubule failure
- idiopathic oligospermia
- idiopathic azospermia
- testicular mosaicism with infertility
- Kartagener's syndrome
- myotonia dystrophica
- cystic fibrosis

Acquired testicular disorders
- orchitis
  - mumps
  - tuberculosis
  - leprosy
  - gonorrhoea
  - Brucella
  - syphilis
  - hyperpyrexia
  - irradiation
  - neoplasm
- surgical castration
- trauma

Enzyme defects in androgen synthesis
- 20-alpha-hydroxylase deficiency (lipoid adrenal hypoplasia)
- 17,20-desmolase deficiency
- 3-beta-hydroxysteroid hydrogenase deficiency
- 17-hydroxylase deficiency
- 17-ketosteroid reductase deficiency
- 5-alpha-reductase deficiency

Defect in androgen action
- Complete androgen insensitivity: testicular feminization
- Incomplete androgen insensitivity: testicular feminization

Congenital anomaly
- Persistent Müllerian duct syndrome

Differential Diagnosis of Male Hypogonadism

Abnormalities of semen
- gonadotrophin and/or tubular insufficiency
- eunuchoidism
- varicocele
- testicular maldescent
- mumps
- traumatically blocked vasa deferentia
- venereal disease

Impotence
- psychosexual
- neurological

drug-induced
eunuchoidism

Abnormality in female partner

Poor sexual technique

Impaired Leydig cell function

Primary testicular failure
genetic
Klinefelter syndrome
Ullrich–Turner syndrome
developmental
anorchia
cryptorchia
acquired
castration

Gonadotrophin failure
delayed puberty
selective gonadotrophin deficiency
panhypopituitarism

THYROID DISORDERS

Thyroiditis

Acute thyroiditis: due to bacterial invasion
Subacute thyroiditis: de Quervain's granulomatous thyroiditis ? due to viral infection
Chronic thyroiditis
Hashimoto's lymphadenoid lymphocytic thyroiditis: autoimmune disease affecting the thyroid
Riedel's ligneous thyroiditis [R]
Focal thyroiditis
lymphoid foci in gland ? significance
tuberculosis
secondary carcinoma
sarcoidosis
mycoses
amyloid deposits

Hypothyroidism

Primary
Non-goitrous
idiopathic atrophy
congenital cretin
adult
thyroiditis
postoperative thyroidectomy

post ^{131}I, post-irradiation
thyroid dysgenesis
Goitrous
inherited defects: six specific defects described
acquired
iodide deficiency myxoedema
drug-induced hypothyroidism
chronic lymphoid thyroiditis

Secondary
Anterior pituitary hypothyroidism: TSH deficiency
primary pituitary atrophy
pituitary ablation
tumours, granulomas, vascular accidents damaging anterior pituitary
Hypothalamic hypothyroidism: TRH deficiency
pituitary stalk section
granulomas affecting pituitary stalk, etc.
Peripheral tissue resistance to thyroid hormone

Hypothyroidism in Childhood

With goitre
enzyme deficiency
drug-induced
iodine-induced
chronic lymphocytic thyroiditis

Without goitre
congenital absence of thyroid
thyroid hypoplasia
ectopia
secondary hypothyroidism

Thyrotoxicosis

T4-T3 thyrotoxicosis
diffuse toxic goitre with ophthalmopathy (Graves' disease)
toxic uninodular or multinodular goitre (Plummer's disease)
thyrotoxicosis following excess thyroid, L-thyroxine, thyroglobulin, or liotrix
ectopic thyrotoxicosis
hydatidiform mole
chorioncarcinoma
struma ovarii
metastatic thyroid carcinoma

T3 thyrotoxicosis
nodular goitre with preferential T3 secretion
T3 thyrotoxicosis from excess tri-idothyronine
T3 thyrotoxicosis following radioactive iodine treatment of Graves' disease

T4 thyrotoxicosis
increased serum T4 with decreased serum T3 due to metabolic diversion

Hyperthyroidism

Diffuse toxic goitre
Toxic nodular goitre
1. Solitary autonomous toxic adenoma
2. Toxic multinodular goitre
Thyroiditis with thyrotoxicosis
1. Subacute thyroiditis
2. Chronic lymphocytic thyroiditis
3. Hashimoto's disease
4. Post-irradiation
deep X-ray
^{131}I
Neonatal thyrotoxicosis
Exogenous iodine-induced thyrotoxicosis (Jod–Basedow)
Factitious hyperthyroidism
Toxic struma ovarii
Metastatic toxic thyroid carcinoma
Thyrotropin-producing pituitary tumour
Tumours producing circulating TSH-like thyroid stimulation
1. Chorioncarcinoma
2. Embryonal cell carcinoma of testis
3. Hydatidiform mole

Goitre

Iodine deficiency
Due to goitrogens
Nodular goitre
toxic
non-toxic
Graves' disease
Hashimoto's disease
Viral thyroiditis
Carcinoma of the thyroid
Familial goitre

Familial Goitre

Iodine is normally transported into the thyroid gland from plasma, where it undergoes oxidation and progressive build-up into mono- and di-iodotyrosines, then T3 and T4 biochemical defects can occur anywhere along the chain of production
Iodide transport defect [R]
Organification, peroxidase defect [R]
Familial goitre and deaf-mutism (Pendred's syndrome) [R]
Cretinism with failure of coupling of iodotyrosines [R]

Cretinism from failure of iodotyrosine deiodinase activity [R]
Familial goitre with diminished or altered thyroglobulin synthesis [R]
Cretinism with abnormal iodinated polypeptides in serum [R]
Cretinism with impaired thyroid response to thyrotropin
Hypothyroidism with possible target-organ refractoriness to thyroid hormone [R]
Undefined cases [R]

GASTROINTESTINAL TRACT

Small intestinal villous atrophy
Tumours of small intestine
Some diseases presenting as 'appendicitis'
Large bowel
Polyps of colon and rectum
Proctitis
Anal incontinence

GENERAL SIGNS AND SYMPTOMS

Disorders of Appetite

Increased appetite
- (rarely the primary complaint made by a patient)
- psychoneurotic disorder
- central nervous system disease (rare)
- diabetes mellitus, accompanied by thirst
- hyperthyroidism (some cases)
- pregnancy (some cases)
- ? infestation with intestinal worms (round worm, tape worm)

Diminished appetite
- any chronic disease process
- gastrointestinal disease
- liver disease
- chronic alcoholism
- uraemia
- congestive cardiac failure
- depressive states
- anorexia nervosa

Perverted appetite
- may occur in normal pregnancy
- mentally retarded patients
- psychosis

Possible Complications of Elemental Diet

Unpalatability
Gastrointestinal
- nausea
- delayed gastric emptying
- vomiting
- diarrhoea

Aspiration of food into respiratory tract

Water balance
- hyperosmolar dehydration
- hypertonic non-ketotic coma

Hyperglycaemia
Skin rashes

Vomiting

The vomiting centre is in the reticular core of the medulla

Psychological stimuli
- sights
- smells
- sounds
- associations

Reflex vomiting via the vagal and sympathetic afferent nerves: from the abdominal organs

Reflex vomiting via the vestibular organs
- motion sickness
- labyrinth disease

Drugs capable of causing vomiting
- apomorphine
- morphine
- ergot derivatives
- digitalis glycosides
- nitrogen mustard
- high salt concentrations in fluid drunk

Bowel Sounds

Increased:
- borborygmi
  - physiological: diet
  - pathological
    - carcinoid syndrome
    - Jeghers' syndrome
    - post-gastrojejunostomy

Decreased or absent
- paralytic ileus
- peritonitis

Diarrhoea

True diarrhoea: increased stool volume
- steatorrhoea
- watery diarrhoea
- watery diarrhoea with blood and/or mucus

Spurious diarrhoea: normal or decreased stool volume
- spurious diarrhoea associated with faecal impaction
- faecal frequency with passage of small fragments of stool
- frequent passage of blood and/or mucus without faecal material
- passage of large volume of mucus

True Diarrhoea

Adults
- infection
  - bacteria
    - Shigella
    - Salmonella
    - *Cl. welchii* and *Cl. perfringens*
    - *B. cereus*
    - Enteropathic *E. coli*
    - *Vibrio cholerae*
    - *Vibrio parahaemolyticus*
    - *Staph. pyogenes*
  - virus: especially Echo virus
  - protozoa: amoebic dysentery
  - parasites
    - giardiasis
    - worms
      - hookworms
      - round worms
      - strongyloides
    - schistosomiasis
  - postenteritic malabsorption
- pancreatitis
- Crohn's disease
- ulcerative colitis
- stagnant loop syndrome – postgastrectomy
- neoplasm
  - carcinoma of colon
  - lymphoma in small bowel
- irritable colon syndrome
- diverticulitis
- drugs
  - abuse of purgatives
  - antibiotics
  - colchicine etc.
- loss of absorptive surface of small bowel
  - malabsorption syndromes
  - following resection of small bowel
- associated with
  - thyrotoxicosis
  - uraemia
  - carcinoid syndrome
  - Zollinger–Ellison syndrome
  - anxiety states

Infants
- unsuitable feeds, e.g. excessive sugar in feed
- infection
  - infantile gastroenteritis
  - systemic infection
    - urinary tract infection
    - upper respiratory tract infection

carbohydrate intolerance
Hirschsprung's disease
pancreatic disorders
coeliac disease
fibrocystic disease
protein-losing enteropathy
drugs: including antibiotics
metabolic disorders

Constipation

Common causes
inadequate bulk in the diet
lack of exercise
failure and/or inability to answer the call to stool
part of the stool may be retained, resulting in cumulative constipation
painful anal conditions interfere with regular habits
Secondary to motility disorders of unknown origin
irritable bowel syndrome
diverticular disease
slow transit constipation
idiopathic megabowel
aged bowel
obstetric bowel
Secondary to psychiatric states
depression and chronic psychoses
anorexia nervosa
Secondary to known causes
colonic disease, rectal disease, anal disease } including Hirschsprung's disease and systemic sclerosis affecting the bowel
Neurological disease
Endocrine disorder: hypothyroidism
Metabolic
dehydration
hypercalcaemia
Drug-induced, with decreased peristalsis
hypotensives
antacids
anticholinergics

Malnutrition

Diet
insufficient intake
inappropriate diet
Malabsorption syndrome, with consequent excessive elimination
Increased dietary requirement
(Blockade of utilization)

Patients liable to suffer from Malnutrition
(excluding malabsorption syndrome etc.)

Refugees
Vagrants
Alcoholics
Elderly living alone
Mentally ill
Children of recent immigrants from the developing countries
Pregnant women

CIRCULATORY PROBLEMS

Medium and Large Vessel Disease affecting the Alimentary Tract

Visceral circulation: large vessel occlusion
- tumour
- fibrous band
- embolism

Input trunks
- acute mesenteric occlusion
- mesenteric infarction
- chronic intestinal ischaemia
- coeliac axis compression syndrome

Arteries of distribution
- atheroma
- Buerger's disease
- polyarteritis nodosa
- trauma
- hernia
- volvulus

Venous occlusion
- volvulus
- blood dyscrasia

Non-occlusive intestinal ischaemia
- hypotension
- cardiac failure
- splanchnic vasoconstriction
  - trauma
  - drugs

Small Vessel Disease which can affect the Alimentary Tract

Inflammatory
- Adjacent to ulcer
- Ulcerative colitis
- Crohn's disease

Infective angiitis
- typhoid
- tuberculosis
- syphilis
- dysentery
- leprosy

Radiation damage
Specific arteritis: in Crohn's disease
Arteritis
- Takasayu's disease
- giant cell arteritis
- malignant hypertension
- amyloidosis

Benign focal arteritis (in appendix)
Buerger's disease

Vasospastic
- Malignant hypertension
- Post-coarctation syndrome
- Arteriolitis associated with phaeochromocytoma
- Vasopressive drug therapy

Immune complex and connective tissue disease
- Systemic lupus erythematosus
- Polyarteritis nodosa
- Rheumatoid arthritis
- Dermatomyositis
- Sjögren's syndrome
- Wegener's granuloma
- Anaphylactoid purpura (Schönlein–Henoch)
- Progressive systemic sclerosis

Degenerative: atherosclerosis, e.g. in diabetes mellitus

Miscellaneous
- Hereditary haemorrhagic telangiectasia
- Amyloidosis
- Pseudoxanthoma elasticum
- Ehlers–Danlos syndrome
- Malignant atrophic papulosis (Köhlmeier Degos disease)
- Fabry's syndrome
- Local potassium salts
- Thrombotic thrombocytopenic purpura

Anaemia and the Gastrointestinal Tract

Iron deficiency
- bleeding
  - peptic ulcer
  - small intestine
    - neoplasm
    - lymphoma
    - hamartogenous polyps

- Meckel's diverticulum
- Crohn's disease
- vascular occlusion
- intussusception

large intestine
- ulcerative colitis
- diverticulitis
- carcinoma
- amyloidosis
- haemorrhoidal haemorrhage

primary haemorrhagic disease
- haemophilia
- von Willebrand's disease
- other plasma clotting defects
- haemorrhagic telangiectasia
- thrombocytopenia

malabsorption
defective diet

Vitamin B_{12} deficiency
- defective diet
- pernicious anaemia
- gastric surgery
- stagnant intestinal loop, syndrome
- ileal resection
- Imerslund's disease
- fish tapeworm
- tropical sprue
- coeliac disease

Folate deficiency
- coeliac disease
- tropical sprue
- major small intestinal resection
- drugs – phenytoin and phenobarbitone
- Crohn's disease
- lymphoma of small intestine
- amyloidosis
- Whipple's disease

Protein-losing Gastroenteropathy in Cardiac Disease

Congestive cardiac failure, especially associated with constrictive pericarditis

Right-sided heart failure
- tricuspid valve regurgitation and rheumatic heart disease
- pulmonary stenosis
- Lutembacher syndrome
- atrial septal defect
- cardiomyopathy

Possible causes of hypoproteinaemia
- protein loss into gut
- increased urinary protein loss

defective protein synthesis due to liver dysfunction
increase in plasma volume has a dilution effect

INHERITED GASTROINTESTINAL NEOPLASMS

Oesophageal carcinoma with plantar and palmar keratosis (AD)
Colonic carcinoma without polyposis (AD)
Colonic carcinoma with polyposis
  Familial polyposis coli (AD)
  Gardner's syndrome (AD)
  Turcot's syndrome (AD)
  Discrete solitary polyp (AD)
Adenocarcinomatosis occurring in several members of the same family (AD)
Multiple mucosal neuromas with medullary thyroid carcinoma (AD)

UNUSUAL BOWEL DISORDERS

Endometriosis of the bowel: rare complication of pelvic endometriosis
Eosinophilic infiltration of the gut
  with eosinophilia and diffuse infiltrating or ulcerating lesion
  without eosinophilia. Localized lesions, which are polypoid, confined to the submucosa and commonest in the stomach
Familial Mediterranean fever (AR)
Gastrointestinal carcinoid tumour
Megacolon
  congenital: faulty enervation of distal colon and rectum (Hirschsprung's disease)
  acquired idiopathic
  acquired secondary to
    laxative overdose
    geriatric faecal impaction
    Chagas' disease with damage to mesenteric plexus
    diffuse scleroderma with damage to colonic muscle
Pneumatosis cystoides intestinalis
  infants under 1 year
    with pyloric stenosis
    intestinal obstruction
    colitis
  adults – associated with
    colitis
    infarction
Pseudomembranous enterocolitis
Solitary ulcer of rectum

MOUTH

Cheilitis

Angular cheilitis: occurs especially in the edentulous and aged. Senile retraction and atrophy of mandible with overclosure of upper and lower jaws and excessive salivation

Exfoliative cheilitis
- prolonged exposure to the sun
- skin disease, e.g. atopic eczema
- lip-licking habit
- heavy pipe smoking

Oral Pigmentation

Melanotic pigmentation – physiological, racial

Exogenous
- intestinal polyposis associated with freckle-like pigmentation in the mouth, on lips, hands and face. Peutz–Jegher's syndrome
- post-inflammatory hyperpigmentation
- drugs and poisons
  - antimalarials, bismuth, mercury, lead } blue-line gums
- Addison's disease: patches of brown pigmentation in adrenocortical insufficiency

Fordyce's disease: small yellow submucosal spots

malignant melanoma

black hairy tongue

Burning Sensation in the Mouth
(*excluding trauma, noxious substances etc.*)

Wearers of dentures
Women after the menopause
Vitamin B deficiency
Malabsorption
Diabetes mellitus
Cancerophobia

Aphthae on Tongue and Lower Lip

Aphthous ulcer

Trauma from habit tic

Virus
- herpes simplex
- herpangina
- hand-foot-mouth disease

Treponemal infection: syphilis

Infections secondary to:
- leukaemia
- lymphosarcoma

agranulocytosis
Stevens–Johnson syndrome
Behçet's syndrome
Methotrexate stomatitis

Disorders of Teeth

Dental erosion
- industrial: acidic fumes or droplets
- regurgitation of stomach contents (repeated)
- acid medicines
- diet
  - apples
  - grapefruit
  - lemons
  - Cola drinks
  - vinegar
  - etc.

Dental attrition
- diet
- resistance of dental enamel
- bruxism

Dental abrasion
- excessive use of toothbrush and pastes
- habits, e.g. biting threads
- dental: deliberate abrasion

Dental staining
- intrinsic
  - single tooth: following trauma
  - all teeth
    - infantile jaundice
    - tetracycline therapy during formative years
    - high content of fluoride in drinking water (natural)

Gingivitis

Acute
- Acute herpetic gingivostomatitis: primary herpes virus infection
- acute necrotizing ulcerative gingivitis: Vincent's angina
- desquamative gingivitis

Chronic
- localized: epulis
- generalized gingival enlargement
  - due to chronic inflammation
  - during puberty and in normal pregnancy (hormonal)
  - leukaemia
  - drugs, e.g. phenytoin
  - inherited [R]

Ptyalism

Apparent or real excess of saliva

1. Difficulty in swallowing, resulting in dribbling
    - bulbar palsy
    - pseudobulbar palsy
    - bilateral facial palsy
    - myasthenia gravis
    - paralysis of the hypoglossal nerve
    - diphtheritic palsy
    - Parkinsonism
    - botulism
    - rabies

2. Excess production of saliva
    - drugs
        - mercury
        - iodides
        - pilocarpine
        - bromides
        - excessive smoking
    - generalized stomatitis
        - jagged carious tooth
        - broken or ill-fitting dental plate
        - foreign body embedded in gum
        - gumboil
        - tumour in oral cavity
    - excessive salivation arising from gastric reflex
        - duodenal ulcer
        - dilatation of stomach
        - pancreatitis
        - nausea from any cause

THROAT

Dysphagia

Due to discomfort
- stomatitis
- ulcerated tongue, swollen tongue
- sore throat: due to tonsillitis, etc.
- laryngitis
    - infection
    - inflammation
    - neoplasm

Pharyngeal symptoms
- difficulty in initiating swallowing
    - emotional
    - nerve lesion
    - motor neuron disease
- with coughing, choking and regurgitation
    - bilateral upper motor neuron lesion
        - bilateral hemiplegia
        - multiple sclerosis

lower motor neuron lesion (nucleus ambiguus or Xth nerve)
  motor neuron disease
  bulbar poliomyelitis
  syringomyelia
  polyneuropathy
  familial dystrophia myotonica
myasthenia gravis
lump or obstruction in throat
  pharyngeal pouch
  postcricoid carcinoma
  thyroid enlargement
  globus hystericus
  foreign body
  Plummer–Vinson syndrome

Oesophageal symptoms
  food held up in chest
    mechanical block
      carcinoma of oesophagus
      carcinoma of cardia
      oesophageal stricture
      oesophageal atresia
      mediastinal tumour
      aortic aneurysm
    muscular incoordination
      achalasia cardia
      Chagas' disease
      diffuse muscle spasm
      systemic sclerosis
    chest pain on swallowing
      oesophagitis
        monilial infection
        gastric content reflux
      diffuse muscle spasm
      achalasia
  mechanical defect: cleft palate

Lower Oesophageal Sphincter

Decreased lower oesophageal sphincter pressure
  lower sphincter incompetence with or without hiatus hernia
  pregnancy
  post-vagotomy
  neuropathy
    diabetes mellitus
    alcoholism
  infantile chalasia
  progressive systemic sclerosis

Increased lower oesophageal sphincter pressure
  achalasia

diffuse oesophageal spasm
malignancy
Chagas' disease

Gastro-oesophageal Reflux

May occur in
- infancy
- pregnancy
- old age
- hiatus hernia
- post-surgery
  - partial gastrectomy
  - vagotomy
  - cardiomyotomy and resection of the cardia
- systemic sclerosis

STOMACH

Peptic Ulceration
(*Gastric Ulcer – Duodenal Ulcer*)

Including:
- Social and genetic factors
- Effects of smoking, alcohol, diet and life-style
- Drug-induced
- Hyperparathyroidism – hypercalcaemia induces gastrin release
- Acute burns
- Renal dialysis patients
- Zollinger–Ellison syndrome

Post-gastrointestinal Surgery Dumping Syndromes

Late Dumping Syndrome
Insulin-type hypoglycaemia, with weakness, faintness and occasionally unconsciousness develops 1½–3 hours after meals. The condition is relieved by oral sugar and frequent small meals

Early Dumping Syndrome
Gastrointestinal symptoms, including fullness, abdominal cramps and diarrhoea, with vasomotor symptoms including, headache, fainting, tachycardia, changes in blood pressure, and light-headedness, occur soon after meals
Follows subtotal gastrectomy in up to 50% of cases, and follows total gastrectomy in 100% of cases. Relieved by avoiding carbohydrate-rich meals and eating 'dry' meals

Infiltrative processes affecting the Stomach

Malignant: carcinoma

Non-malignant:
- Chronic granulomatous conditions
  - Crohn's disease
  - granulomatosis gastrica
  - syphilis
  - sarcoidosis
  - tuberculosis
  - histoplasmosis
  - chronic granulomatous disease of childhood
- Acute inflammatory infiltration
  - eosinophilic gastroenteritis
  - pseudolymphoma
  - amyloidosis
  - corrosive ingestion
  - peptic ulcer
  - chronic gastritis
  - perigastric inflammation
  - perigastric adhesions
  - perigastric bands
  - gastric spasm
  - post-irradiation

Gastric Polypoid Masses

- Carcinoma
- Varices
- Hereditary haemorrhagic telangiectasia
- Haematoma
- Gastritis
- Benign ulcer
- Pseudolymphoma
- Postoperative defects
  - Fundoplasty
  - Gastrostomy
- Gastritis cystica polyposa
- Extrinsic inflammatory processes
- Amyloidosis

UPPER GASTROINTESTINAL HAEMORRHAGE

Gastric ulcer
  acute
  chronic
Duodenal ulcer
Erosive gastritis
	} the common causes	N.B. patients with no dyspeptic history may bleed from peptic ulcer. Patient with known peptic ulcer may bleed from other sites

- Mallory–Weiss tear
- Hiatus hernia with
  - oesophagitis
  - oesophageal ulceration
- Oesophageal varices
- Carcinoma of stomach

Less common causes

- Stomal ulceration
- Oesophageal carcinoma
- Haemobilia
- Stomach
  - benign tumour
  - foreign body
- Duodenum
  - benign tumour
  - duodenitis
- Bleeding disorders
  - plasma coagulation defect
  - platelet deficiency or thrombocytopenia
  - tissue abnormality
    - hereditary haemorrhagic telangiectasia
    - pseudoxanthoma elasticum
- Rupture of aortic aneurysm into gastrointestinal tract

Other causes of haematemesis

- Vomiting of swallowed blood from
  - epistaxis
  - haemoptysis
  - bleeding from mouth or throat lesion

SMALL INTESTINE

Malabsorption

- Mucosal lesion
  - gluten sensitivity enteropathy
  - alactasia
  - a-β-lipoproteinaemia
  - tropical sprue
  - Whipple's disease
  - intestinal lymphangiectasia
- Metabolic disorders
  - thyrotoxicosis
  - Addison's disease
  - hypoparathyroidism
  - connective tissue diseases
  - hypogammaglobulinaemia
  - malignant disease
  - widespread skin disease
- Infection
  - acute enteritis

viral
bacterial
parasites, e.g. giardiasis
chronic enteritis: tuberculosis
Structural intestinal defects
Crohn's regional ileitis
gastrointestinal resection, or bypass operations
small bowel malignancy
arterial insufficiency in vessels supply the gut
defective intestinal motility
blind loop syndrome
diverticula
fistulas
partial obstruction
systemic sclerosis
pseudo-obstruction
pneumonia
pancreatitis
congestive cardiac failure
systemic sclerosis
amyloid infiltration of intestines
hypothyroidism
Maldigestion
liver disease } leading to bile salt deficiency in gut
biliary tract disease }
pancreatic enzyme deficiency
Zollinger–Ellison syndrome
Iatrogenic
drugs
surgery
radiotherapy to abdomen

Small Intestinal Lesions causing Malabsorption

Mucous membrane damage
Non-specific
gluten intolerance
chronic infection
Giardia lamblia infection
post-gastroenteritis
cow's milk protein allergy
tropical sprue
immune deficiency states
severe iron deficiency
dermatitis herpetiformis
intestinal drugs – neomycin
ionizing radiation
Lymph drainage obstruction
intestinal lymphangiectasis
Whipple's disease
Deficiency states
Disaccharidase deficiency
sucrose-isomaltose

primary congenital alactasia
adult lactase deficiency
trehalase deficiency
Monosaccharide transport defect: glucose-galactose malabsorption
Chloride exchange defect: familial chloride diarrhoea
Defective zinc absorption: acrodermatitis enteropathia
Amino-acid transport defects rarely cause diarrhoea
Vitamin B_{12} malabsorption: multiple causes
Folate malabsorption – multiple causes
a-β-lipoproteinaemia
Enterokinase deficiency
Secondary malabsorption associated with mucosal damage: multiple causes
Exocrine pancreatic insufficiency
Cystic fibrosis
Pancreatic achylia and neutropenia (Schwachman–Diamond syndrome)
Specific lipase deficiency
Malnutrition
Cholestasis: multiple causes
Bacterial overgrowth in intestinal lumen causing bile-salt deconjugation
Overgrowth of bacteria in upper small intestine
Contaminated small bowel syndrome
Intestinal obstruction
Intestinal anastomoses, blind loops, fistulas
Surgical resection of small intestine, malabsorption proportional to length of gut resected
Any chronic diarrhoea

Selective Inborn Errors of Absorption

Protein: enterokinase deficiency
Aminoacids
Cystinuria: cystine, lysine, arginine
Iminoaciduria: proline
Hartnup's disease: tryptophan, histidine, phenylalanine
Blue diaper syndrome: tryptophan
Methionine malabsorption: methionine
Lowe's syndrome: lysine, arginine
Carbohydrate
glucose-galactose malabsorption
lactase deficiency
sucrose-isomaltase deficiency
trehalase deficiency
Lipids
a-β-lipoproteinaemia
Lipase deficiency
Vitamins
Vitamin B_{12}
gastric intrinsic factor deficiency
biologically inert gastric intrinsic factor

congenital selective vitamin B_{12} malabsorption
transcobalamin I deficiency
transcobalamin II deficiency
Folate: congenital folate malabsorption
Chloride: congenital chloridorrhoea (stool chloride exceeds the sum stool sodium and potassium)
Familial hypomagnesaemia
Familial hypophosphataemic rickets

Malabsorption of Fat-soluble Vitamins
(vitamins A, D, E and K)

Small bowel disease producing steatorrhoea
coeliac disease
fibrocystic disease of the pancreas
Absence of bile in the gut lumen
obstructive jaundice
liver disease with reduced bile salt excretion into the small intestine
blind-loop syndrome with bacterial deconjugation of bile salts
cholestyramine therapy: with removal of bile salts
Failure of lipid transfer across intestinal mucosa
a-β-lipoproteinaemia

Malabsorption in Children

Neonatal period
congenital lactase deficiency
secondary disaccharidase deficiency
congenital glucose-galactose malabsorption
congenital chloridorrhoea
enterokinase deficiency
cow's milk protein intolerance
soya bean protein intolerance
primary immunological defects: Wiskott–Aldrich syndrome
cystic fibrosis
short bowel syndrome
neonatal hepatitis – biliary atresia
primary hypogammaglobulinaemia
1 month–2 years
sucrose-isomaltase deficiency
secondary disaccharidase deficiency
secondary monosaccharidase deficiency
enterokinase deficiency
cow's milk protein sensitivity
soya bean protein sensitivity
primary immune defects
Wiskott–Aldrich syndrome
thymic aplasia with agammaglobulinaemia
cystic fibrosis
neonatal hepatitis

biliary atresia
choledochal cyst
intestinal parasites
pancreatic insufficiency
coeliac sprue
a-β-lipoproteinaemia
Intestinal lymphangiectasia
Whipple's disease [R]
Wolman's disease [R]
aminoacid malabsorption syndromes [R]
vitamin B_{12} malabsorption syndromes [R]
congenital malabsorption of folic acid [R]
intestinal stasis syndrome

Steatorrhoea

Intestinal mucosal lesion
Gluten sensitivity enteropathy
Tropical sprue
Dermatitis herpetiformis (histological lesion as in gluten sensitivity)
Collagenous sprue
Hypogammaglobulinaemia
Coeliac disease
Structural lesions of the intestine
Congenital
congenital short intestine
primary intestinal lymphangiectasis
Acquired
Crohn's disease
lymphoma
amyloidosis
secondary lymphangiectasia and lymphatic obstruction
arterial insufficiency
atheroma
polyarteritis nodosa
systemic mast cell disease
macroglobulinaemia
pneumatosis intestinalis
radiotherapy affecting small intestine
Infection within the gut
Acute enteritis, especially in children
Parasites
Tuberculosis
Whipple's disease [R]
Small intestinal stasis
anatomical abnormality
jejunal diverticula
obstructive lesion in gut wall
surgical 'blind loop'
fistulas
defective intestinal motility

intestinal pseudo-obstruction
systemic sclerosis

Maldigestion
- Bile salt deficiency
  - obstructive jaundice
  - acute liver disease
  - chronic liver disease

  } diseases of the liver and biliary tract
- Pancreatic enzyme deficiency
  - pancreatitis
  - cystic fibrosis
  - congenital pancreatic hypoplasia
  - congenital pancreatic enzyme deficiencies
  - carcinoma of pancreas
  - postoperative pancreatic insufficiency
  - pancreatectomy
  - malnutrition
  - atrophy of the pancreas
- Spurious steatorrhoea, e.g. large intake of nuts: nut lipids are not all completely absorbed

Surgery
- Gastric surgery
- Intestinal resection, especially ileal resection

Biochemical abnormalities
- Alactasia with intestinal hurry
- Lipoprotein deficiency
  - a-β-lipoproteinaemia [R]
  - a-alpha-lipoproteinaemia [R]
- Zollinger–Ellison syndrome: inactivation of pancreatic lipase and intestinal hurry
- Macroamylasaemia

Diseases which may present with steatorrhoea
- Thyrotoxicosis
- Addison's disease (adrenocortical insufficiency)
- Hypoparathyroidism
- Renal tumours
- Carcinoid syndrome

Diseases in which steatorrhoea may occur
- Hypothyroidism
- Hyperparathyroidism
- Diabetes mellitus
- Ulcerative colitis
- Collagen diseases
- Paget's disease of bone
- Vascular congestion of the gut occurring in
  - congestive cardiac failure
  - constrictive pericarditis
- Widespread skin disease
- Severe anaemia
- malnutrition
- Allergic conditions
- Malaria (acute malignant tertian – *M. falciparum*)

Drug-induced steatorrhoea (probably dose-dependent)
- Neomycin

Kanamycin
Tetracycline
Polymyxin
Bacitracin
Calcium carbonate
Cholestyramine
Colchicine
PAS (para-aminosalicylate)
Liquid paraffin
Phenoformin
Phenolphthalein
Triparanol
Quinacrine (in large doses)
Clofibrate (interferes with absorption of sterols)

PANCREAS

Acute Pancreatitis in Adults

'Idiopathic': over one-third of all cases: ? 'vascular' subgroup
12–20 year age group
Biliary tract disease: over half of all cases
Chronic alcoholism
Mumps (uncommon)
Coxsackie-B virus
Hyperparathyroidism [R]
Carcinoma of head or ampulla of pancreas
Hypothermia
Drugs
- steroid therapy (long-term: uncommon)
- chlorothiazides
- azathioprine
- oral contraceptive pill

Secondary acute pancreatitis

Upper abdominal injury with blunt instrument
Penetrating abdominal injury
Post-partial gastrectomy
Post-biliary tract surgery
Post-endoscopic choledochopancreatography
Post-translumbar aortography

Chronic Pancreatitis

Primary calcifying chronic pancreatitis
- temporal zone – alcohol
- tropics – low protein intake in childhood

Hereditary chronic pancreatitis [R]
Chronic pancreatitis in hyperparathyroidism
Mucoviscidosis in adults
Gallstones and chronic pancreatitis

Obstruction of pancreatic ducts
Primary inflammatory pancreatitis in old people

Pancreatic Disorders in Childhood

- Malformations
  - ectopic pancreas (in mucosa of stomach, duodenum, jejunum)
  - pancreas annulare – leading to duodenal stenosis
- Primary congenital hypoplasia of pancreas (lipomatosis) [R]
- Isolated congenital pancreatic enzyme deficiencies
  - lipase deficiency [R]
  - amylase deficiency [R]
- Deficiency in proteolytic zymogen activation
  - pancreatic trypsinogen deficiency
  - lack of intestinal enterokinase leading to apparent pancreatic insufficiency
  - pancreatic deficiency with bonemarrow dysfunction [R]
- Pancreatitis
  - acute
    - idiopathic
    - steroid-induced
    - traumatic pancreatitis
    - ascaridiasis
    - cystic fibrosis
    - congenital malformation of pancreas and biliary tract
  - chronic
    - sporadic
    - familial
      - pancreas alone affected
      - Type I, hyperlipoproteinaemia induced by fat
      - pancreatitis with hyperlipaemia
      - pancreatitis with hyperparathyroidism
      - hereditary pancreatitis
- Systemic disease affecting the pancreas
  - acute
    - mumps pancreatitis
    - viral encephalopathy with pancreatitis
    - graft-versus-host reaction with pancreatitis
  - chronic
    - cystic fibrosis
    - Schwachman syndrome (? the same condition as primary congenital hypoplasia of pancreas)
    - protein-calorie malnutrition leading to pancreatic insufficiency
- Pancreatic pseudocysts
  - secondary to acute or chronic pancreatitis
  - secondary to traumatic pancreatitis

Hormone-producing Pancreatic Tumours

Solitary adenoma
Diffuse adenomatosis
Carcinoma
  Classification by hormone-produced
    insulinoma
    gastrin-secreting (Zollinger–Ellison syndrome)
    glucagonoma
    diarrhoeogenic (watery diarrhoea hypokalaemic achlorhydric – WDHA syndrome)

Pancreatic Cysts

Pseudocysts
  collection in lower sac
  pseudocysts in the head or tail
True pancreatic cysts (with epithelial lining)
  congenital
    simple
    polycystic
    dermoid
  parasitic, e.g. hydatid
  neoplasm
    benign: cystadenoma
    malignant
      cystadenocarcinoma
      teratoma

SMALL INTESTINAL VILLOUS ATROPHY

Tropical sprue
Crohn's disease
Ulcerative colitis
Cystic fibrosis
Whipple's disease
Zollinger–Ellison syndrome
Intestinal stasis
Hypogammaglobulinaemia with giardiasis, or other parasitic infections
Ischaemia of small intestine
Irradiation of small intestine
Small intestinal lymphoma
Eosinophilic gastroenteritis
Soy protein sensitivity
Skin diseases
  dermatitis herpetiformis
  other dermatoses
Vitamin B_{12} deficiency
Folate deficiency
Tuberculosis
Hepatitis
Drugs
Macroamylasaemia
Hypothyroidism

TUMOURS OF SMALL INTESTINE

Malignant (less than 1% of all gastrointestinal tract tumours)
- carcinoma
- lymphoma
- carcinoid
- leiomyoma

Benign (50% of malignant tumours of small intestine)
- adenoma
- lipoma
- myxoma
- fibroma
- angioma (very rare)

APPENDIX

Some Diseases Presenting as 'Appendicitis'

Appendicitis
Sigmoid diverticulitis
Perforated duodenal ulcer
Meckel's diverticulum, strangulated small bowel
Meckel's diverticulitis
Carcinoid of appendix
Cholecystitis
Ruptured uterus
Regional enteritis
Rupture of the spleen
Haematocolpos
Infarcted caecum

Indications for Appendicectomy

Acute appendicitis
Resolved appendix abscess
Chronic or recurrent appendicitis
Mucocele, associated with
- obstruction of lumen of the appendix
- faecolith
- caecal diaphragm

Carcinoid tumour
Carcinoma (very rare)
Parasitic infestation, e.g. threadworm
Foreign body, e.g. metal object (very rare)
'Routine' appendicectomy during abdominal surgery

LARGE BOWEL

Polyps of Colon and Rectum

Hamartomatous polyps (growth anomaly)

Juvenile polyposis (familial)
distal colon
rectum
Peutz–Jeghers polyposis associated with mucocutaneous pigmentation (AR): affecting stomach, duodenum, small intestine, and less commonly colon and rectum
retention polyp (juvenile)
Inflammatory polyps
inflammatory polyp associated with
ulcerative colitis
regional ileitis
inflammatory bowel disease
pseudopolyposis
cystic pneumatosis
lymphoid polyps and polyposis
'metastatic' polyps: ? viral in origin
colon
rectum
Hyperplasia
hyperplastic (metaplastic)
related to haemorrhoids
Neoplastic
Adenoma
adenomatous polyp
mixed villoglandular polyp
villous (papillary) adenoma
adenomatous familial polyposis syndrome (AD)
Usually very large numbers in rectum and colon. Carcinoma develops 10 years after adenoma
Lipoma
Leiomyoma
Gardner's syndrome: rare familial polyposis with
osteoma
osteosclerosis
dental abnormalities
soft-tissue tumours (lipoma and dermoid tumours)
Carcinoid tumour
Metastatic
carcinoma
leukaemia
lymphoma
Polypoid carcinoma

Proctitis

Idiopathic: commonest form
Crohn's disease
Solitary ulcer of rectum (occurring especially in young adults)
Radiation proctitis
Traumatic proctitis
Infections
- Gonorrhoeal proctitis
- Tuberculosis
- Rectal syphilis
- Amoebic proctitis
- Lymphogranuloma venereum
- Rectal actinomycosis
- Bilharziasis of rectum
- Antibiotic proctocolitis

Anal Incontinence

Rectum: loss of nervous connections of rectum
Anal canal: loss of sensitivity of upper anal canal, e.g. in chronic constipation
Anal muscles
- incontinence at times of stress, due to weak muscles
- absence of reflex activities of stretch reflex of muscles
- voluntary muscles around anal canal act as emergency controllers of passage of faeces. If these fail, then incontinence may occur

Rectal contents: difficult to contain, if too liquid

HAEMATOLOGY

Anaemia
- anaemia
- iron deficiency
- failure to respond to iron therapy in hypochromic anaemia
- megaloblastic anaemia
- drugs which may be associated with megaloblastosis
- sideroblastic anaemia
- refractory normocytic normochromic anaemia
- refractory anaemia with hyperplastic bonemarrow
- anaemia in the tropics
- aplastic anaemia
    - pancytopenia
    - pure red cell aplasia
    - neutropenia
    - thrombocytopenia
- bonemarrow transplantation failure
- haemolytic anaemia
- haemolytic anaemia causes
    - microangiopathic haemolytic anaemia

Haemoglobins
- reduced or absent synthesis of haemoglobin
- thalassaemia
- haemoglobinopathies
- methaemoglobinaemia
- sulphaemoglobinaemia
- porphyria
- leucoerythroblastic anaemia

White blood cells
- immunological causes of neutropenia
- neutropenia due to causes other than marrow aplasia
- biochemical disorders of granulocytes
- impaired phagocytosis in humoral abnormalities
- acquired myeloidysplastic syndrome

Spleen
- conditions associated with splenomegaly
- chronic splenomegaly with neutropenia and/or pancytopenia
- common causes of splenomegaly in the tropics
- indications for splenectomy
- hyposplenism
- asplenia
- diseases associated with hyposplenism

Myeloproliferative disorders
- myeloproliferative disorders
- increased risk of development of leukaemia
- myelofibrosis
- polycythaemia
- renal polycythaemia

Lymphoproliferative disorders
- primary reticuloendothelial neoplasia
- lymphoproliferative disorders

classifications of non-Hodgkin's lymphomas
T-cell neoplasms
B-cell neoplasms

Haemorrhagic disorders

haemorrhagic disorders
purpura
purpura fulminans
congenital abnormalities of vessel walls
acquired abnormality of vessel walls
thrombocytopenia
marrow suppression
other than marrow aplasia
inherited disorders of platelet function
acquired reduction in platelet function
hereditary disorders of haemostasis
acquired plasma coagulation factor defects
disseminated intravascular coagulopathy

Conditions predisposing to thrombosis

Blood transfusion

infectious diseases which can be transmitted in transfused blood
blood transfusion hazards
iron overload
indications for therapeutic plasmapheresis

ANAEMIA

Deficiency anaemia
- Iron deficiency
  - defective diet
  - defective absorption
- Vitamin B_{12} deficiency
  - defective diet
  - defective absorption
- Folate deficiency
  - defective diet
  - defective absorption
  - excessive utilization
- Pyridoxine deficiency
  - defective diet [R]
  - defective metabolism
- Severe protein-calorie deficiency
- Vitamin C deficiency

Depression of erythropoiesis
- Aplastic and hypoplastic anaemia
- Refractory anaemia

primary
secondary
Marrow replacement, e.g. malignancy
Blood loss
Haemolytic anaemia
intravascular
extravascular
Haemorrhage

Iron Deficiency Anaemia

Poor dietary intake
Growth (with excessive iron utilization)
Loss
Physiological
infants and children – rate of growth exceeds available iron
menstruation
pregnancy
Pathological
menorrhagia
gastrointestinal bleed
haematuria
haemoglobinuria
Malabsorption

Failure to respond to Iron Therapy in Hypochromic Anaemia

Failure to take medicine
Malabsorption
Continuing blood loss
Refractory anaemia
infections } failure of utilization of iron stored in
uraemia } reticuloendothelial system
hypochromic anaemia associated with chronic disease
connective tissue disorders
malignancy
sideroblastic anaemia, presenting as hypochromic anaemia
thalassaemia

Megaloblastic Anaemia

Vitamin B_{12} deficiency
inadequate intake: very low B_{12} content in diet
gastric faults
pernicious anaemia: late onset of failure to produce intrinsic factor
gastrectomy affecting intrinsic-factor-producing area of stomach
congenital intrinsic factor deficiency or abnormality
intestinal faults
part of general malabsorption syndrome

specific abnormality of B_{12} absorption sites in terminal ileum (very rare)
fish tape worm removing B_{12} from food in intestine
Folate deficiency
inadequate diet
part of general malabsorption syndrome
increased usage and turnover of folate in the body
pregnancy and lactation
prematurity
haemolytic diseases
malignancies
chronic inflammatory disease, e.g. rheumatoid arthritis
excessive losses
chronic dialysis
congestive cardiac failure
active liver disease
metabolic: homocystinuria
interference by drugs
anticonvulsants
alcohol
(oral contraceptives: very rare)
some cytotoxics, e.g. methotrexate
Defects in DNA synthesis
congenital
orotic aciduria [R]
Lesch–Nyhan syndrome
transcobalamin II deficiency [R]
inborn errors of folate metabolism [R]
congenital dyserythropoietic anaemia [R]
acquired
antimetabolic drugs, e.g. methotrexate, cytosine arabinoside etc.)
erythroleukaemia
in some cases of myeloid leukaemias

Drugs which may be associated with Megaloblastosis

Anticonvulsants
phenytoin
primidone
phenobarbitone
amylobarbitone
quinalbarbitone
phenylmethybarbituric acid
Antimetabolites
azathioprine
6-mercaptopurine
methotrexate
pyrimethamine
cyclophosphamide
homofolic acid
5-fluorouracil
vitamin B_{12} antagonists
cytosine arabinoside

Antituberculous
- para-aminosalicylate (PAS)
- pyrazinamide
- cycloserine

Antibacterial
- nitrofurantoin
- cotrimoxazole

Others
- phenylbutazone } very rare
- arsenic }

Sideroblastic Anaemia

- Hereditary
  - X-linked recessive
    - pyridoxine responsive
    - pyridoxine unresponsive
    - anaemia hypochromica sideroblastica hereditaria, with increased coproporphyrin and decreased protoporphyrin levels
  - Autosomal: pyridoxine responsive
- Acquired
  - Primary idiopathic
    - pyridoxine refractory
    - pyridoxine responsive
  - Secondary
    - specific
      - defects in vitamin B_6 metabolism
        - vitamin B_6 deficiency
        - antituberculous drugs, e.g. cycloserine
      - interference with haem and/or globin synthesis
        - lead poisoning
      - defects in DNA synthesis
        - vitamin B_{12} deficiency
        - folate deficiency
        - folate antagonists and other chemotherapeutic agents
      - some drugs
        - phenacetin
        - chloramphenicol
        - chlorambucil
        - alcohol
      - chronic neoplastic conditions and inflammatory disorders
        - rheumatoid arthritis (may be underlying folate deficiency)
        - myelomatosis
        - agnogenic myeloid metaplasia
      - haemolysis
    - non-specific
      - myeloproliferative disorders
      - leukaemia

Refractory Normocytic Normochromic Anaemia

Aplastic or hypoplastic anaemia
Thalassaemia (hypochromic cells)
Pyridoxine deficiency [R]
Sideroblastic anaemia
Anaemia associated with infection
Anaemia associated with uraemia
Anaemia associated with connective tissue disease, e.g. rheumatoid arthritis
Anaemia following burns
Refractory anaemia with dysproteinaemia in the elderly
'Preleukaemic Phase' in patients who eventually present with frank acute leukaemia

Refractory Anaemia with Hyperplastic Bonemarrow

Congenital
- Thalassaemia syndromes
- Sideroblastic anaemia
- Congenital dyserythropoietic anaemia, Types 1, 2 and 3 [R]
- Refractory megaloblastic anaemia [R]
  - orotic aciduria [R]
  - rare inherited enzyme deficiencies concerned with folate metabolism [R]

Acquired
- Sideroblastic anaemia
- Myeloproliferative disorders
  - erythraemic myelosis
  - di Guglielmo's disease
- Refractory anaemia with pancytopenic syndrome
- Goldberg's chronic anaemia in the elderly, responsive to steroids
- (Random hyperplastic marrow aspirate samples may be obtained unpredictably in cases of hypoplastic anaemia)

Anaemia in the Tropics

Deficiency anaemia
- Iron deficiency
  - dietary deficiency
  - blood loss due to parasites
- Vitamin B_{12} deficiency
  - dietary deficiency
  - malabsorption syndrome
- Folate deficiency
  - can develop during pregnancy
  - malabsorption syndrome
  - chronic haemolysis uses up folic acid
- Ascorbic acid deficiency: dietary deficiency
- Pyridoxine deficiency: dietary deficiency may be associated with a microcytic anaemia

Protein deficiency: anaemia develops in kwashiorkor

Haemolytic anaemia
- Infections
  - direct invasion of the erythrocytes
    - e.g. malaria, Bartonellaceae
  - kala azar } associated with splenomegaly
  - African trypanosomiasis } associated with splenomegaly
- Haemoglobinopathies
  - sickle cell anaemia
  - sickle cell-haemoglobin C disease
  - sickle cell-haemoglobin D disease

Thalassaemia

Glucose-6-phosphate dehydrogenase deficiency: Haemolytic anaemia may develop when certain drugs are given

Aplastic Anaemia: I

Idiopathic
- Constitutional: Fanconi's syndrome
- Acquired

Secondary
- Chemical and physical agents
  - drugs
  - non-pharmacological substances
  - irradiation
- Infections
  - virus, e.g. hepatitis
  - bacterial, e.g. miliary tuberculosis
- Metabolic
  - acute pancreatitis
  - pregnancy
- Immunological
  - graft-versus-host reaction
- Neoplasm
  - bonemarrow invasion
- Marrow 'exhaustion'
  - paroxysmal nocturnal haemoglobinuria

Aplastic Anaemia: II

Pancytopenia
- Acquired
  - Acute transient: infections, especially viral
  - Chronic
    - idiopathic
    - drugs and toxic agents
      - dose-dependent
      - idiosyncrasy
    - radiation
    - thymoma
    - aplastic-paroxysmal nocturnal haemoglobinuria syndrome

Primary
- Fanconi's anaemia
- Familial aplastic anaemia [R]
- Schwachman–Diamond–Blackfan syndrome [R]

(? preleukaemic syndrome)

Pure red cell aplasia
- Acquired
  - thymoma
  - idiopathic
  - autoimmune
  - drugs (much less frequent than pancytopenia, agranulocytosis or thrombocytopenia)
- Congenital Diamond–Blackfan hypoplastic anaemia

Neutropenia (agranulocytosis)
- Acquired
  - idiopathic
  - drugs
    - dose-related, e.g. cytotoxic drugs
    - potentially toxic, e.g. gold
    - possible toxin, e.g. phenylbutazone
  - irradiation
  - infections
    - bacterial
    - viral
    - Rickettsia
    - malaria
    - kala azar
    - toxoplasmosis
- Congenital
  - Hereditary neutropenia
    - autosomal recessive (Kostmann syndrome) [R]
    - autosomal dominant [R]
  - Reticular dysgenesis
  - Familial granulocytopenia with immunological deficiencies
  - Chronic hypoplastic neutropenia
  - Familial cyclical neutropenia [R]

Thrombocytopenia
- Acquired
  - Idiopathic
  - Drugs leading to suppression of formation
  - Marrow infiltration
- Congenital
  - Wiskott–Aldrich syndrome
  - Fanconi syndrome
  - May–Hegglin anomaly
  - Other varieties of familial thrombocytopenia, including amegakaryocytic thrombocytopenia with absent radii

Bonemarrow transplantation failure

Too few marrow cells given
Patient dies before the marrow cells graft can be established
Failure to produce a close match of the major histocompatibility antigens, leading to rejection
Possible: reaction against host tissues by immunocompetent cells (T-cells) transferred with the marrow graft

Haemolytic Anaemia Causes

- Red cell defects
  - red cell membrane abnormality
    - paroxysmal nocturnal haemoglobinuria
    - vitamin E deficiency [R]
  - red cell sodium pump defects
    - congenital spherocytic haemolytic anaemia (AD)
    - elliptocytosis
    - stomatocytosis [R]
  - other rare enzyme deficiencies
  - defects in the red cell glycolytic enzymes
    - glucose-6-phosphate dehydrogenase deficiency
      - Negro form
      - Mediterranean form, e.g. favism
      - Canton variety
      - Northern European – severe
      - non-spherocytic haemolytic anaemia
    - pyruvate kinase deficiency (used to be Type II non-spherocytic inherited haemolytic anaemia)
    - other very rare enzyme deficiencies
  - deficiencies in red cell membrane glutathione metabolism [R]
  - Haemoglobinopathies
    - thalassaemia
      - alpha-thalassaemia
      - beta-thalassaemia
    - abnormal haemoglobins
      - haemoglobin S disease
      - haemoglobin C disease
      - haemoglobin D disease
      - haemoglobin E disease
      - haemoglobin M disease
      - etc.
    - combinations of thalassaemia, sickle Hb, etc.
- Extracorpuscular factors
  - Iso-immune haemolysins
    - incompatible blood transfusion
    - haemolytic disease of the newborn, erythroblastosis fetalis
  - autoimmune
    - 'warm' antibodies
      - idiopathic, primary
      - secondary, including

lymphoproliferative disorders
systemic lupus erythematosus
carcinoma
'cold' antibodies
idiopathic
secondary, including
lymphoma
mycoplasma pneumonia
infectious mononucleosis [R]
paroxysmal cold haemoglobinuria
viral infection
syphilis
drug haemolysis associated with immune reactions
immune complex (antigen-antibody) adsorbed onto red cell, complement activated haemolysis, e.g. quinidine
drug adsorbed onto red cell and circulating antibody reacts, leading to red cell lysis, e.g. cephalosporins
red cell membrane altered by drug, antibodies react with drug bound to red cell, leading to lysis, e.g. cephalothin
drug causes formation of antibodies against normal red cell group substances, e.g. anti-Rh from α-methyldopa
toxins and drugs which cause haemolysis in proportion to dose
e.g. phenylhydrazine
snake venom
certain spider bites
infections
Oroya fever
clostridial infection, septicaemia
malaria
hypersplenism, *see* Hypersplenism
microangiopathic haemolytic anaemia (*see below*)

Microangiopathic Haemolytic Anaemia

Haemolytic-uraemic syndrome
Thrombotic thrombocytopenic purpura
Renal vein thrombosis
Renal transplant rejection
Radiation nephritis
Chronic renal failure
Renal cortical necrosis
Malignant hypertension
Severe hepatocellular disease
Giant haemangioma
Coarctation of the aorta
Severe valvular heart disease
Artificial heart valve replacement
Bacterial endocarditis affecting the aortic valve

Severe burns
Disseminated herpes infection
Meningococcal septicaemia
Malignant cerebral malaria (falciparum)
Any cause of disseminated intravascular coagulopathy (DIC)
Purpura fulminans
Eclampsia
Abruptio placentae
Widespread adenocarcinoma
Procoagulant snake venom (snakebite)
Traumatic arteriovenous fistula

HAEMOGLOBINS

Normal haemoglobins
- HbA (major adult haemoglobin): $alpha_2$ $beta_2$
- HbA_2 (minor adult haemoglobin): $alpha_2$ $delta_2$
- HbF (fetal haemoglobin): $alpha_2$ $gamma_2$
- Hb Gower 1 (embryonic haemoglobin): $epsilon_4$
- Hb Gower 2 (embryonic haemoglobin): $alpha_2$ $epsilon_2$
- Hb Portland (embryonic haemoglobin): $gamma_2$ $zeta_2$

Abnormalities involving normal haemoglobins
- Thalassaemias

Reduced or absent synthesis of haemoglobin
1. Beta-thalassaemia
   - Beta-thalassaemia with or without beta-chain production
   - Delta-beta-thalassaemia
   - Haemoglobin Lepore thalassaemia
   - Hereditary persistence of fetal haemoglobin (HbF)
   - Beta-thalassaemia plus beta-chain haemoglobin variants
2. Alpha-thalassaemia
   - Alpha-thalassaemia with or without alpha-chain production
   - Alpha-thalassaemia with an alpha-chain variant with reduced synthesis rate
   - Alpha-thalassaemia in combination with alpha-chain variants

(Delta-thalassaemia and Gamma-thalassaemia)
Abnormal persistance of HbF

Abnormal haemoglobins – haemoglobinopathies
- Haemoglobin S
  - Heterozygote: sickle trait
  - Homozygote: sickle cell anaemia
  - Sickle cell: HbC disease (SC disease)
  - Sickle cell: thalassaemia
  - Sickle cell: HbD disease [R]
- Haemoglobin C
  - Heterozygote: symptomless trait
  - Homozygote: HbC disease

Haemoglobin D
 Heterozygote: symptomless trait
 Homozygote: HbD disease [R]
Haemoglobin E
 Heterozygote: symptomless trait
 Homozygote: HbE disease: not serious
Rare haemoglobins: unstable haemoglobins, e.g. haemoglobins M

Methaemoglobinaemia

Secondary methaemoglobinuria, occurring most commonly in the newborn
 nitrite and nitrate ingestion, e.g. food preservatives, overfertilized spinach
 aniline dyes
 sulphonamides
 antimalarials
 anaesthetics, e.g. benzocaine
 vitamin K analogues in excessive doses
 resorcin
 phenacetin
 chlorates
 naphthalene, e.g. moth balls
Rarely: primary methaemoglobinaemia
 inherited enzyme deficiency – NADH-methaemoglobin reductase deficiency (AD)
 M-haemoglobinopathies (AD)

Sulphaemoglobinaemia [R]

Whole blood sulphaemoglobin levels rarely exceed 10% of total haemoglobin. Probably sulphaemoglobin formation is preceded by methaemoglobin. The reason for the formation of sulphaemoglobin is unknown
 phenacetin
 sulphonamides
 acetanelide
 nitrates
 nitrites
 etc.

Porphyria

Erythropoietic porphyria
(Bulk of excessive porphyrin production occurs in the bone-marrow)

Erythropoietic protoporphyria: (AD). The enzyme defect is of reduced ferrochetolase activity. Photosensitivity. Red cell protoporphyrin increased. Stool protoporphyrin, and to a lesser extent stool coproporphyrin increased in attacks

Congenital porphyria: (AR) [R]. The enzyme defect is uroporphyrinogen III cosynthetase reduction. Photosensitivity. Urine uroporphyrin I and to a lesser extent urine coproporphyrin I increased in attacks. Red cell protoporphyrin and coproporphyrin increased

Erythropoietic coproporphyria: [R]. Only one case as yet described

Hepatic porphyria
(Bulk of excessive porphyrin production occurs in the liver)

Acute intermittent porphyria (Swedish type): (AD). The enzyme defect is reduction in activity of uroporphyrinogen-l-synthetase and of hepatic δ-5-alpha-reductase. Urine delta-aminolaevulinic acid, porphobilinogen, and uroporphyrin increased

Variegate porphyria (South African type): (AD). The enzyme defect is reduction in activity of ferrochetolase with reduced activity of protoporphyrinogen oxidase in leucocytes and normoblasts (?). Urine delta-aminolaevulinic acid, and porphobilinogen increased markedly in attacks, with faecal porphyrins increased. Photosensitivity

Porphyria cutanea tarda (cutaneous hepatic porphyria): (AD). The enzyme defect is reduction in activity of liver uroporphyrinogen decarboxylase. Urine uroporphyrin greatly increased. Photosensitivity

Hereditary coproporphyria: (AD). The enzyme defect is reduction in activity of hepatic and leucocyte coproporphyrinogen oxidase in some cases and of uroporphyrinogen decarboxylase in others. Photosensitivity. Urine coproporphyrin, delta-aminolaevulinic acid and porphobilinogen increased in attacks

Leucoerythroblastic Anaemia
(Immature red cells and white cells in the peripheral blood)

Acute severe infection: one-third of cases (a few primitive cells seen only)
Haemolytic anaemia: one-third of cases (more early red cells than early white cells)
Marrow infiltration: one-third of cases
- metastatic carcinoma, especially
  - breast
  - prostate
  - lungs
  - thyroid
  - adrenal
- leukaemia
  - acute
  - chronic
- erythraemic myelosis
- myelosclerosis, myelofibrosis, agnogenic myeloid metaplasia
- marble bone disease [R]

myeloma
Hodgkin's disease
Gaucher's disease
Niemann–Pick's disease
Hand–Schüller–Christian disease } some cases

Occasional
severe haemorrhage
irradiation
poisoning
benzene
carbon tetrachloride
fluorine
phosphorus

Nucleated Red Cells in the Peripheral Blood

Untreated megaloblastic anaemia
Severe oxygen lack
congestive cardiac failure
severe pulmonary disease
Haemolytic anaemia
(Leucoerythroblastic anaemia)

WHITE BLOOD CELLS

Immunological Causes of Neutropenia

Fetal-maternal incompatibility
Primary autoimmune neutropenia in infants
Primary autoimmune neutropenia in adults (may cause transient neutropenia in the newborn of affected mothers)
Neutropenia associated with cold-reacting antibodies
Primary cold agglutinin neutropenia
Secondary cold agglutinin neutropenia in
lymphoma
infectious mononucleosis
Mycoplasma pneumonia
Neutropenia in other immunological disorders
systemic lupus erythematosus
Felty's syndrome
Drug-associated neutropenia: aminopyrine

Neutropenia due to Causes other than Marrow Aplasia

Overdestruction
Immune
Isoantibody
neonatal
blood transfusion
autoimmune
systemic lupus erythematosus

rheumatoid arthritis
lymphoma
drug-dependent
anaphylaxis
serum sickness
Mechanical destruction
haemodialysis
cardiac bypass
Infections

Biochemical Disorders of Granulocytes

Pharmacological agents interfere with granulocyte chemotaxis
chlorpromazine
amphotericin B
tetracyclines, etc.
Inherited defects
mannosidosis [R]: accumulated mannose in leucocytes interferes with reception of chemotactic stimulants on granulocytes
chronic granulomatous disease
defective activation of 'respiratory burst'
oxygen-independent granulocyte microbicidal mechanism defects
Chediak–Higashi anomaly
protein-calorie malnutrition

Impaired Phagocytosis in Humoral Abnormalities

Antibody deficiency syndromes
Normal early infancy
Genetic
Acquired idiopathic
Secondary to lymphatic neoplasia
Complement deficiency
C4 deficiency: genetic absence [R]
C3 deficiency
genetic absence [R]
genetic hypercatabolism [R]
Properdin factor B deficiency: some neonates
Depletion of many factors
Inhibition of activation of many factors
rheumatoid arthritis
systemic lupus erythematosus
sickle cell anaemia
inflammatory states

Acquired Myeloidysplastic Syndrome

Secondary myeloidysplasia
Deficiency of
vitamin B_{12}
folate

combined vitamin B_{12} and folate
Secondary sideroblastosis
Secondary to drug action
Idiopathic myeloidysplasia
Acquired idiopathic sideroblastic anaemia
Refractory anaemia with excess of 'blast cells'
Chronic myelomonocytic leukaemia
Aplastic anaemia
Paroxysmal nocturnal haemoglobinuria
Bonemarrow failure with cellular marrow

SPLEEN

Conditions associated with Splenomegaly

Circulatory
- Chronic passive congestion
  - congestive cardiac failure
  - constrictive pericarditis
- Portal hypertension
  - intrahepatic: cirrhosis, etc.
  - extrahepatic: splenic vein obstruction, etc.

Increased haematopoietic activity
- Granulopoieses
  - reactive hyperplasia
    - acute infection
    - chronic infection
  - myeloproliferative disorders
    - myeloid leukaemia
    - myelosclerosis
    - polycythaemia vera
- Lymphopoiesis
  - virus infection, e.g. infectious mononucleosis
  - lymphoproliferative disorders
    - lymphatic leukaemia
    - lymphosarcoma
- Erythropoiesis
  - haemolytic anaemia
    - autoimmune
    - hereditary haemolytic anaemia
    - haemoglobinopathy
  - polycythaemia vera
  - extramedullary haemopoiesis

Reticuloendothelial system disorders
- Lymphoma
- Lymphadenoma
- Reticuloendothelial overactivity
  - idiopathic thrombocytopenic purpura
  - lipid storage disease
  - mucopolysaccharidosis
  - amyloidosis

Reticuloendothelial overactivity associated with chronic infection
- malaria
- kala azar
- leishmaniasis
- schistosomiasis
- etc.

Tropical splenomegaly syndrome
- with hepatic sinusoidal lymphocytosis
- without hepatic sinusoidal lymphocytosis

Splenic neoplasm
- primary: lymphangioma, haemangioma, haemangiosarcoma
- secondary metastases [R]

Splenic cyst, abscess

Chronic Splenomegaly with Neutropenia and/or Pancytopenia

Congestive splenomegaly
Malignant lymphoma
Leukaemia
Myelosclerosis
Systemic lupus erythematosus
Bacterial endocarditis
Chronic brucellosis
Sarcoidosis
Lipid storage diseases
- Gaucher's disease
- Niemann–Pick's disease

Kala azar (leishmaniasis)
Chronic malarial splenomegaly
Felty's syndrome

Common Causes of Splenomegaly in the Tropics

Parasites
- malaria
- leishmaniasis
- schistosomiasis

Infection
- virus
- Rickettsia
- bacteria
- fungus

Blood disorders
Infiltrative conditions of the spleen
Congestive splenomegaly
Tropical splenomegaly syndrome
- with hepatic sinusoidal lymphocytosis
- without hepatic sinusoidal lymphocytosis

Indications for Splenectomy

Usual
- Portal hypertension due to splenic vein thrombosis

Hypersplenism causing symptoms: chronic idiopathic thrombocytopenia
Congenitally defective red cells removed prematurely by normal spleen: hereditary spherocytic anaemia
Sometimes
Acquired haemolytic autoimmune anaemia: 'warm' antibody type
Hereditary elliptocytosis: if associated with haemolytic anaemia
Acute idiopathic thrombocytopenia: unsuccessful attempts at control with steroids
Tropical splenomegaly
Occasional
Chronic myeloid leukaemia (splenectomy appears to improve response to treatment)
Chronic lymphatic leukaemia: if splenic enlargement causing discomfort
Myelosclerosis: if evidence of hypersplenism, and no evidence of erythropoiesis in spleen
Malignant lymphoma
Hodgkin's disease: as part of staging during treatment
(Thalassaemia major, aplastic anaemia)

Hyposplenism

Congenital absence of spleen [R]. Usually associated with cardiac anomalies
Splenic hypoplasia: Fanconi's anaemia
Atrophy of spleen
Idiopathic steatorrhoea
Essential thrombocythaemia
Sickle cell disease
Systemic lupus erythematosus

Asplenia

Congenital asplenia
Surgical splenectomy
Splenic atrophy: repeated infarcts: occurring in
sickle cell disease (haemoglobin SS)
haemoglobin SC disease
small intestine disease, e.g. non-tropical sprue
haemorrhagic thrombocythaemia
Functional asplenia: immature newborn infant

Diseases associated with Hyposplenism

Normal sized or large spleen
sickle cell anaemia
sarcoidosis
amyloidosis
Atrophic spleen
coeliac disease

ulcerative colitis
dermatitis herpetiformis
thyrotoxicosis
haemorrhagic thrombocythaemia
Thorotrast poisoning

MYELOPROLIFERATIVE DISORDERS

Myeloproliferative Disorders

Proliferation of red cell precursors
  Polycythaemia rubra vera
  Erythraemic myelosis – acute and chronic, *see below*
Proliferation of granulocyte precursors
  Acute myelogenous leukaemia
    acute myeloblastic leukaemia
    acute myelomonocytic leukaemia
    acute promyelocytic leukaemia
    hypoplastic leukaemia
    erythroleukaemia (erythraemic myelosis)
  Chronic myeloid leukaemia
Proliferation of platelet precursors
  Essential thrombocythaemia
Proliferation of precursors of fibroblasts and osteoblasts in marrow
  Primary myelofibrosis
  Primary myelosclerosis

Increased Risk of Development of Leukaemia

High-risk families
Bloom's syndrome
Fanconi's syndrome
Ataxia telangiectasia
Down's syndrome
Inherited immunodeficiency disorders
External agents
  irradiation: linear increase in incidence with exposure exceeding 100 rads
  chemicals
    benzene [R]
    drugs that can cause marrow aplasia
  ? viruses
'Preleukaemic' conditions
  sideroblastic anaemia
  hypoplastic anaemia
  paroxysmal nocturnal haemoglobinuria
  marrow hypoplasia with leucopenia
  marrow hypoplasia with thrombocytopenia
  myelosclerosis
  polycythaemia vera

Myelofibrosis

Primary
- acute
- chronic

Secondary
- malignant infiltration of marrow
- renal osteodystrophy with osteosclerosis
- post-irradiation
- marble bone disease
- fluorosis
- Hodgkin's lymphadenoma
- Rare
  - toxic, benzene poisoning, tuberculosis, syphilis, secondary to other myeloproliferative disorders

Polycythaemia

1. Polycythaemia vera
2. Secondary polycythaemia, with increased erythropoietin production
   a. Physiologically appropriate, with decreased oxygen saturation
      - high altitude
      - chronic obstructive pulmonary disease
      - postural hypoxia
      - cardiovascular shunt, from right to left side
      - congenital methaemoglobinopathy
      - Pickwickian syndrome, with massive obesity
      - high oxygen affinity haemoglobinopathy
        - HbM variant
        - increased sulphaemoglobin
        - congenital decreased red cell DPG concentration

   b. Physiologically inappropriately increased erythropoietin production
      i. Tumour
         - renal carcinoma
         - cerebral haemangioblastoma
         - hepatoma
         - uterine fibroid
         - adrenal cortical adenoma
           - with hyperplasia
           - without hyperplasia
         - ovarian carcinoma
         - bronchogenic carcinoma [R]

      ii. Renal
         - renal cysts
         - hydronephrosis
         - Bartter's syndrome
         - transplantation

      iii. Excessive intake of cobalt salts

   c. Familial polycythaemia, recessive inheritance

3. Relative polycythaemia: decreased plasma volume, with relative increase in haematocrit, but without absolute increase in red cell mass
   - Hypertension, especially when treated with thiazide diuretics
   - Gaisböck's syndrome
   - 'Stress, spurious, pseudopolycythaemia'
   - Dehydration

Renal Polycythaemia

Related to increased production of erythropoietin
- Increased intrarenal pressure
  - hydronephrosis
  - multilocular cysts of kidney
  - polycystic kidney
  - solitary renal cyst
  - renal tumour
- Compression on renal blood supply leading to renal tissue anoxia
- Tumours producing erythropoietin, or erythropoietin-like substance [R]
  - renal tumour: hypernephroma, Wilm's tumour
  - cerebellar haemangioblastoma
  - hepatoma
  - myxoma
  - uterine fibroids

LYMPHOPROLIFERATIVE DISORDERS

Primary Reticuloendothelial Neoplasia

- Reticulosarcoma
- Mycosis fungoides
- Hodgkin's lymphadenoma
- Lymphosarcoma
- Giant follicular lymphoma
- Chronic lymphatic leukaemia
- Thymoma
- Malignant paraproteinaemia
  - myeloma
  - macroglobulinaemia

Lymphoproliferative Disorders

- Leukaemia
  - Acute lymphoblastic leukaemia
  - Chronic lymphocytic leukaemia
- Lymphoma
  - Hodgkin's disease
    - Stage I – Involvement of a single lymph gland (I) or of a single extralymphatic organ or site (IE)

Stage II – Involvement of two or more lymph node regions on the same side of the diaphragm (II) or localized involvement of extralymphatic organ or site and of more lymph node regions on the same side of the diaphragm (IIE)

Subclassified

A: none of B

B: unexplained weight loss of more than 10%, unexplained fever above 38 °C, and night sweats

Stage III – Involvement of lymph node regions on both sides of the diaphragm (III) which may be accompanied by localized involvement of extralymphatic organ or site (IIIE) or by involvement of the spleen (IIIS) or both (IIISE)

Stage IV – Diffuse or disseminated involvement of one or more extralymphatic organs or tissues with or without associated lymph node enlargement. (Classify by N = nodes, H = liver, M = marrow, P = pleura, S = spleen, L = lung, O = bone, D = skin.)

Hodgkin's disease – histological classification

Lymphocytic predominance
Nodular sclerosis
Mixed cellularity
Lymphocytic depletion } 5% of all cases
Unclassified }

Non-Hodgkin's disease

1. Nodular non-Hodgkin's lymphoma
   a. Lymphocytic, well differentiated
   b. Lymphocytic, poorly differentiated
   c. Histiocytic
   d. Mixed, histiocytic and lymphocytic
2. Diffuse non-Hodgkin's lymphoma
   a. Lymphocytic, well differentiated
   b. Lymphocytic, poorly differentiated
   c. Histiocytic
   d. Mixed, histiocytic and lymphocytic
3. Totally undifferentiated non-Hodgkin's lymphoma

(*See also next page*)

T-cell Neoplasms

20% of all cases of acute lymphoblastic leukaemia
Sezary's syndrome
Mycosis fungoides (probably)
T-cell chronic lymphatic leukaemia [R]
T-cell lymphocytic leukaemia [R]

B-cell Neoplasms

Stem cell (B_0). Combined T + B cell acute lymphoblastic leukaemia

Classifications of non-Hodgkin's Lymphomas

Lymphocytic malignant lymphoma	Well-differentiated lymphocytic diffuse	Lymphatic lymphoma
Lymphoplasmactoid malignant lymphoma	Lymphoproliferative disease with dysproteinaemia	Lymphocytic lymphoma
Centrocytic malignant lymphoma	Poorly differentiated lymphocytic diffuse	Lymphocytic lymphoma
Centroblastic centrocytic, follicular/ diffuse malignant lymphoma	Poorly differentiated lymphocytic and mixed L- and H-nodular (follicular) and diffuse	Follicular lymphoma
Centroblastic malignant lymphoma	Histiocytic – nodular and diffuse	Follicular lymphoma
Lymphoblastic malignant lymphoma	Undifferentiated malignant lymphoma	
B type		
Burkitt	Burkitt	Stem cell lymphoma
Non-Burkitt	Non-Burkitt	Lymphoblastic lymphoma
T type		
U type		
Immunoblastic malignant lymphoma	Histiocytic diffuse	Clasmatocytic lymphoma

Virgin lymphocyte (B_1):
  chronic lymphatic leukaemia
Immunoblast (B_2)
  Poorly differentiated lymphocytic lymphoma (PDLL)
  Burkitt's lymphoma
Memory cell (B_3): a few cases of chronic lymphatic leukaemia
Lymphocytoid-plasma cells (B_4): Waldenströms's macroglobulinaemia
Plasma cell (B_5): myeloma
Other
  'Hairy cell' leukaemia
  cold agglutinin disease

HAEMORRHAGIC DISORDERS

Haemorrhagic Disorders

Abnormal blood vessels
  Platelets
    thrombocytopenia
    qualitative platelet function defect
  Plasma coagulation factors
    deficiency
    circulating anticoagulant
  (Singly or in combination)

Purpura

Thrombocytopenia
  Decreased platelet production } singly or combined
  Increased platelet loss }
Platelet dysfunction
  With normal platelet count
    Congenital
      thrombasthenia
      platelet release reaction defects
      Bernard–Soulier syndrome
    Acquired
      uraemia
        defect on platelet Factor 3 release
        prolonged bleeding time
      fibrin degradation products
      paraproteinaemia
      aspirin and other drugs
  With increased platelet count
    thrombocythaemia
Vascular purpura
  Vasculitis
    'allergic purpura' – Henoch–Schönlein syndrome
    allergic vasculitis
    periarteritus nodosa
    systemic lupus erythematosus
    rheumatoid arthritis
    drugs

DNA hypersensitivity – painful ecchymoses with haematoxylin bodies in skin biopsy
Amyloid: deposition of amyloid around small blood vessels in some cases
Atrophy
senile purpura
scurvy: defect in collagen synthesis affecting small blood vessels. Platelet Factor 3 release reduced, and platelet adhesiveness reduced
corticosteroid-induced atrophy of skin
Cushing's syndrome
Ehlers–Danlos syndrome
Anoxic
hyperglobulinaemia, and cryoglobulinaemia. (Platelets may also be coated by these proteins, with reduction in function)
fat embolism
Gardner–Diamond syndrome – autoerythrocyte sensitivity. Painful ecchymoses and purpura in females

Purpura Fulminans

May follow
Scarlet fever (27%)
Varicella (20%)
Unspecified upper respiratory disease (23%)
Other streptococcal infections
Roseola
Vaccination
Smallpox
etc.
resulting in
cutaneous ecchymoses
hypotension and fever
disseminated intravascular coagulopathy

Congenital Abnormality of Vessel Walls

Hereditary haemorrhagic telangiectasia (AD)
Vascular pseudohaemophilia (?AD) Prolonged bleeding time [R]
Pulmonary haemosiderosis
Idiopathic haematemesis and melaena
Ehlers–Danlos syndrome (AD)
Osteogenesis imperfecta
Pseudoxanthoma elasticum

Acquired Abnormality of Vessel Walls

Purpura fulminans Haemolytic uraemic syndrome Non-thrombocytopenic purpura* Symptomatic purpura e.g. infections uraemia macroglobulinaemia	there is a platelet function element, in all these conditions except*

Thrombocytopenia

Thrombocytopenia due to causes other than marrow aplasia
- Isoantibody – following blood transfusion
- Immune
  - drug-dependent
  - autoimmune: idiopathic thrombocytopenic purpura
- Intravascular coagulation
- Thrombotic thrombocytopenic purpura
- Haemolytic-uraemic syndrome
- Alcoholism

Thrombocytopenia without suppression of thrombopoieses
- Immunological, e.g. quinidine
- Blood transfusion
  - post-transfusion, with dilution of circulating platelets by donor blood
  - intravascular coagulopathy during transfusion
- Infections: ? intravascular coagulopathy with toxin
- Malignancy: intravascular coagulopathy
- Drugs: direct action on circulating platelets, e.g. ristocetin

Inherited Disorders of Platelet Function

Defective adhesion to subendothelium
- plasma abnormality: von Willebrand's disease
- platelet abnormality: Bernard–Soulier syndrome

Defective adhesion to collagen
- collagen abnormality: Ehlers–Danlos syndrome

Defective platelet aggregation in response to ADP
- plasma abnormality: afibrinogenaemia
- platelet abnormality: thrombasthenia (Glanzmann's disease

Defective release reaction
- platelet storage pool deficiency
  - idiopathic disorder
  - Hermansky–Pudlak syndrome
  - Wiskott–Aldrich syndrome
  - Chediak–Higashi syndrome
- defective platelet release mechanism
  - cyclo-oxygenase deficiency
- defective platelet nucleotide metabolism
  - glycogen storage disease Type I
  - fructose-1,6-diphosphatase deficiency

Acquired Reduction in Platelet Function

Uraemia: reduced availability of platelet Factor 3, inhibition of platelet aggregation by methylcreatine accumulation
Fibrin degradation products: developing in disseminated intravascular coagulopathy
Paraproteinaemia: e.g. coating of platelets by IgM in Waldenström's macroglobulinaemia
Iatrogenic reduction in platelet function
- aspirin: inhibition of platelet release reaction
- clofibrate: weak inhibition of ADP-induced platelet aggregation
- dipyridamole: inhibition of primary and secondary ADP-induced platelet aggregation
- hydroxychloroquine: antimalarial drug which inhibits ADP-induced platelet aggregation
- sulphinpyrazone: non-steroidal anti-inflammatory drug which inhibits platelet release reaction

Hereditary Disorders of Haemostasis

*Factor VIII deficiency
- True haemophilia (XR)
- von Willebrand's disease (AD) – Factor VIII reduced and plasma platelet factor deficiency

*Factor IX deficiency: Christmas disease (XR)
Factor I deficiency:
- Afibrinogenaemia (AR)
- Dysfibrinogenaemia (AD)

Factor II deficiency: true prothrombin deficiency (AR) [R]
Factor V deficiency: (AR) [R]
Factor VII deficiency: (AR) [R]
Factor X deficiency: (Stuart–Prower deficiency): (AR) [R]
Factor XI deficiency: dominant inheritance with variable penetrance [R]
Factor XII deficiency: Hageman's disease: (AR) [R]
Factor XIII deficiency: Inheritance autosomal incompletely recessive [R]
Fletcher Factor [R]
*The commonest cause of clinical haemophilia in Europe. Incidence – perhaps True Haemophilia 10 times more frequent than Christmas disease

Acquired Plasma Coagulation Factor Defects

Acquired
- liver disease (reduced factor V, VII, VIII, IX, X)
- vitamin K deficiency – reduced Factors II, VII, IX and X
- excessive consumption of coagulation factors
  - disseminated intravascular coagulopathy
- defective activity
  - circulating anticoagulants
  - dysproteinaemia
  - interference by fibrin-fibrinogen degradation products

Disseminated Intravascular Coagulopathy

Infection
- bacterial, especially Gram negative septicaemia
- viral
- rickettsial
- protozoal, especially malaria

Injury
- trauma, including major surgery
- near-drowning
- heat stroke
- burns
- envenomation

Circulation
- shock
- pulmonary embolism
- dissecting aneurysm
- cyanotic heart disease

Obstetric
- amniotic fluid embolism
- abruptio placentae
- retained dead fetus

Immunological
- incompatible blood transfusion
- allograft rejection
- immune complex disease
- anaphylactic drug reaction

Metabolic
- diabetic ketoacidosis
- acute fatty liver of pregnancy

Neoplasm
- leukaemia
- solid tumours

CONDITIONS PREDISPOSING TO THROMBOSIS

Increasing age
Prolonged bed rest
Venous stasis – sitting in one position for a long time, e.g. deck chair, aircraft seat
Trauma, especially below diaphragm
Surgery, especially below diaphragm
Carcinoma, e.g. thrombophlebitis migrans associated with pancreatic carcinoma
Chronic infection
Pregnancy
Oral contraceptive pill
Congestive cardiac failure
Blood changes
- polycythaemia causing whole blood hyperviscosity
- plasma hyperviscosity, hence whole blood hyperviscosity e.g. myeloma

Inherited
- congenital antithrombin III deficiency
- homocystinuria (arterial platelet thrombi)
- Blood group A_1 – a higher incidence of thrombotic incidents
- unexplained familial tendency

BLOOD TRANSFUSION

Infectious Diseases which can be transmitted in Transfused Blood

Viral hepatitis A, B, others } probably the most important hazard

Malaria: a hazard where selection of non-infected donors is impracticable. Antimalarial drugs can be given with a suspect blood transfusion

American trypanosomiasis (Chagas' disease): an important cause in South America

Possible causes
- Cytomegalovirus (CMV)
- Epstein–Barr virus
- Post-vaccination, Measles, Influenza } theoretically possible if donor in prodromal stage of the disease

Unlikely causes
- Syphilis, Yaws, Relapsing fever, Kala azar, Brucellosis, Toxoplasmosis } unless a direct donor-to-recipient transfusion with fresh blood from donor with active infection

Blood Transfusion Hazards

Incompatibility (ABO, Rh, etc.)

Haemolysed blood
- blood overheated before transfusion
- blood frozen and thawed by accident before transfusion
- blood too old, i.e. stored too long before transfusion
- blood infected – organisms growing in blood during storage

Presence of pyrogens

Disease transmitted from donor
- hepatitis
  - hepatitis A
  - hepatitis B
  - hepatitis non-A, non-B
- other viruses
  - post-vaccination
  - measles

influenza
glandular fever
cytomegalovirus
protozoa
malaria
American trypanosomiasis (Chagas' disease in S. America)
sporadic disease
syphilis
yaws
relapsing fever
kala azar
brucellosis
African trypanosomiasis
Other transfusion hazards
overtransfusion
air embolism
potassium overload
transfusion with 'old' blood
patient with poor renal function
renal disease
newborn infant
citrate overload: massive blood transfusion
thrombophlebitis related to the transfusion site
haemosiderosis: in patients requiring repeated blood transfusion without blood loss, e.g. aplastic anaemia
excessive depression of patient's body temperature
massive transfusion of cold blood straight from storage
newborn infant, exchange transfusion with cold blood

Iron Overload

Diet: Very high inorganic iron content of diet. Absorption increases with amount ingested
Idiopathic haemochromatosis – inherited
Alcoholic cirrhosis – with high dietary iron intake
Siderosis following portocaval anastomosis
Transfusion haemosiderosis
Chronic anaemia with hypercellular marrow and disturbed iron metabolism
sideroblastic anaemia
thalassaemia
Congenital
iron overload
atransferrinaemia (very rare)
Local
idiopathic pulmonary haemosiderosis: lung
paroxysmal nocturnal haemoglobinuria: kidney
rheumatoid arthritis: joints

Indications for Therapeutic Plasmapheresis

Removal of excessive amounts of abnormal plasma paraproteins, to reduce dangerously high whole blood viscosity
- Waldenström's macroglobulinaemia – high IgM
- Myeloma
  - high IgG
  - high IgA

Reduction of dangerously high whole blood platelet levels in thrombotic essential thrombocythaemia

Removal of dangerous circulating antibodies
- Antibodies against red cells
  - maternal rhesus sensitization
  - cold agglutinin haemolytic anaemia
- Antibodies against platelets
  - autoimmune idiopathic thrombocytopenia (ITP)
  - ? thrombotic thrombocytopenic purpura (success not yet reported)
- Antibodies against coagulant factors: anti-Factor VIII antibody

Removal of other antibodies
- Myasthenia gravis: 90% of cases have circulating antibodies which can be removed temporarily in emergency pending treatment with steroids and/or cyclophosphamide. (Congenital myasthenia gravis does not respond to plasmapheresis, as it is an end-organ abnormality)
- Raynaud's disease: plasmapheresis can be used to reduce the level of circulating cryofibrinogen and vasoactive substance

Removal of circulating immune complexes
- systemic lupus erythematosus
- allergic and necrotizing vasculitis
- ? Felty's syndrome
- Goodpasture's syndrome: plasmapheresis rapidly stops lung haemorrhages, and may allow some improvement in renal function unless there is total renal failure

IMMUNOLOGY

CLINICAL CONDITIONS ASSOCIATED WITH ANERGY

(Technical errors in skin testing to be excluded)
- Immunological deficiency states
  - Congenital
    - mixed
      - ataxia telangiectasia
      - thymic alymphoplasia (X-linked)
      - agammaglobulinaemia (AR)

cell
- thymic aplasia with lymphopenia (Nezeloff)
- thymic aplasia with parathyroid aplasia (diGeorge)

variable
- mucocutaneous candidiasis
- Wiskott–Aldrich disease

Acquired
- sarcoidosis
- chronic lymphatic leukaemia
- carcinoma
- immunosuppressive therapy
- connective tissue vascular disorders
- uraemia
- alcoholic cirrhosis
- pregnancy
- old age
- post-surgery, post-trauma
- Hodgkin's lymphadenoma
- lymphoma

Associated with infections

Viral
- influenza
- mumps
- measles
- viral vaccination

Rickettsia: typhus

Bacterial
- miliary and active tuberculosis
- disseminated mycotic disease
- lepromatous leprosy
- scarlet fever

ANAPHYLAXIS TRIGGERS

Foods
Hormones
Sera, vaccines, etc.
Drugs

Aminopyrine Aspirin Dextran Procaine Penicillin Streptomycin Cephalothin	among many

Diagnostic materials acting as antigens (e.g. used in diagnostic X-ray investigations)

Venoms

Insects
- bee
- wasp
- hornet

Arachnid: spiders
Snakes
Jelly fish

ALLERGIC DISEASES

Atopic disease
- allergic rhinitis
- asthma
- urticaria and angioneurotic oedema
- anaphylaxis

Serum sickness
Extrinsic allergic alveolitis
- farmer's lung
- ventilation pneumonitis
- mushroom worker's lung
- bagassosis
- malt worker's lung
- suberosis (from mouldy cork)
- cheese worker's lung
- bird fancier's lung
- wheat weevil's disease
- fishmeal worker's lung
- pituitary snuff taker's lung

Pulmonary eosinophilia
Allergic contact dermatitis
Allergic drug reactions

HYPERSENSITIVITY

Anaphylactic
- local: exposure of tissue mast cells in sensitized individuals to specific antigens
  - respiratory
    - allergic rhinitis
    - extrinsic asthma
  - intestinal: food allergy
  - skin: urticarial reactions
- systemic: large doses of antigen after a small sensitizing dose

Cytotoxic: antibody–antigen combination on cell surface, leading to cell death, e.g. haemolysis resulting from antibodies directed against red cell antigens, or other antigens on the red cell surface
Complement-mediated
- antigen and antibody react in an excess of antigen, and antigen–antibody complex is carried to other sites, e.g. capillary plexuses in renal glomerulus, skin, etc.
- where antigen and antibody react in an excess of antibody, the complexes remain at the site of formation

1. antibody excess
   Arthus reaction: acute vasculitis
   allergic alveolitis
2. antigen excess
   glomerulonephritis
      post-streptococcal
      systemic lupus erythematosus
      quartan malaria
      drug-induced
   skin: erythema multiforme
   rheumatic fever

Delayed-type hypersensitivity
   mediated by T lymphocytes
   e.g. caseation in tuberculous infection
   tuberculoid in leprosy
   contact dermatitis
   homograft rejection

AUTOIMMUNE DISEASE – POSSIBLE INITIATORS

Expression of new antigens
   virus infection
   hereditary factors
   malignant transformation
   somatic mutation
Alteration of normal antigens by haptens
   drugs
   environmental substances
   virus infection
Exposure of hidden antigens (unmasking)
   after injury
   infection
Loss of tolerance of self-antigens

AUTOIMMUNE DISEASES

Systemic lupus erythematosus: autoantibody formation to double-stranded DNA, single-stranded DNA, RNA, histone and other nuclear components.
Rheumatoid arthritis: rheumatoid factor is an IgM antibody reactive against native IgG, with high synthesis in synovial membranes, and reaction with complement in joints
Polymyositis: ? antigen is myosin
Sjögren's syndrome: ? antigens of salivary glandular tissue
Scleroderma
Polyarteritis nodosa
Rheumatic fever: probable antigens are sarcolemma and sarcoplasm in cardiac myofibrils, skeletal muscle, smooth muscle of vessel walls, and endocardium
Polymyalgia rheumatica
Ankylosing spondylitis

Autoimmune Diseases of the Kidney

Immune complex nephritis
Goodpasture's syndrome: autoimmunity develops against the glomerular basement membranes

Endocrine Autoimmune Diseases

Thyroid
- hypothyroidism
- lymphocytic thyroiditis
- thyrotoxicosis (Graves' Disease)

Adrenal: idiopathic Addison's disease
Pancreas: autoimmune diabetes mellitus
Parathyroid: idiopathic hypoparathyroidism
Gonads
- female
  - gonadal failure
- male
  - gonadal failure
  - allergic orchitis: may follow
    - vasectomy
    - injury

Autoimmune Diseases of the Central Nervous System
(*See also* Muscle Section, p. 344)

Acute idiopathic polyneuritis

Autoimmune Diseases of the Gastrointestinal Tract

Gastric atrophy and pernicious anaemia
? Ulcerative colitis

Autoimmune Diseases of the Liver

Chronic active hepatitis
Primary biliary cirrhosis

Autoimmune Diseases of Muscle

Dermatomyositis
Myasthenia gravis (muscle end plate)

Autoimmune Disease of Heart

Postcardiotomy syndrome
Post-myocardial infarction syndrome (Dressler's syndrome)

Ophthalmic Autoimmune Diseases

Sympathetic ophthalmia
Phagogenic uveitis

Autoimmune Disease of Skin

Pemphigoid
Pemphigus vulgaris

Autoimmune Diseases of the Blood

Cold haemagglutinin disease: caused by IgM antibodies reacting optimally at 0–4 °C
Paroxysmal cold haemoglobinuria: cold antibodies of IgG class
Warm-type autoimmune haemolytic anaemia: antibodies of IgG class
Idiopathic thrombocytopenia: IgG antibodies react with surface antigens of platelet
Neutropenia: antibodies react with surface antigens of neutrophil
Lymphopenia: antibodies react with lymphocyte specific surface antigens
Autoimmune aplastic anaemia: ? T cell-mediated immunity reaction

IMMUNE COMPLEX DISEASE

Immune Complex Pathogenesis in Microbial Disease

Local formation of complexes
- allergic bronchopulmonary aspergillosis
- pulmonary lesions
  - after respiratory
  - syncytial virus
  - after measles immunization

Localization of complexes from circulation
- nephropathy
  - post-streptococcal infection
  - bacterial endocarditis
  - quartan malaria
- cutaneous vasculitis
  - post-streptococcal infection
  - candidiasis
  - *Mycobacterium leprae* (erythematosum nodosum leprosum)
- polyarteritis: hepatitis B
- chronic angiitis: trypanosomiasis

Diseases associated with Circulating Immune Complexes

Serum sickness
Drug sickness, e.g. associated with penicillin, insulin, etc.
Specific infections
- viral
  - hepatitis B
    - polyarthralgia
    - urticaria

dengue haemorrhagic fever
Mycoplasma pneumoniae
measles
bacteria: glomerulonephritis
bacterial endocarditis
infected ventriculo-atrial shunts
parasites
schistosomiasis
malaria
? nephrotic complications
? cerebral complications
Non-specific with infections
myalgia
arthralgia
haematuria
albuminuria
fleeting skin rashes
Connective tissue disease
systemic lupus erythematosus
rheumatoid arthritis: immune complexes may be restricted to synovial fluid
Wegener's granulomatosis
Malignancy
some cancers, Hodgkin's disease, leukaemia } immune complexes have been demonstrated

Immune Complex Disease

Endogenous antigens
autoimmunity
rheumatoid arthritis
systemic lupus erythematosus
neoplasm: tumour antigens
carcinoma
lymphoma
Exogenous antigens
dietary: gluten sensitivity
infection
bacterial
bacterial endocarditis
meningococcal infections
mycobacterial infection (leprosy)
viral
hepatitis B
dengue fever
protozoal: malaria
occupational: chronic allergic alveolitis
drugs
serum sickness
penicillin
sulphonamides
systemic lupus erythematosus syndrome

procainamide
hydralazine

HYPERSENSITIVITY REACTIONS TO DRUGS

Anaphylaxis
Serum sickness
Drug fever
Bronchospasm
Angioneurotic oedema
Skin eruptions, rashes
- urticaria
- exanthemas
- contact dermatitis
- photoallergic rashes
- fixed eruptions
- exfoliative dermatitis
- Stevens–Johnson syndrome

Blood dyscrasias
- agranulocytosis
- thrombocytopenia
- aplastic anaemia
- haemolytic anaemia

Vasculitis
- acute
- chronic

Drug-induced lupus erythematosus (genetic predisposition plus ? allergy)
Allergic pulmonary reactions
Iatrogenic jaundice
Nephritis
Allergic parotitis
Lymphadenopathy ('pseudolymphoma')

IMMUNOGLOBULIN DISORDERS

Immunocytomas and Immunoglobulin Disorders

Myeloma
- May be
  - multiple
    - symptomatic
    - asymptomatic
  - localized plasmacytoma
- Immunoglobulin types
  - IgG (50% +)
  - IgA (20% +)
  - IgD (1·5%)
  - IgM (0·5%)
  - IgE (less than 0·1%)
  - 1% of all cases have no detectable paraprotein in the serum

Immunocytoma with excess production of light chains only (20%)
Plasma cell leukaemia: some of these may be IgE myeloma
Soft tissue plasmacytoma: paraproteins may be found in many after concentration of urine

Heavy chain disease
- gamma-chain [R]
- alpha-chain ('Arabian lymphoma')
- mu-chain [R]

IgM paraproteins
- Waldenström's disease: monoclonal IgM
- malignant lymphoma
- primary cold agglutinin disease
- chronic lymphatic leukaemia
- IgM myeloma (*see above*)
- rheumatoid factor paraproteins
- IgM paraproteins associated with carcinoma
- benign IgM paraproteinaemia

Monoclonal Gammopathy

Plasma cell myeloma
- multiple myeloma
- localized plasmacytoma

Waldenström's macroglobulinaemia
Heavy chain disease [R]
Light chain disease: a more malignant form of myeloma
Primary amyloidosis in the absence of myeloma [R]
Idiopathic non-myeloma gammopathy

Lymphadenopathy with Dysgammaglobulinaemia

1. Connective tissue disease
   Rheumatoid arthritis
   - rheumatoid arthritis
   - Felty's syndrome
   - juvenile rheumatoid arthritis

   Systemic lupus erythematosus
   Arthralgia – purpura-weakness syndrome (Peetoom–Meltzer disease)
   Sjögren's syndrome
   Mixed connective tissue disease (specific antibody to extractable nuclear antigen – ENA – present)

2. Malignant disease
   multiple myeloma (some cases)
   Waldenström's macroglobulinaemia
   heavy chain disease
   - heavy chain
     - γ chain
     - α chain
     - μ chain (very rare)

heavy chain fragments
leukaemia (especially in chronic lymphocytic leukaemia, and myelomonocytic leukaemia)
lymphoma
Kaposi's sarcoma

3. Chronic lymphadenopathy with systemic signs and symptoms
Angio-immunoblastic lymphadenopathy
Sinus histiocytosis with massive lymphadenopathy
Giant lymph node hyperplasia

4. Others
infectious disease
infectious mononucleosis
cytomegalic inclusion virus
toxoplasmosis
syphilis
sarcoidosis
vaccination and immunization responses
amyloidosis (primary generalized amyloidosis)
drug-induced hypersensitivity
graft-versus-host reaction

Immunodeficiency

Primary

Infantile X-linked agammaglobulinaemia
Selective immunoglobulin deficiency (IgA)
Transient hypogammaglobulinaemia of infancy
Thymic hypoplasia (pharyngeal pouch syndrome, DiGeorge's syndrome)
Episodic lymphopenia with lymphocytotoxin
Antibody deficiency syndrome with normal or raised immunoglobulin concentration
Immunodeficiency with ataxia telangiectasia
Immunodeficiency with thrombocytopenia and eczema (Wiskott–Aldrich syndrome)
Immunodeficiency with thymoma
Immunodeficiency with short-limbed dwarfism
Immunodeficiency with generalized haematopoietic hypoplasia
Severe combined immunodeficiency (autosomal or X-linked)
Variable immunodeficiency (common, largely unclassified, appearing from 2 years onwards)
Neutrophil abnormalities
chronic granulomatous disease
Chediak–Higashi anomaly
myeloperoxidase deficiency
chronic mucocutaneous candidiasis
Complement deficiencies

Secondary

- physiological
  - newborn, pregnancy, old age
- pathological
  - infection
    - bacteria
      - leprosy, tuberculosis
    - virus, e.g. measles
    - protozoa
    - syphilis
  - chronic inflammation
    - rheumatoid arthritis
    - Sjögren's syndrome
    - biliary cirrhosis
    - multiple sclerosis
  - granulomatous conditions
    - sarcoidosis
    - Whipple's disease [R]
    - Crohn's regional enteritis
    - Wegener's granulomatosis
  - metabolic disorders
    - uraemia
    - diabetes mellitus
    - iron deficiency
    - protein–calorie malnutrition
    - protein-losing and hypercatabolic states
      - nephrotic syndrome
      - protein-losing enteropathy
      - intestinal lymphangiectasia
      - dystrophia myotonica
  - lymphoid and myeloid proliferative disorders
    - leukaemia
      - chronic lymphatic leukaemia
      - acute leukaemia
    - lymphosarcoma
    - myloma
    - macroglobulinaemia
    - lymphoma
    - lymphadenoma
  - congenital
    - Down's syndrome
    - Gaucher's disease
  - drugs

Immunosuppression

Physiological: normal pregnancy

Surgery

- Major surgery
- Major trauma
- Splenectomy
- Thoracic duct drainage
- Thymectomy in newborn

Irradiation: of lymphoid tissue and bonemarrow
Drugs
- Corticosteroids: depress cell-mediated immunity
- Alkylating agents: cyclophosphamide
- Folic acid antagonists: methotrexate
- Purine analogues: 6-mercaptopurine, azathioprine } inhibit the proliferation of lymphoid cells in the immune response

Diseases associated with immunosuppression
- Congenital immunological deficiencies
- Malignancy
- Severe infection
- Uraemia
- Malnutrition
- Severe vitamin deficiencies
- Connective tissue disease
  - rheumatoid arthritis
  - Sjögren's syndrome
  - primary biliary cirrhosis
- Sarcoidosis
- Crohn's regional enteritis

Consequences of Immunosuppression

Increased incidence and severity of infection, especially
- varicella
- measles
- herpes zoster
- cytomegalovirus
- *Pneumocystis carinii*
- opportunistic organisms
- fungus infection

Patient with Defective Immunity, Fever and Abnormal Appearances on Chest X-ray

(*i.e. during course of malignant disease, autoimmune disease, and/during their treatment, or during other severe illness*)

Progression of disease process
- Hodgkin's lymphoma
- Non-Hodgkin's lymphoma
- Leukaemia
- Myeloma

Pneumonia
- Gram-negative septicaemia
- Gram-positive septicaemia
- Tuberculosis
- Viraemia

Fungus
- Pathogenic fungi
  - histoplasmosis
  - coccidioidomycosis

cryptococcus
nocardiosis
actinomycosis
blastomycosis
Opportunistic fungi
candidiasis
aspergillosis
phycomycoses
Pneumocystis carinii
cytomegalovirus
Drug reactions
Steroids
Busulphan
Cytoxan
Methotrexate
Bleomycin

SYSTEMIC NON-SUPPURATIVE NECROTIZING ANGIITIS

Periarteritis nodosa
Hypersensitivity angiitis
Granulomatous angiitis
Wegener's granulomatosis
Malignant nephrosclerosis
Giant cell arteritis
Malignant atrophic papulosis
Schönlein–Henoch purpura
Arteritis associated with
systemic lupus erythematosus
rheumatoid arthritis
rheumatic fever
dermatomyositis

CELL-MEDIATED IMMUNITY DETECTABLE BY SKIN TESTING IN INFECTIOUS DISEASE

Brucellosis: Brucellin skin test
Candidiasis: Candidin skin test
Leprosy: Lepromin skin test
Lymphogranuloma inguinale: Frei test
Tuberculosis: PPD (tuberculin test)
Histoplasmosis: Histoplasmin skin test
Trichophyton: Trichophyton skin test in ringworm, etc.
Vaccinia virus: reaction to vaccinia vaccination to produce immunity to smallpox
Mumps: mumps antigen skin test

SARCOID-LIKE GRANULOMA

Sarcoid
Infections
Myobacterial infection

- Cat scratch fever
- Toxocara infection
- Histoplasmosis
- Helminth infestation

Gastrointestinal tract
- Ulcerative colitis
- Crohn's disease, regional ileitis

Autoimmunity, allergy, etc.
- Primary biliary cirrhosis
- Farmer's lung

Others
- Hypogammaglobulinaemia
- Neoplasm

Irritant substances
- Beryllium
- Zirconium
- Silica
- Talc

INFECTION

SEPTICAEMIA – PREDISPOSING FACTORS

Skin lesions, e.g. severe burns
Focal infection
Instrumentation of bladder
Intravenous catheter

Leucocyte abnormalities
- Leucopenia
- Neutropenia
- Functional neutrophil defects

Immunological deficiencies
- Primary
  - humoral
  - cellular
- Secondary
  - humoral
  - cellular
- Including –
  - disease
  - drugs (especially cytotoxic and immunosuppressive)
  - ionizing radiation
  - dialysis
  - organ transplantation with steroid and immunosuppression
  - malignancy, leukaemia, lymphoma } chemotherapy enhances risk of infection
  - cirrhosis of the liver
  - diabetes mellitus
  - post-splenectomy
  - post-surgical operation

'Opportunistic' infection with 'non-pathogenic organisms' occurs in:
- malignancy
- cytotoxic therapy
- immunosuppression
- intensive antibiotic therapy

OPPORTUNISTIC BACTERIAL INFECTIONS

Occur especially in Intensive Care Units
- associated with
  - tracheostomy
  - respiratory ventilators
  - intravenous catheters
  - humidifiers
  - 'routine' administration of antibiotics in
    - urethral catheterization
    - acute respiratory infection
    - acute leukaemia

ACUTE HAEMORRHAGIC FEVERS

Bacteria: septicaemia, e.g. septicaemic plague in Africa

Protozoal:
- Trypanosomiasis
- Malaria

Viral
- Yellow fever
- Smallpox
- Tick-borne
  - Kyasanu Forest fever
  - Omsk haemorrhagic fever
  - Congo viruses
  - Crimean haemorrhagic fever
- Rodent-borne
  - Lassa fever
  - lymphochoriomeningitic virus
  - Junin virus (Argentine)
  - Machupo virus (Bolivia)
- Mosquito-borne from sick animals
  - Marburg virus (usually affects cattle)
  - Dengue haemorrhagic fever (sensitizing infection followed by second infection with immunological disaster ? mosquito-borne)
- Chikungunya virus
- Rift Valley fever
- etc.

MASSIVE INTRAVASCULAR COMPLEMENT ACTIVATION

Gram-negative septicaemia
- Schwartzman phenomenon
- Waterhouse–Friderichsen's syndrome

Viraemia
- Yellow fever
- Dengue haemorrhagic fever

Parasitaemia
- Malaria

COMPLICATIONS AND SEQUELAE OF INFECTIONS

Complications and Sequelae of Strept. pyogenes Lancefield Group A Infection

Direct infection
- septicaemia
- scarlet fever
- erysipelas
- tonsillitis
- etc.

Sequelae
- otitis media
- renal – nephritis
- rhinitis
- adenitis
- arthritis

multiple
septic
cardiac
myocarditis
endocarditis

Complications and Sequelae of Bacillary Dysentery

Arthritis
Iritis and iridocyclitis – especially with arthritis
Haemorrhoids
Boils
Peripheral neuritis [R]
Peritonitis [R]
Stenosis: healing of ulcer encircling the gut [R]
'Carrier' state

Complications and Sequelae of Amoebic Dysentery

Amoebic hepatitis
Liver abscess: may perforate into
lung
pleural cavity
pericardium
externally
stomach
peritoneum
Appendicitis
'Carrier' state

Complications and Sequelae of Diphtheria

Vomiting (danger signal)
Cardiac damage
Proteinuria
Bronchitis and bronchopneumonia
Erythematous rash
Periadenitis and cellulitis of neck
Later – Post-diphtheritis paralysis
palate
eye
limbs
trunk muscles
diaphragm
intercostal muscles
(Desert sore – diphtheritic infection in skin ulcer)
(N.B. Toxin production related a phage-like infection of the diphtheria bacillus)

Complications and Sequelae of Meningococcal Meningitis

Central nervous system

facial paralysis, hemiplegia, paraplegia } Rare, and may recover
Arthritis, Synovitis } 5 – 10 % of cases
Ear: deafness, which may be permanent
Rarely
- pericarditis
- pneumonia
- epididymitis

Complications and Sequelae of Gonococcal Infection

Arthritis – may lead to
- fibrous adhesions
- flat foot
- bursitis
- painful heels

Myositis
Iritis
Meningitis
Endocarditis
Pleurisy
Keratodermia blenorrhagica [R]

Post-Infection Syndromes

Breaking of tolerance, with development of autoimmune disease
- may occur after
  - glandular fever (infectious mononucleosis)
  - *Mycoplasma pneumoniae*
  - measles
  - leprosy
- (The condition may cease with elimination of the precipitating cause)

Following infection with Beta-haemolytic streptococcus Group A
- rheumatic fever, Sydenham's chorea, rheumatic heart valve damage
- glomerulonephritis

DIFFERENTIAL DIAGNOSIS OF TETANUS

Tetanus: onset in jaw and posterior neck muscles. Early abdominal rigidity. Body temperature raised above normal in most cases
Trismus: spasm of jaw muscles, with no rigidity of the neck muscles
Tetany: extremities mainly affected, with characteristic posture
Rabies: spasm especially affects the larynx

Hysteria
Strychnine poisoning: the jaw and neck muscles are not especially affected. There is complete relaxation between attacks of spasm. Body temperature normal

LEPROSY – CLINICAL VARIETIES

Tuberculoid: occurs in those with high resistance to *Mycobacterium leprae*
Lepromatous: attacks
- face
- mucous membranes
- limbs, with nerve fibrosis and damage
- eyes
  - conjunctivitis
  - keratitis
  - iritis

Dimorphous type: may regress to lepromatous type
Reactional states: swelling and possibly ulceration in lesions especially in tuberculoid and dimorphous types shortly after starting treatment
- lepra reaction: in lepromatous lesions after much treatment (probably due to absorption of dead lepra bacilli)

VENEREAL DISEASES

Syphilis
Gonorrhoea
Lymphogranuloma inguinale
Chancroid
Granulosum inguinale
Non-specific genital infections
- Chlamydia (Bedsonia)
- Mycoplasma
- Bacteria
- Trichomoniasis
- Candidiasis
- Genital warts (condylomata acuminata)
- Genital herpes (herpes simplex Type II)
- Genital molluscum contageosum
- Genital scabies
- Genital lice (pediculosis pubis)

ACTINOMYCOSIS

Three main sites of infection
- jaw and neck
- intestine, especially appendix
- lung

Secondary abscesses occur in
- liver
- cerebrum
- skin
- kidney, etc.

CHLAMYDIAL DISEASES

(*Organisms which are placed between bacteria and viruses*)

Psittacosis (ornithosis): spread to man by inhalation of infected material from birds
Lymphogranuloma venereum: a venereal disease seen in the tropics, and occasionally elsewhere – females usually having symptomless infections
Trachoma: a major cause of blindness in tropical countries
Inclusion conjunctivitis (inclusion blenorrhoea)

RICKETTSIAL DISEASES

(*More like small Gram-negative bacteria than true viruses – contain DNA and RNA*)

Typhus: caused by *Rickettsia prowazekii.* Vector: lice
Brill's disease: caused by *R. prowazekii.* A mild form of typhus due to reactivation of a latent infection, after a primary attack of classic typhus
Murine typhus: caused by *R. mooseri.* Vector: fleas from rats
Rocky Mountain fever, and other tick-borne fevers: due to *R. rickettsii.* Vector: ticks from rodents, rabbits, dogs
Scrub typhus (Tsutsugamushi group): caused by *R. orientalis.* Vector: mites from ? small rodents and birds
Q fever: caused by *Coxiella burnetii.* Sporadic fever first described in Queensland, Australia

VIRUSES

Australia Antigen – Hepatitis B

HBV = virus causing Hepatitis B (cf. HAV causing infective hepatitis A)
Dane particle = large double-shelled spherical particle, thought to be HBV
HB_cAg = antigen in the core of HBV
HB_sAg = antigen on the surface of HBV. Also found in small 20 nm particles and long tubular structures seen on electron microscopy
Anti-HB_c = antibody against core antigen = carrier state. This is not associated with resistance of infection or any indicator of recovery
Anti-HB_s = antibody against coat antigen

HBIG = hepatitis B immune globulin for short-term protection

e antigen = antigen found in HBV infection, probably host antigen. This may be a bad prognostic sign, and is associated with chronic and aggressive hepatitis

anti-e = antibody which has a good prognostic significance. When it is found in an HB_SAg carrier stringent precautions can be relaxed

Positive Australia Antigen Test

Australian aborigine
Carriers: varying throughout the world
Pathological conditions associated with long-term carriage of hepatitis B
- Down's syndrome (22% positive)
- leukaemia – especially during cytotoxic therapy, and treatment with immunosuppressives
- following blood transfusion (i.e. from donor)
- hepatitis B
- renal dialysis cases
- during and following immunosuppressive therapy
- lepromatous leprosy

Arthropod-borne Virus Infections

Togaviruses: multiply in arthropod vectors without causing disease and may be excreted for months after the initial infection

1. Alphaviruses (formerly group A arboviruses)
   - Eastern equine encephalitis
   - Western equine encephalitis
   - Venezuelan equine encephalitis
   - O'nyong-nyong
   - Chikungunya

   } vector: mosquito
2. Flaviviruses (formerly group B arboviruses)
   - St Louis encephalitis
   - Japanese B encephalitis
   - Murray Valley encephalitis
   - Yellow fever
   - Dengue

   } vector: mosquito
   - Tick-borne encephalitis
   - Louping Ill
   - Kyasanur Forest fever

   } vector: tick
3. Bunyaviruses
   - California encephalitis. Vector: mosquito
   - Crimean haemorrhagic fever. Vector: tick
4. Orbivirus: Colarado tick fever. Vector: tick

PARASITES

Major Causes of Parasitic Disease in the World

Malaria: 25% of the world population live in areas where malaria is transmitted

Trypanosomiasis
African: in rural Africa
South America
Leishmaniasis: 1 million affected
Filariasis: 300 million affected
Schistosomiasis: 200 million infected
Ascariasis: 25 % of the world's population
Hookworm: 400 million
Trichuris trichiura: 350 million

Malaria – Varieties

Plasmodium vivax: benign tertian: temperate, subtropical and tropical distribution
P. ovale (ovale tertian): East, central and West Africa
P. malaria – quartan malaria: widespread, but less common
P. falciparum – malignant tertian, Distribution tropics and subtropics

Complications of Severe Malaria
(i.e. with more than 5% of all red cells affected)

Algid type: vomiting, diarrhoea, anuria
Cardiac: congestive failure or sudden death
Gastrointestinal tract
'gastric malaria'
'choleraic malaria'
Renal: renal tubular damage, anuria, blackwater fever
Cerebral malaria
amnesia, blindness, psychosis
paralyses
ataxia
Ocular
corneal ulceration
iritis
retinal haemorrhage
Spleen: rupture
Hepatitis and gallstones occur in malignant tertian, as does blackwater fever

Differential Diagnosis of Blackwater Fever

Blackwater fever: pyrexia, haemoglobinuria, jaundice, oliguria, and malarial parasites in the blood
Yellow fever
'Bilious remittent fever' of malaria
Haemolytic anaemia with haemoglobinuria caused by administration of an oxidant drug to a subject deficient in red cell glucose-6-phosphate dehydrogenase

Leishmaniasis

Visceral leishmaniasis
- Kala azar
- infantile kala azar

Cutaneous leishmaniasis
- oriental sore
- mucocutaneous leishmaniasis
- lupoid leishmaniasis
- diffuse cutaneous leishmaniasis
- local ulcer
  - Chiclero's ulcer, affecting ear
  - Peruvian cutaneous leishmaniasis

Metazoan Parasites

Trematode fluke infection (distomiasis)

Pulmonary fluke
- Paragonimiasis: in China, Far East and West Africa

Hepatic fluke
- Clonorchiasis: in China and Far East
- Fascioliasis: worldwide

Intestinal flukes
- Fasciolopsiasis: Far East, especially China
- Heterophyiasis: Egypt, Middle and Far East
- Schistosomiasis
  - *Sch. haematobium* – in Africa, Mediterranean coast, African east coast, Congo, Niger, Natal, Cape, Iraq and Yemen
  - *Sch. mansoni* – in Africa, Nile delta, a belt from Zanzibar to Sierra Leone, north of South America
  - *Sch. japonicum* – in Japan, Philippines and parts of South-east Asia

Sites of disease
- *Sch. haematobium*
  - genito-urinary tract: lower end of ureter and bladder
- *Sch. mansoni*
  - intestine invaded
  - later, liver invaded, leading to portal hypertension and splenomegaly
  - cardiopulmonary schistosomiasis
- *Sch. japonicum*
  - intestine invaded, later hepatosplenomegaly

Cestodes (taeniasis)

Intestinal tapeworm
- *T. solium* – pork
- *T. saginata* – beef
- *Hymenolepis nana* – rats and mice

Diphyllobothrium latum – hosts are dog and man intermediate hosts are pike and other fish. Occurs in Finland, Baltic and Switzerland, Central Asia and Far East

Cysticercosis: presence of the larval form in man of *T. solium*

Cysticercus cellulosae

- subcutaneous
- muscles
- central nervous system
- eye
- tongue
- skin

Taenia echinococcus hydatid cysts: presence of larval form in man of *T. echinococcus*

primary cysts: lead to secondary cysts and may lead to free tertiary cysts

- liver cysts
- lung cysts
- pleural cysts
- less commonly
  - bone
  - kidney
  - central nervous system
  - omentum

Differential diagnosis of hydatid cyst in the liver

Hydatid cyst in the liver

Carcinoma of the liver

Amoebic abscess of the liver

Pleural effusion

Hydronephrosis

Dilated gallbladder

Pancreatic cysts

Syphilitic liver

Nematodes

Ascaris lumbricoides: roundworm. Infest intestines

Enterobius (*Oxyuris*) *vermicularis:* threadworm. Infest caecum + rectum

Trichiniasis: muscles most affected

- diaphragm
- intercostals
- muscles of neck
- eye muscles
- the larger voluntary muscles

Ancylostomiasis

Hookworm

Ancylostoma duodenale
Necator Americanus } Infest the jejunum

Strongyloidiasis: *Strongyloides stercoralis:* Far East and tropics. Invades intestinal mucosa

Trichuris trichiura: Whipworm: Infest caecum + large intestine

Filariasis

Bancroftian filariasis: *Wuchereria bancrofti.* Invades lymphatics

Loasis: infection with *Loa loa.* Invades subcutaneous tissues

Acanthocheilonema perstans: Invades serous cavities, mesentery and connective tissue

Onchocerciasis: *Onchocerca volvulus.* Invades subcutaneous and connective tissue

Dracontiasis: *Dracunculus medinensis.* Invades subcutaneous tissue

Animal Vectors of Human Disease

- Domestic
  - Dog
    - Virus: Rabies
    - Leptospirosis
      - *L. canicola*
      - *L. icterohaemorrhagiae*
    - Rickettsia
    - Protozoa
      - Leishmaniasis
        - visceral
        - kala azar
      - Toxoplasmosis
    - Fungus: *Microsporum canis*: ringworm
    - Helminth
      - *Echinococcus granulosus* (hydatid disease)
      - *Dipylidium caninum*
      - *Toxocara canis*
      - *Ancylostoma canicorum*
      - *Ancylostoma Braziliense*
    - *Sarcoptes scabei* var. *canis*
  - Cat
    - virus: lymphogranuloma-psittacosis infection
    - leptospirosis
    - *Spirillum minus* (rat bite fever)
    - (risks less than with dogs, as cats are cleaner)
  - Birds
    - ornothosis/psittacosis
    - aspergillosis (from oral feeding of pigeons)
  - Allergy disease
    - Bird fanciers' lung disease
    - reactions to animal danders, etc.
  - Cattle and horses and sheep, etc.
    - bacterial
      - brucellosis
      - anthrax
      - tuberculosis
      - Salmonellosis
      - Erysipeloid
      - Tetanus

Leptospirosis
Virus
encephalitis
hand-foot-and-mouth disease (Coxsackie A)
Cow pox
Rickettsial infections
Fungus: trichophyton
Helminths
T. saginata (beef)
T. solium (pork)
Liver fluke (sheep)
Trichinella (pork)

Poultry
salmonella
tuberculosis

Wild animals
Plague
Salmonella
Yellow fever
Lassa fever
Spirillum minus: soduku in Japan
Streptobacillus moniliformis: Haverhill fever
Leptospirosis (rats)
Virus infections
Rickettsia
Helminths
Trypanosomiasis
etc.

Human Disease from Shellfish

Viral hepatitis
Neuroparalytic disorders: caused by photosynthesizing marine diflagellates ingested by the shellfish
Allergic reactions
urticaria
rashes
abdominal cramps and vomiting
Gastrointestinal disorders: from faecal pollution of shellfish beds
typhoid
cholera
Esch. coli
Vibrio parahaemolyticus

ANTIBIOTICS

Antibiotic Action

Interfere with cell wall synthesis
Benzyl penicillin
Ampicillin

Cloxacillin
Carbenicillin
Cephalothin
Cephaloridine
Cephalexin
Cycloserine
Bacitracin A
Phosoponomycin

Interfere with protein synthesis in the ribosome
Clindamycin
Neomycin
Streptomycin
Kanamycin
Gentamicin
*Tetracycline
*Lincomycin
*Erythromycin
Fusidic acid
*Chloramphenicol

Interfere with nucleic acid synthesis
Nalidixic acid
Actinomycin
Rifampicin

Interfere with DNA replication
Nalidixic acid
Novobiocin
*Chloramphenicol

Interfere with cell membrane barrier function
Polymyxin
Gramicidine
Chlorhexidine
Cetrimide

Alter the biochemical environment of the bacteria
*Sulphonamides: interfering with *p*-aminobenzoic acid
*Trimethoprim: interfering with folic acid metabolism
Isoniazid: ? interfering with pyridoxal metabolism
Nitrofurans

* = bacteriostatic – all others bacteriocidal

During therapy
Bacteriostatic + bacteriostatic = additive action
Bacteriocidal + bacteriostatic = may be antagonistic
Bacteriocidal + bacteriocidal = may be synergistic

Complications of Antibiotic Therapy

Allergy and hypersensitivity reactions
rashes
erythema multiforme
Stevens–Johnson syndrome
exfoliative dermatitis
bonemarrow depression

thrombocytopenia
neutropenia
Reactions related to dosage
renal damage, e.g. gentamicin
ototoxicity, e.g. streptomycin
liver damage
Host–drug interactions
'grey syndrome' in premature infants and neonates receiving chloramphenicol, due to low activity of hepatic glucuronyl transferase
mild folate deficiency increased by co-trimoxazole
Hepatotoxicity developing during pregnancy – tetracyclines
Discoloration of teeth, e.g. tetracyclines
Growth of organisms resistant to antibiotic administered
Pseudomembranous enterocolitis, e.g. clindamycin
Drug interaction
suppression of gut vitamin K formation, leading to warfarin overaction
hypoglycaemia in diabetics on tolbutamide if sulphonamides given
anticonvulsives potentiated by chloramphenicol

JOINTS

Arthropathy
- classification of arthropathy
- infective arthritis
- variants of rheumatoid arthritis
- seronegative arthritis
- arthritis in children
- osteoarthrosis
- unusual arthropathy

Soft tissue rheumatism

Joints
- monarticular joint disease
- hypermobile joints
- joint crepitus
- joint pain

Back
- scoliosis
- low back pain
- back pain
- sacro-iliitis
- pain in hip

Hands and feet
- carpopedal tunnel syndrome
- contractures
- deformity of hand and/or feet

ARTHROPATHY

Classification

Include

Congenital

1. By contraction, e.g. arthrogryposis multiplex congenita and Hurler's syndrome
2. Following increased laxity and hyperextensibility of joints, e.g. Ehlers–Danlos syndrome
3. Failure to appreciate pain, e.g. congenital indifference to pain
4. Premature osteoarthrosis, e.g. osteodysplasty
5. Abnormal tissue fragility, e.g. osteogenesis imperfecta

Acquired

degenerative, traumatic, occupational

dietetic, e.g. following severe rickets deformity

- endocrine
    - acromegaly
    - myxoedema
    - hyperparathyroidism
- haematological
    - clinical haemophilia with haemarthrosis
    - sickle cell disease – with aseptic necrosis on bone in heads of femur or humerus
- connective tissue disorders
    - rheumatoid arthritis
    - ankylosing spondylitis
    - Felty's syndrome
    - Still's disease
    - Sjögren's syndrome
    - palindromic rheumatoid arthritis
- infective
    - virus
    - bacteria
    - fungi
    - Treponema
    - protozoa (amoebiasis)
- post-infective arthritis
- post-inflammatory arthritis
- metabolic, e.g. gout, renal transplant syndrome, etc.
- vascular, e.g. avascular necrosis in caisson disease
- neoplasm affecting joint
- neuropathy
- pharmacology, e.g. excessive corticosteroid therapy

Infective Arthritis

- Gonococcal arthritis
- Meningococcal arthritis
- Osteomyelitis
- Acute hip synovitis
- Post-trauma
- Virus
    - Rubella
    - Mumps
    - Chickenpox
    - Infective hepatitis
    - Infectious mononucleosis
    - Echo virus
    - Arbovirus
    - Mycoplasma

Variants of Rheumatoid Arthritis

- Clinical
    - episodic
    - monoarticular
    - asymmetrical
    - arthritis mutilans

multinodular

Radiological
- diffuse osteoporosis
- osteoarthropathy
- mixed arthritis
- bone cysts
- bony ankylosis

Serological
- seronegative
- highly seropositive
- rheumatoid arthritis with antinuclear factor
- rheumatoid arthritis with arteritis

Eponymous variants
- Still's disease
- Felty's syndrome
- Sjögren's syndrome

Episodic arthritis
- true episodic rheumatoid arthritis
- palindromic
  - two-thirds eventually 'true rheumatoid arthritis'
  - one-third 'true palindromic arthritis'
- crystal arthritis
  - urate (gout)
  - pyrophosphate (chondrocalcinosis)
- others
  - pigmented villonodular synovitis

(Palindromic arthritis: different joints affected at different times and not associated with positive X-ray changes)

Seronegative Arthritis (SCAT –ve)

Psoriatic arthritis
- distal
- deforming
- identical with rheumatoid arthritis

} may all be complicated by sacro-iliitis and spondylitis

Ankylosing spondylitis

Reiter's syndrome triad (HLA–B27. 75%+ve)
- urethritis
- conjunctivitis
- arthritis
  - post-dysenteric
  - post-sexual

Gastrointestinal tract disease
- enteropathic arthritis
- ankylosing spondylitis

Whipple's disease [R]

Behçet's disease
- recurrent oral and genital ulceration
- iritis
- arthralgia with or without arthritis

Seronegative spondyloarthritis

Arthritis in Children

Bacterial infection

Viral infection
Rheumatic fever
Henoch–Schönlein purpura
Juvenile chronic polyarthritis (Still's disease)
Chronic inflammatory bowel disease
Psoriatic arthritis
Connective tissue disease
- systemic lupus erythematosus
- polyarteritis nodosa
- scleroderma

Blood dyscrasia
- haemophilia
  - Factor VIII deficiency
  - Factor IX deficiency
- sickle cell disease
- leukaemia
- bone tumours
  - primary
  - secondary

Rare
- drug sensitivity
- serum sickness
- erythema nodosum
- sarcoidosis
- congenital syphilis
- cat scratch fever
- Ehlers–Danlos syndrome
- Marfan's syndrome
- pseudoxanthoma elasticum
- arthrogryphosis multiplex congenita
- familial Mediterranean fever [R]
- primary hypertrophic pulmonary osteoarthropathy (affecting knees and wrists, with finger clubbing)
- Lesch–Nyhan syndrome

Osteoarthrosis

Primary
- hereditary
- related to use of joints
- ? related to diet
- part of natural ageing process
- biochemical changes

Secondary
- Previous damage
  - trauma (e.g. acrobat)
  - infection
  - inflammation
    - rheumatoid arthritis
    - gout
  - dysplasia
- endocrine
  - diabetes mellitus

acromegaly
hyperparathyroidism
obesity
occupation
hypermobility of joints
avascular necrosis
familial Mediterranean fever [R]
Kaschin–Beck disease

Unusual Arthropathy

Viral
- Rubella
- Mumps
- Varicella
- Variola
- Vaccinia
- Infective hepatitis
- Infectious mononucleosis
- Arbovirus
- Adenovirus
- Enterovirus
- Parainfluenza A

(all of the above: transient arthropathy may occur)

Bacterial
- Salmonella, especially typhimurium (*N.B. Salmonella osteomyelitis* in sickle cell disease)
- Shigella
- *Yersinia enterocolitis*
- 'Travellers' diarrhoea

Endocrine
- Acromegaly
- Hypothyroidism
- Hyperparathyroidism
- Hypoparathyroidism [R]

Metabolic
- Pyrophosphatic arthropathy
- Ochronosis
- Hyperlipidaemia, especially
  - Type II
  - Type IV

Malignancy

Also
- Sarcoidosis
- Wegener's granulomatosis
- Amyloidosis
- Polychondritis
- Osteochromatosis
- Pigmented villonodular synovitis

SOFT TISSUE RHEUMATISM

Muscle disease
- local myositis

polymyositis
myalgia
polymyalgia rheumatica
minor muscle injuries
muscle spasm
prodromal phase of fevers and connective tissue diseases

Tendon and tendon sheath
tendonitis
tenosynovitis (tenovaginitis)
tenoperiostitis
calcified tendonitis

Bursitis
simple
calcific

Capsulitis (periarthritis): capsulitis of shoulder and hip

Fasciitis
primary plantar fasciitis
secondary fasciitis

Fibrositis
muscle spasm
calcium deposits in soft tissue
fibrositic nodules

Panniculitis
simple benign
Weber–Christian disease

Neuritis
disc lesion
brachial neuralgia
sciatic neuralgia
mononeuritis multiplex
polyneuritis
entrapment neuropathies

Non-articular rheumatism associated with systemic disease
infection
endocrine disorders
metabolic disorders
systemic connective tissue diseases

Psychological

JOINTS

Monoarticular Joint Disease

Inflammatory arthritis
rheumatoid arthritis
seronegative arthritis

Osteoarthrosis

Crystal synovitis

Infection

Trauma and meniscular tears

Hypermobile Joints

Marfan's syndrome

Homocystinuria
Ehlers–Danlos syndrome
Osteogenesis imperfecta
Charcot's arthropathy
Idiopathic

Joint Crepitus

Osteoarthrosis
Rheumatoid arthritis (late)
Tenosynovitis
Fracture
Skull
- hydrocephalus
- craniotabes
- congenital syphilis
- severe rickets in infants

Joint Pain

- Joint structures
  - Inflammatory
    - rheumatoid arthritis and variants
    - post-viral arthritis
    - rheumatic fever arthritis
    - septic
      - pyogenic
      - tuberculous
  - Degenerative changes
    - osteoarthrosis
    - chondromalacia (depending on joint)
    - osteochondritis
      - osteochrondritis dissecans
      - Osgood–Schlatter's disease
    - loose bodies in the joint cavity
  - Metabolic disorders
    - gout
    - pseudogout
  - Neoplasm
    - bone ends
      - sarcoma
      - osteoclastoma
    - synovium
      - synovitis
      - synovioma
      - synovial chondromatosis
  - Trauma
    - dislocation
    - fracture
    - meniscus injury
    - ligament sprain or rupture
    - synovial contusion
    - tendon rupture

Periarticular structures
- bursitis
- capsulitis
- tendinitis

Referred pain from lesions away from the painful joint

Systemic disease often associated with joint pain
- sarcoidosis
- carcinomatosis
- hypertrophic pulmonary osteoarthropathy
- leukaemia

BACK

Scoliosis

Congenital
- Idiopathic
- Congenital: due to vertebral anomalies
- Inherited myopathies
- Inherited neuropathies

Low back pain

Trauma
Intervertebral disc lesion
Renal disease
Sacro-iliac strain
Ankylosing spondylitis
Osteochondritis
Coccygodynia

Back Pain

Congenital
- transitional vertebrae
- spondylosis
- spondylolisthesis
- abnormalities of posterior articular facets
- short leg syndrome

Trauma
- damage to soft tissues, mucles, ligaments, etc.
- fracture of body or transverse process of vertebra
- prolapse of inverterbral disc

Inflammation
- Anklyosing spondylitis
- Sacro-iliitis
    - Reiter's syndrome
    - ulcerative colitis
    - psoriasis

Osteomyelitis
staphylococcus
brucellosis
Salmonella typhi
tuberculosis
Osteochondritis
Neoplasm
Bone
primary tumour
secondary invasion
Intrathecal tumour
Metabolic disorders
causing osteoporosis
causing osteomalacia
ochronosis
Paget's disease of bone
Degeneration
spondylosis
ankylosing hyperostosis
'Referred' pain
pelvic and abdominal disease
postural strain
gynaecological disorders
('psychological')

Sacro-iliitis

Ankylosing spondylitis
Reiter's syndrome
Rheumatoid arthritis
adult
juvenile form
Psoriatic arthritis
Sacro-iliitis complicating
ulcerative colitis
regional ileitis (Crohn's disease)
Rheumatic fever
Scheuermann's disease
Trauma
Metastases
Myelomatosis
Spinal tuberculosis
Brucellosis
Whipple's disease

Pain in Hip
(*due to disease in hip*)

Osteochondritis of femoral capital epiphysis (Perthes' disease)
Avascular necrosis of femoral head
idiopathic
haemophilia
sickle cell disease
Gaucher's disease

Osteochrondritis of femoral capital epiphysis following treatment of congenital dislocation of the hip

Fragmented epiphyses

hypothyroidism chondrodystrophies osteodystrophies	bilateral. Other epiphyses may be affected

HANDS AND FEET

Carpopedal Tunnel Syndrome

Idiopathic
Complicating
- myxoedema
- acromegaly
- arthritis of wrist joints
- previous scaphoid fracture
- intermittent trauma

Contractures

Following disuse of limb or limbs, without adequate care
Acute anterior poliomyelitis
Motor neuron disease
Neuritis
- neglected alcoholic neuritis
- diphtheritis neuritis
- lead poisoning
- diabetes mellitus (uncommon)

Diseases affecting bones and joints
- rheumatism
- rheumatoid arthritis
- spondylitis defermans
- tuberculosis
- gonorrhoea

Dermatomyositis
Trauma
- burns contractures
- following severe trauma

Following varicose ulcers
(Dupuytren's contracture affecting the finger)

Deformity of hand and/or feet

Claw foot
- disease or injury of second sacral segments of spinal cord or of corresponding spinal nerve roots
- poliomyelitis
- peroneal atrophy (Tooth's paralysis), with atrophy of leg muscles beginning in muscles supplied by the peroneal nerve

Claw hand
- progressive muscular atrophy
- amyotrophic lateral sclerosis
- ulnar paralysis
- syringomyelia
- cervical pachymeningitis
- acute poliomyelitis
- accessory rib
- spondylosis

Club foot – talipes
- talipes equinus: forepart of foot not raised
- talipes calcaneus: heel of foot depressed and forepart of foot elevated
- talipes valgus: foot everted and abducted at ankle joint
- talipes varus: foot inverted and abducted at ankle joint
- talipes cavus: the arch of the foot is too high or hollow

Talipes
- congenital
- acquired
  - spastic paralysis
  - flaccid paralysis
  - cerebellar ataxia
  - muscular dystrophy
  - cerebral defects
  - meningeal haemorrhage
  - poliomyelitis
  - spinal cord injury

LIVER AND BILIARY TRACT

Jaundice
- Jaundice: classification
- Persistent or recurrent jaundice with minimal structural liver change
- Postoperative jaundice
- Complications of jaundice
- Jaundice in infancy and childhood
- Aggravating factors in physiological jaundice of the newborn

Hepatitis
- Clinical varieties of acute viral hepatitis
- Post-transfusion hepatitis
- Hepatitis B
- Groups positive for Hepatitis B antigen
- Chronic hepatitis
  - chronic persistent hepatitis
  - chronic active hepatitis

Liver disease
- Enlargement of the liver
- Nutritional depletion in liver disease
- Hepatotoxic activity of drugs
- Immune-mediated liver disease
- Arthropathy and liver disease
- Parasites causing liver disease
- Liver biopsy
- Liver tumours
- Hepatic calcification

Cirrhosis
- Portal hypertension
- Cirrhosis
- Complications of cirrhosis
- Cirrhotic fluid formation
- Sodium retention in cirrhosis
- Hepatic coma during treatment of ascites with diuretics
- Hepatic precoma in cirrhosis
- Hepatic coma
- Hepatic encephalopathy
- Heart disease developing in cirrhotics after portacaval shunt operation
- Inborn errors of metabolism with associated hepatic enlargement and cirrhosis

Biliary tract
- Intrahepatic biliary obstruction
- Extrahepatic biliary obstruction, related to the portal vein
- Intrahepatic biliary tract disorders
- Intrahepatic cholestasis
- Chronic cholangitis
- Sclerosing cholangitis
- Fibro-polycystic disease of the liver and biliary tract

Gallstones
    diseases associated with
    risk factor

JAUNDICE (a)

Haemolytic
Liver cell damage
Obstruction
  intrahepatic
  extrahepatic

JAUNDICE (b)

Premicrosomal
  Haemolysis – increased bilirubin production
  Acquired: drugs
    novobiocin, rifamycin } competition with bilirubin for liver cell uptake and impaired bilirubin conjugation
  Congenital: Gilbert's syndrome:
    partial lack of glucuronyl transferase
    defective hepatic uptake of bilirubin
Postmicrosomal
  Acquired
    biliary obstruction: impaired bilirubin excretion
    cirrhosis, viral hepatitis, drugs, toxins } impaired bilirubin transport
  Congenital
    Dubin–Johnson syndrome, Rotor syndrome [R] } impaired bilirubin transport and excretion

JAUNDICE (c)

Predominant increase in unconjugated bilirubin
1. Increased production of bilirubin
    ineffective erythropoiesis
    haemolysis
2. Familial
    Crigler–Najjar syndrome, Gilbert's syndrome } impaired conjugation

3. Milk-steroid jaundice in newborn: Lucey–Driscoll syndrome
4. Drug action

novobiocin, rifamycin, etc. — competition with bilirubin for hepatic uptake, and impaired bilirubin conjugation

Predominant increase in conjugated bilirubin

1. Familial and inherited disorders of bilirubin secretion

Dubin–Johnson syndrome, Rotor syndrome [R] — impaired transport and excretion of bilirubin into canaliculi

2. Cholestasis
    - canalicular cholestasis
        - idiopathic recurrent intrahepatic cholestasis
        - pregnancy
        - oral contraceptives
        - hepatitis
            - viral
            - drugs, e.g. testosterone
            - alcoholic
        - cirrhosis
    - intrahepatic bile duct cholestasis
        - primary biliary cirrhosis
        - biliary atresia
        - primary sclerosing cholangitis
    - extrahepatic cholestasis
        - biliary obstruction from any cause
3. Hepatocellular jaundice
    - infection
        - viral: hepatitis
        - bacterial, e.g. septicaemia
        - Oroya fever
        - malaria
        - Weil's disease
    - drugs, e.g. paracetamol in large doses
    - toxins, e.g. *Amanita phalloides*, etc.

Persistent or Recurrent Jaundice with Minimal Structural Liver Change

Increased bilirubin production
- haemolysis
- posthepatitis hyperbilirubinaemia
- shunt hyperbilirubinaemia

Defective uptake of bilirubin by hepatocytes
- Gilbert's disease (AD)

Defective conjugation of bilirubin in hepatocytes
- Arias Type I, Crigler–Najjar syndrome
- Arias Type II

Defective transport of conjugated bilirubin out of hepatocytes
- without true cholestasis
    - Dubin–Johnson syndrome

Rotor syndrome
with true cholestasis: canalicular defect (AR)

Postoperative Jaundice

1. Increased pigment load
    Blood transfusion, especially of stored blood
    Resorption of haematoma or haemoperitoneum
    Haemolytic anaemia
2. Impaired hepatocellular function
    a. Hepatitis-like
        halothane
        drugs
        shock
        infection
            hepatitis A
            hepatitis B (N.B. long incubation period)
    b. Cholestatic
        hypotension
        hypoxaemia
        drugs
        sepsis
3. Extrahepatic obstruction
    Bile duct injury
    choledocholithiasis
    postoperative cholecystitis

Complications of Jaundice

Chronic biliary obstruction
    pruritus
    haemorrhagic tendency leading to frank haemorrhage
    osteoporosis
    postoperative oliguric failure
    xanthomatosis
    secondary liver cell damage
Chronic liver cell jaundice
    fluid retention (steroid imbalance)
    encephalopathy
    haemorrhagic tendency leading to frank bleeding
    portal hypertension
    sepsis
Haemolytic jaundice
    brain damage
    cerebral infarction
    gallstones possibly resulting in biliary obstruction and/or cholangitis

Jaundice in Infancy and Childhood

Physiological jaundice
    Increased production of bilirubin
    Impaired hepatic uptake of bilirubin

Deficiencies in glucuronide formation
Transient poor hepatic excretion of bilirubin diglucuronide
Increased enteric reabsorption of unconjugated bilirubin

Unconjugated hyperbilirubinaemia
- Haemolytic anaemia
- Infection
- Aggravation of physiological jaundice
- Breast milk syndrome: steroid interferes with bilirubin conjugation
- Crigler–Najjar syndrome
- Transient familial neonatal hyperbilirubinaemia (starts in the first few days after birth and lasts 2–3 weeks)

Conjugated hyperbilirubinaemia
- Hepatitis
  - intrauterine infection
    - rubella
    - cytomegalovirus
    - herpes simplex
    - Coxsackie
    - adenovirus
    - syphilis
    - listeriosis
    - *Toxoplasma gondii*
  - inherited metabolic defect

Aggravating Factors in Physiological Jaundice of the Newborn

Prematurity: reduced levels of activity of conjugated enzyme
Dehydration
Hypoglycaemia
Hypoxia
Haemolytic disorders: excess blood pigment to eliminate
Excessive bruising: excess blood pigment to eliminate
Infection
Drugs conjugating with glycuronic acid (the substance normally conjugating with bilirubin)
Breast milk jaundice: conjugating enzyme inhibited
Transient familial neonatal hyperbilirubinaemia
High intestinal obstruction
Hypothyroidism
Crigler–Najjar syndrome [R]

HEPATITIS

Clinical Varieties of Acute Viral Hepatitis

Viruses involved
- Hepatitis A
- Hepatitis B
- Hepatitis non-A, non-B

Anicteric
1. Risk in blood donors to recipients

2. Increased incidence in immunosuppressed patients
    a. Renal transplant cases
    b. Myeloproliferative disorders under treatment
    c. Cytotoxic therapy in other malignancies

Classic acute hepatitis
Cholestatic viral hepatitis. Uncommon
Relapsing hepatitis
    ? following excessive exercise in convalescence
    ? following excessive alcohol in convalescence
Fulminant acute liver failure
Subacute hepatic necrosis
Chronic sequelae

1. Chronic persistent hepatitis
2. Chronic active hepatitis
3. Carrier state (especially in immunosuppressed patients)

Post-transfusion Hepatitis

Hepatitis B: incubation period up to 3 months
Hepatitis A: incubation period about 30 days
Herpes simplex } rarely transmitted via adult blood
Epstein–Barr virus }
Cytomegalovirus: incubation period 2–4 weeks
Differential diagnosis
    mechanical obstruction of the intrahepatic biliary ducts
    benign intrahepatic cholestasis
    halothane 'hypersensitivity'

Hepatitis B

Acute hepatitis
    sporadic or endemic (insect bite, etc.)
    post-transfusion
    drug addicts
Chronic hepatitis
    e.g. haemodialysis patients without acute hepatitis

Groups Positive for Hepatitis B Antigen

Acute hepatitis
Subclinical infections
Long-term carriers
Late manifestation of antigenaemia, e.g. chronic hepatitis
Polyarteritis nodosa

Chronic Hepatitis

(A) Chronic Persistent Hepatitis (benign)
    Infection
        virus
            post-acute Type A Hepatitis
            post-acute Type B Hepatitis
            post-acute Type Non-A, Non-B Hepatitis
        schistosomiasis (*Sch. mansoni*)

associated with inflammatory bowel disease
excessive alcohol intake

(B) Chronic Active Hepatitis (aggressive)
Unknown: majority of cases
Infection
previous Hepatitis B
previous Hepatitis A
previous Hepatitis Non-A, Non-B
rubella
cytomegalovirus
schistosomiasis
inflammatory bowel disease
Other diseases
hepatolenticular degeneration
homozygous $alpha_1$-antitrypsin deficiency
galactosaemia
alcoholic liver disease
primary biliary cirrhosis
Drugs
methyldopa
nitrofurantoin
oxyphenisatin

LIVER DISEASE

Enlargement of the Liver

Vascular
Cardiac failure
Pericarditis, constrictive
Tricuspid stenosis
} causing reduction in outflow
Infection
Viral hepatitis
Malaria
Schistosomiasis
Infiltration
Myeloid metaplasia
Leukaemia
Lymphoma
Hodgkin's disease
Space-occupying lesions
Secondary carcinoma
Hepatic carcinoma
Liver abscess
Liver cyst
Metabolic
Cirrhosis – early stages, and nodular proliferative hyperplasia
Fatty infiltration
Secondary amyloidosis

Inherited storage disorders
- Glycogen storage disease
  - Type I glucose-6-phosphatase deficiency
  - Type III amylo-1, 6-glucosidase deficiency
  - Type IV alpha-1, 4-glucose transferase deficiency
  - Type VI phosphorylase deficiency
  - Type VIII phosphorylase kinase deficiency
- Familial hyperlipidaemia
  - Type I
  - Type IV
  - Type V
- Lipid storage disorders
  - Tay–Sachs disease
  - GM1 gangliosidosis
  - Gaucher's disease
  - Niemann–Pick's disease
  - Wolman's disease
  - Cholesterol storage disease
- Mucopolysaccharidosis
  - Type I
  - Type II
  - Type VI

Nutritional Depletion in Liver Disease

Decreased nutritional intake
- due to anorexia
- due to decrease in sense of taste (zinc depletion)
- unavailability of nutritious food

Malabsorption
- toxic injury to intestinal mucosa
- decreased availability of endogenous substances necessary for solubilization of nutrients or intestinal transport
- diarrhoea
- steatorrhoea
- intestinal mucosal damage secondary to folate deficiency

Malutilization due to decreased conversion of nutrients to metabolically active forms
- decreased assimilation
- reduced hepatic uptake

Excess loss in urine

Hepatotoxic Activity of Drugs

Interference with bilirubin metabolism
- Haemolysis via drug action, leading to increased bilirubin production
- Competition with bilirubin for albumin-binding sites
  - sulphonamides
  - salicylates
- Interference with transport of bilirubin through liver cells: toxins

Interference with conjugation of bilirubin: novobiocin

Interference with excretion into biliary canalicule (cholestasis)
- methyl testosterone
- thorazine
- phenothiazines
- meprobamate
- thiacetasone

Cytotoxic action (hepatocellular damage)
- paracetamol overdose
- spoilt tetracyclines
- nitrogen mustard
- cytotoxics, e.g. methotrexate
- para-aminosalicylate (PAS)
- hepatitis-like reaction
  - isoniazid
  - iproniazid
  - halothane

Combined cytotoxic damage and hepatocanalicular flow reduction
- methyltestosterone
- phenylbutazone
- iproniazid

Cytotoxic damage with lipofuscin in the Kupffer cells
- chlorpropamide
- tolbutamide

Toxic substances
- carbon tetrachloride
- chlorophenothane (DDT)
- benzene derivatives
- tannic acid
- muscarine
- aflatoxin
- metals
  - organic arsenic
  - very rarely
    - manganese
    - gold
    - mercury
  - phosphorus
  - vinyl chloride
  - Thorotrast

Immune-mediated Liver Disease

Active chronic hepatitis
- autoimmune, lupoid hepatitis
- B-antigen-related hepatitis
- drug-induced
- cryptogenic

Non-suppurative cholangitis: primary biliary cirrhosis

Cryptogenic cirrhosis

Arthropathy and Liver Disease

Active chronic hepatitis: arthralgia
Haemochromatosis
  acute arthropathy (pseudogout)
  chronic arthropathy
Hepatolenticular degeneration (Wilson's disease): bone fragmentation at the elbows and wrists
Viral hepatitis: arthralgia may occur in hepatitis B

Parasites causing Liver Disease

Malaria
  Plasmodium falciparum
  Pl. vivax
  Pl. malaria
  Pl. ovale
Trypanosomiasis
  African { *Tr. brucei gambiense*, *Tr. brucei rhodiense*
  S. American { *Tr. cruzi*
Leishmaniasis: *L. donovani*
Amoebiasis: *Ent. histolytica*
Giardiasis: *Giardia intestinalis*
Toxoplasmosis: *Tox. gondii*
Schistosomiasis
  Sch. mansoni
  Sch. haematobium
  Sch. japonicum
Clonorchiasis: *Clonorchis sinensis*
Opisthorchiasis:
  O. felineus
  O. viverrini
Fascioliasis
  Fasc. hepatica
  Fasc. gigantica
Paragonomiasis: *P. westermani*
Echinococcus infestation
  Ech. granulosus
  Ech. multilocularis
Ascariasis: *Ascaris lumbricoides*
Toxocariasis
  T. canis
  T. cati
Capillariasis: *Capillaria hepatica*
Strongyloidiasis: *Str. stercoralis*
Pentastomiasis
  Linguatula serrata
  Porocephalus armillatus

Liver Biopsy

Useful in
  Diagnosis of acute and chronic jaundice

Acute hepatitis and its sequelae
Cirrhosis
Portal hypertension
Drug-induced liver damage
Alcohol-induced liver damage
Hepatomegaly due to storage diseases
Unexplained abnormalities of liver function
Infective diseases, e.g. brucellosis
Connective tissue diseases affecting liver, e.g. systemic lupus erythematosus
Tumour in liver
Screening of relatives of patients with known familial diseases of liver

Liver Tumours

Primary [R]
Malignant
1. Hepatocellular carcinoma
   producing alpha-fetoprotein
   may be induced by androgenic anabolic steroids
2. Cholangiocarcinoma
3. Hepatoblastoma: occurring in infants, and producing alpha-fetoprotein
4. Haemangiosarcoma
   rarely primary
   associated with thorium oxide
   may be associated with arsenicals
   associated with vinyl chloride
5. Leiomyosarcoma – very rare, as primary tumour

Benign
1. Haemangioma
2. Focal nodular hyperplasia
3. Hepatic adenoma
4. Mesenchymal hamartoma of infancy
5. Non-parasitic cyst
6. Bile duct
   adenoma
   cholangioadenoma

Secondary
1. Carcinomatous metastases
2. Carcinoid metastases
3. Sarcoma
4. Lymphoma

Hepatic Calcification

Intrahepatic calculi
Hepatic artery aneurysm
Infections
  Hydatid cysts
  Old pyogenic abscesses
  Old amoebic abscesses

Brucellosis
Histoplasmosis
Tuberculosis
Syphilitic gumma
Tumours
Primary hepatic tumours
cholangiocarcinoma
hepatocellular carcinoma
haemangioma
malignant haemangioendothelioma
Secondary tumour
metastatic tumours, especially from –
carcinoma of colon
carcinoma of ovary

CIRRHOSIS

Portal Hypertension

Increased resistance to flow
Prehepatic portal hypertension
portal vein thrombosis
neonatal umbilical sepsis
exchange transfusion via umbilical vessels
suppurative pyelophlebitis associated with
acute appendicitis
chronic pancreatitis
thrombosed portacaval shunt
myeloid metaplasia
hepatic malignancy
hepatoportal sclerosis
Hepatic portal hypertension
cryptogenic
chronic active hepatitis
chronic progressive hepatitis
alcoholic cirrhosis
primary biliary cirrhosis
haemochromatosis
hepatolenticular degeneration
congenital hepatic fibrosis
schistosomiasis
fibrocystic disease
hydatid disease
sarcoidosis
Posthepatic portal hypertension
obstruction to hepatic veins
congestive cardiac failure
congestive pericarditis
pulmonary hypertension
Budd–Chiari syndrome
spread from renal carcinoma
oral contraceptives

thrombophlebitis migrans
polycythaemia rubra vera
post-trauma
Jamaican veno-occlusive disease (Bush tea)

Increased hepatic blood flow
With enlarged spleen
tropical splenomegaly syndrome
blood dyscrasias with splenomegaly
cirrhosis with congestive splenomegaly
With arteriovenous fistulas: post-trauma

Cirrhosis

Infection
virus hepatitis B
virus hepatitis A
virus hepatitis non-A, non-B
? other viruses
congenital syphilis
schistosomiasis

Toxins and drugs
alcohol
methyldopa
oxyphenisatin
methotrexate
trichlorethylene [R]
? mycotoxins

Disturbed immunity
chronic active hepatitis } autoimmune disease
primary biliary cirrhosis }

Prolonged cholestasis
biliary tract
atresia
stones
strictures
tumours
ulcerative colitis (long-standing)
Indian childhood cirrhosis

Vascular factors
prolonged congestive cardiac failure
chronic venous outflow obstruction
veno-occlusive disease (Jamaica)
sickle cell disease
thalassaemia major

Inherited metabolic disorders
hepatolenticular degeneration
galactosaemia
fructosaemia
tyrosinosis [R]
glycogen storage disease Types III and IV
Niemann–Pick's disease
Gaucher's disease
cholesterol ester storage disease
cystinosis

cystic fibrosis (fibrocystic disease)
alpha-1 antitrypsin deficiency
hepatic porphyria
Hurler's disease (mucopolysaccharidosis)
Byler's disease
haemochromatosis
hereditary haemorrhagic telangiectasis [R]
Zellweger's syndrome [R]

Metabolic disorders (non-hereditary)
jejuno-ileal bypass operation for obesity relief
malnutrition
cryptogenic

Complications of Cirrhosis

Haemorrhage from varices
Encephalopathy
Infections
Fluid retention
Cholestasis
Hepatoma

Cirrhotic Fluid Formation

Portal hypertension
Lymphatic congestion
Hypoalbuminaemia
Sodium retention

Sodium Retention in Cirrhosis

Reduced glomerular filtration rate
Secondary hyperaldosteronism
physical changes in the kidney, e.g. cortical vasoconstriction
decreased natriuretic substances, e.g. bradykininogen, prostaglandin
increased antinatriureteric substances, e.g. renin

Hepatic Coma during Treatment of Ascites with Diuretics

Gross reduction in total body fluid resulting in falling circulating fluid volume
Blood fluid lost through the kidneys faster than physiological mechanisms can mobilize fluid to replace the loss, from ascites fluid and oedema fluid
Reduced blood flow through the liver, leading to liver cell damage and accumulation of toxic metabolites
Excessive loss of potassium in the urine

Hepatic Precoma in Cirrhosis

Severe damage to the liver cells

Extent of portal collateral shunt
Quantity of protein in the gut } risk of raised
Bacterial flora in the gut } blood ammonia

Hepatic Coma

Fulminant hepatitis (N.B. Severe hypoglycaemia may occur, especially in children)
Hepatic cirrhosis
- acute
- chronic

Precipitating factors
- bleeding, e.g. from oesophageal varices
- narcotic drugs
- electrolyte imbalance, e.g. after rapid response to diuretics
- excessive protein intake (i.e. excessive for the patient)

Hepatic Encephalopathy (a)

Acute liver failure
Cirrhosis: encephalopathy provoked by
- Haemorrhage
- Infection: including infection of ascitic fluid during aspiration
- Surgery and anaesthesia
- Diarrhoea or constipation
- Diuretic therapy producing sodium : potassium imbalance
- Paracentesis of ascitic fluid producing electrolyte and fluid imbalance
- Alcoholic debauch
- Drugs, e.g. sedatives and tranquillizers
- High protein intake

Chronic portasystemic encephalopathy provoked by
- Portacaval shunting
  - natural in course of disease
  - surgical
- Dietary protein intake
- (Ammonium chloride load tests)
- Intestinal bacteria

Hepatic Encephalopathy (b)

? Due to accumulation of
- Ammonia – blood levels exceeding 300 μg/100 ml (17·64 μmol/l) in adults, or exceeding 100 μg/100 ml (5·88 μmol/l) in infants associated with loss of consciousness and fits
- False neurochemical transmitters
- Short-chain fatty acids accumulating
- Increase in blood levels of methionine and other amino-acids
- Increase in blood levels of tryptophan metabolites, including indoles and skatoles

Heart Disease developing in Cirrhotics after Portacaval Shunt Operation

Hypertension
Arteriosclerosis
Cor pulmonale
Haemochromatosis
Bacterial endocarditis
Hyperdynamic circulatory state
Alcoholic cardiomyopathy
Cardiomyopathy of undetermined origin

Inborn Errors of Metabolism with associated Hepatic Enlargement and Cirrhosis

- Aminoacid disorders
  - Argininosuccinic aciduria [R]
  - De Toni Fanconi cystinosis
  - Dibasic aminoaciduria [R]
  - Tyrosinosis [R]
- Lipid metabolism
  - Gaucher's disease
  - Niemann–Pick disease
  - Tay–Sachs disease
  - GM1 gangliosidosis
  - GM3 gangliosidosis
  - Wolman's disease [R]
  - Cholesterol ester storage disease [R]
  - Familial hyperlipoproteinaemia
- Mucopolysaccharidoses
  - Type I. Hurler
  - Type II. Hunter
  - Type IV. Sanfilipo
  - Type VI. Morateaux–Lamy
- Carbohydrate disorders
  - Glycogen storage disease
    - Type I
    - Type III
    - Type IV
    - Type VI
    - Type VIII
  - Fructose intolerance
  - Galactosaemia
- Haematological disorders
  - Thalassaemia major
  - Sickle cell disease
  - Hepatic porphyria
  - Pyruvate kinase deficiency
- Other metabolic disorders
  - Hepatolenticular degeneration (Wilson's disease)
  - Haemochromatosis

BILIARY TRACT

Intrahepatic Biliary Obstruction

Cirrhosis
Non-cirrhotic causes
- Commonly associated with portal hypertension
  - Congenital hepatic fibrosis
  - Hepatic schistosomiasis
  - Nodular regenerative hyperplasia of the liver
  - Primary biliary cirrhosis
  - Alcoholic subacute hepatitis
  - Hepatoportal sclerosis
  - Idiopathic portal hypertension
- Uncommonly associated with portal hypertension
  - Sarcoidosis
  - Steatosis
  - Myeloproliferative syndromes
  - Amyloidosis
  - Gaucher's disease
  - Secondary carcinoma deposits in the liver

Extrahepatic Biliary Obstruction
(related to the portal vein)

Congenital malformation of the portal vein
Compression of the portal vein
- carcinoma of
  - pancreas
  - biliary tract
  - stomach
- chronic pancreatitis
- pancreatic cyst
- hydatid disease
- alveolar hydatid disease
- polycystic disease of liver
- enlarged lymph nodes
  - carcinoma
  - lymphoproliferative syndrome
  - tuberculosis

Invasion of lumen of portal vein by hepatocellular carcinoma
Thrombosis of portal vein
- splanchnic sepsis
- umbilical sepsis
- polycythaemia
- portal vein thrombosis associated with extrasplanchnic venous thrombosis
- portal vein thrombosis secondary to intrahepatic or extrahepatic blocks
- idiopathic portal vein thrombosis
- diseases in which obstruction of the portal vein is recognized but uncommon complication

Intrahepatic Biliary Tract Disorders

Biliary atresia
Biliary ductular proliferation plus ectasia with hepatic fibrosis
Prolonged cholestasis
    Benign recurrent cholestasis (?AR)
    Recurrent cholestasis of pregnancy
    Neonatal hepatitis with persistent cholestasis (AR)
    Fatal progressive intrahepatic cholestasis (Byler's disease) (AR)

Intrahepatic Cholestasis

Familial
    Dubin–Johnson syndrome
    Rotor syndrome
Infection
    viral hepatitis, causing cholangitic cholestasis
    severe systemic infection: causing liver cell damage
Drugs
    e.g. chlorpromazine
    alcoholic steatonecrosis
Postoperative jaundice
Neoplasm
    Hodgkin's disease
    carcinoma of the liver
Benign recurrent intrahepatic cholestasis
Intrahepatic biliary atresia
Sclerosing cholangitis
    primary
    secondary
Idiopathic recurrent cholestasis
Primary biliary cirrhosis – cholestasis in
    ductules
    interlobular space
    septal bile ducts

Chronic Cholangitis

Secondary sclerosing cholangitis: chronic intrahepatic infective cholangitis
Primary sclerosing cholangitis
Primary biliary cirrhosis
Chronic cholangitis due to drugs, e.g. phenothiazines
Biliary atresia
Carcinoma of intrahepatic bile ducts

Sclerosing Cholangitis

Chronic periductal fibrosis with inflammation
1. Small intrahepatic bile ducts affected – pericholangitis

2. Extrahepatic bile ducts affected –
   sclerosing cholangitis

may follow –
- gallstones
- biliary tract surgery
- long-standing ulcerative colitis
- long-standing Crohn's disease
- retroperitoneal fibrosis
- Riedel's thyroiditis
- pseudotumour of the orbit

Fibro-polycystic Disease of the Liver and Biliary Tract

Hepatorenal fibropolycystic disease
- Infancy and childhood
  - Perinatal. Death soon after birth (AR)
  - Neonatal. Death in renal failure in early months (AR)
  - Infantile. Chronic renal failure and gastrointestinal bleeding (AR)
  - Juvenile. Gastrointestinal bleeding (AR)
- Adult – Adult form (AD)

Hepatic fibrosis without associated renal disease. Onset in childhood, with gastrointestinal bleeding (AR)
Congenital intrahepatic biliary dilatation – episodes of cholangitis. Prognosis poor
Choledochus cyst
Solitary non-parasitic liver cyst
Other cysts [R]
(Hamartoma)

Gallstones

Associated with –
- Obesity
- Diabetes mellitus
- Chronic haemolytic anaemia, e.g. congenital spherocytosis
- Hyperlipidaemia: Fredericksen Types IIb and IV
- Disease of terminal ileum
- Resection of terminal ileum
- Parasites
  - *Ascaris lumbricoides*
  - *Clonorchis sinensis*

Risk Factors for Gallstones
Pigment stones
- Oriental more common than Occidental
- Rural more common than urban
- Chronic haemolysis
- Alcoholic cirrhosis
- Biliary tract infection
- Increasing age of subject

Cholesterol stones

Northern Europe, North and South America commoner than the Orient
Obesity
High calorie diet
Clofibrate therapy
Malabsorption of bile acids
- ileal disease
- ileal resection
- ileal bypass
- cystic fibrosis with pancreatic insufficiency

Female sex hormones. More females than males after puberty. Oral contraceptives
Increasing age of subject, especially in males
? In diabetes mellitus
? Associated with high polyunsaturated fat intake

DISORDERS OF METABOLISM

INHERITED DISORDERS

Frequency of Some Inherited Metabolic Disorders in Europe and North America

(*Relevant to screening programmes*)

Phenylketonuria	6·7/100 000 live births
Cystic fibrosis	50/100 000 live births

Hypothyroidism 17/100 000 live births
Galactosaemia 1·5/100 000 live births
Homocystinuria 0·6/100 000 live births
Branched chain amino-acid disorders (including maple syrup disease) 0·6/100 000 live births

Frequencies of such conditions vary throughout the world

Inherited Metabolic Disorders of Carbohydrate Metabolism

Pentosuria: NAD-linked xylitol dehydrogenase deficiency [R]
Galactosaemia: galactose-1-phosphate uridyl transferase reduced
Galactokinase deficiency (AR)
Essential fructosuria (AR) [R]
Hereditary fructose intolerance: fructose-1-phosphate aldolase reduced
Glycogen storage disease
- Type I von Gierke- glucose- 6-phosphatase deficiency
- Type II Pompe – lysosomal- alpha-glucosidase deficiency
- Type III Cori, Forbes: debrancher enzyme deficiency Varieties
  - a. Enzyme deficiency in both liver and muscle
  - b. Enzyme deficiency in liver, but normal in muscle
  - c. Enzyme deficiency in muscle, but normal in liver
- Type IV Andersen – brancher enzyme deficiency
- Type V McArdle – muscle phosphorylase deficiency
- Type VI Hers – liver phosphorylase deficiency
- Type VII muscle phosphofructokinase deficiency [R]
- Type VIII liver phosphorylase kinase deficiency [R]

Lactase deficiency
Fructose and galactose intolerance
Primary hyperoxaluria
- Type I: alpha-ketoglurate: glyoxylate carboligase deficiency (AR) [R]
- Type II: D-glyceric dehydrogenase deficiency (AR) [R]

Oxalosis
(*Deposition of oxalate in tissues*)

Hereditary
- Type I Primary hyperoxaluria [R]
- Type II Primary hyperoxaluria [R]

Acquired
- Exogenous
  - Oxalate poisoning
  - Ethylene glycol poisoning (antifreeze)
  - Xylitol infusion
  - Methoxyflurane infusion
- Enteric: Hyperabsorption of normal dietary oxalate in enteric disease

Uraemia
Dystrophic: local deposition
- in cataracts
- artery wall
- associated with aspergillosis
- giant cells
- thyroiditis

Deficiency: ? hyperoxaluria associated with vitamin deficiencies

Inherited Disorders of Amino-acid Metabolism
(*Disorders in which only one or two cases have been described are not listed*) (*Inheritance is autosomal recessive unless otherwise stated*)

Krebs–Henseleit urea cycle
- Carbamyl phosphate synthetase deficiency [R]
- Ornithine transcarbamylase deficiency [R]
- Citrullinuria [R]
- Argininosuccinic aciduria [R]

Phenylalanine and related compounds
- Phenylketonuria
- Tyrosinaemia [R]
- *Alkaptonuria: homogentisic oxidase deficiency
- *Albinism
  - oculocutaneous
  - ocular (XR)
    - tyrosinase-positive variety
    - tyrosinase-negative variety

Disorders of tryptophan and nicotinic acid metabolism
- Hartnup disease
- Tryptophanuria [R]
- Hydroxykynureninuria [R]

Branched chain amino-acid disorders
- Maple syrup urine disease and variants
- Hypervalinaemia [R]
- Isovaleric acidemia [R]

Disorders of sulphur-containing amino-acids
- Hypermethioninaemia [R]
- Methionine malabsorption [R]
- Cystathionine synthetase deficiency [R]
- Cystathioninuria
- Infantile cystinosis
- *Cystinuria

Others
- Histidinaemia
- Hyperlysinaemia
  - (*a*) periodic hyperlysinaemia with hyperammonaemia [R]
  - (*b*) persistent hyperlysinaemia [R]
- Hydroxyprolinaemia [R]

*Not known to be associated with mental retardation

Hyperprolinaemia
Type I [R]
Type II [R]
Hyperglycinaemia with hyperglycinuria
Type I: ketotic [R]
Type II: non-ketotic [R]
Methylmalonic aciduria
(*a*) responsive to vitamin B_{12} [R]
(*b*) non-responsive to vitamin B_{12} [R]
Various types of hyper-beta-alaninaemia [R]
Monolethrix
Hydroxylysinuria [R]
Pyroglutamate aciduria

Genetic Hyperlipidaemia

Familial
hypercholesterolaemia (monogenic type)
hypercholesterolaemia (polygenic type)
hypertriglyceridaemia
combined hyperlipidaemia (multiple lipoprotein-type hyperlipidaemia)
lipoprotein lipase deficiency (chylomicronaemia)
Familial 'Broad Beta' disease (Fredriksen Type III)

Secondary Hyperlipoproteinaemia

Diet: high fat intake
Diabetes mellitus
Nephrotic syndrome
Myxoedema
Pregnancy
Pancreatitis
Liver disease
Glycogen storage disease
Gout: related to diet
Amyloidosis
Less commonly
Myeloma
Macroglobulinaemia
Thyrotoxicosis
Idiopathic hypercalcaemia

Inherited Lipid Storage Disease

Fabry's disease: ceramide trihexosidase deficiency (X-linked) [R]
Gaucher's disease: glucocerebrosidase deficiency (AR)
clinical varieties
infantile acute neuronopathic
subacute juvenile
adult non-neuronopathic
Tay–Sachs amaurotic familial idiocy: GM2 gangliosidosis: hexosamidase A deficiency

Generalized gangliosidosis GM1: beta-galactosidase deficiency
Juvenile generalized GM1 gangliosidosis: beta-galactosidase deficiency
Niemann–Pick's disease: sphingomyelinase deficiency: various forms
  severe infantile form
  visceral non-neuronopathic form
  subacute form
  Nova Scotia variety
Metachromatic leucodystrophy: acyl sulphatidase deficiency
Krabbe's disease: globoid cell leucodystrophy: beta-galactosidase deficiency (AR) [R]
I-cell disease [R]
Fucosidosis: Alpha-L-fucosidase deficiency [R]
Lactosylceramidosis [R]
Mannosidosis [R]

Inherited Disorders of Lipid Metabolism

A-betalipoproteinaemia
Hypobetalipoproteinaemia
Alpha-lipoprotein deficiency: Tangier disease
Green acyldehydrogenase deficiency [R]
Refsum's disease – phytanic acid oxidase deficiency (AR) [R]

Amaurotic Familial Idiocy
(*abnormal accumulation of GM2 ganglioside*)

Congenital: Norman–Wood disease
Infantile: Tay–Sachs disease
Late infantile: Jansky–Bielschowsky disease
Systemic late infantile form
Juvenile: Vogt–Spielmeyer, Batten's disease
Adult Kuf's disease, Hallervorden–Spatz disease

Mucolipidoses and Oligosaccharidosis

Mannosidosis	alpha-mannosidase activity reduced [R]
Aspartylglucosaminuria	aspartyl glycosamine amidohydrolase [R]
GM1 gangliosidosis (various forms)	beta-galactosidase activity reduced
Sandhoff disease	hexosaminidases A and B activity reduced
Fucosidosis (infantile and adult)	alpha-fucosidase activity reduced [R]
Mucosulphotidosis	multiple sulphatase activities reduced [R]
Mucolipidosis I	*N*-acetyl-neuraminidase activity reduced [R]

Mucolipidosis II multiple lysosomal hydrolase activities reduced [R]
Mucolipidosis III multiple lysosomal hydrolyase activities reduced [R]

Lipomucopolysaccharidosis

Mannosidosis: (AR) [R]
Alpha-fucosidosis: (AR) [R]
Metachromatic leucodystrophy variant: (AR)
Farber's disease: (AR)
Chondroitin-sulphaturia: (AR)

Mucopolysaccharidosis

Type
I–H. Hurler syndrome: (AR). Dwarf, Grotesque face, joint contractures. Mental retardation. Corneal opacity. Marked somatic changes. Alpha-L-iduronidase deficiency.
I–S. Scheie syndrome: alpha-L-iduronidase deficiency
I–H/S Hurler/Scheie compound: alpha-L-iduronidase deficiency (These two latter syndromes are variants of I–H)
II. Hunter syndrome (severe and mild forms): (XR). Dwarf Grotesque face. Somatic changes. Similar to I, but less severe. No corneal changes. Iduronate sulphatase deficiency
IIIA. Sanfilippo A syndrome: (AR). Severe mental retardation. Mild skeletal changes. Heparin sulphate sulphamidase deficiency
IIIB. Sanfilippo B syndrome – Alpha-*N*-acetylglucosaminidase deficiency
IV. Morquio syndrome: (AR) Severe skeletal deformities. No mental retardation. Corneal opacities may occur *N*-acetylgalactosamine-6-sulphatase deficiency
V. This used to be Scheie syndrome, but with enzyme deficiency identification this syndrome has been included as a variety of Type I Hunter syndrome, with no mental retardation, and no corneal opacities, but with alpha-L-iduronidase deficiency
VI. Maroteaux–Lamy syndrome: (AR). Severe and mild forms described. Skeletal changes with gross corneal opacities. No mental retardation. Beta-glucuronidase deficiency
(? I-cell disease should be included here)

Heredofamilial Amyloidoses [R]

Neoropathy
Lower limb neuropathy (AD)
Upper limb neuropathy with carpal tunnel syndrome (AD)
Lower, then upper limb neuropathy with nephropathy (AD)

Nephropathy
  Familial Mediterranean fever (AR)
  Fever with abdominal pain (AD)
  Urticaria, deafness and renal disease (?AD)
  Renal failure, hypertension and amyloid (AD)
Cardiomyopathy: hereditary cardiac amyloid
  Progressive heart failure
  Persistent atrial standstill
Miscellaneous
  Medullary carcinoma of thyroid (AD)
  Lattice corneal hypertrophy (AD)
  Cutaneous amyloidosis

Ehlers–Danlos Syndrome Types

Type I	Gravis: (D)
Type II	Mitis: (D)
Type III	Benign hypermobile: (D)
Type IV	Ecchymotic arterial (Scak–Barabas type)
Type V	X-linked
Type VI	Ocular: (AR)
Type VII	Arthrochalasis multiplex congenita: (AR)

Inherited Disorders due to Disorders of Metal Metabolism

Copper
  Hepatolenticular degeneration: Wilson's disease (AR) abnormally low levels of effective copper-carrying protein in plasma, caeruloplasmin
Iron
  Primary: haemochromatosis
  Secondary iron overload
    excessive iron in diet
    transfusion haemosiderosis

Disorders of Purine and Pyrimidine Metabolism

Gout: Overproduction and/or underexcretion of uric acid. Polygenic
  Normal excretion of uric acid in 85% of gout cases
  Overexcretion of uric acid in 25% of gout cases
Variants:
  Partial deficiency of hypoxanthine-guanine phosphoribosyl transferase
  Severe deficiency of hypoxanthine-guanine phosphoribosyl transferase (XR). Lesch–Nyhan syndrome: with self-mutilation and severe mental retardation
Metabolic disorders with secondary hyperuricacidaemia and gout
  Glucose-6-phosphatase deficiency (AR)
  Hyperuricacidaemia associated with hypertriglyceridaemia which may occur with Types III, IV, and V hyperlipoproteinaemia

Idiopathic familial uric acid nephrolithiasis (AD) with normal serum and urine uric acid levels, occurring in Israel
Secondary hyperuricacidaemia: e.g. following cytotoxic therapy, etc.
Xanthinuria: xanthine oxidase deficiency (AR) [R]
Hereditary orotic aciduria
  Type I [R]
  Type II [R]

Adult Gout – Differential Diagnosis

Gout
Local soft tissue infection
Pyrophosphate arthropathy
Acute calcific periarthritis
Palindromic rheumatism
Ankylosing spondylitis
Reiter's disease
Post-infective arthropathy
Psoriatic arthropathy
Osteoarthrosis
Infective arthritis
Arthritis associated with pancreatic disorders
'Psychogenic' rheumatism (?)

Juvenile Gout – Differential Diagnosis

Primary juvenile gout
Acute Still's disease with monoarticular onset
Pyogenic arthritis (uncommon)
Lesch–Nyhan's disease [R]
Secondary juvenile gout occurring in
  acute leukaemia
  myeloid metaplasia
  congenital haemolytic anaemia
  secondary polycythaemia
  von Gierke's Type I glycogen storage disease
  ? diabetic ketoacidosis might precipitate acute secondary gout in susceptible patient

CHROMOSOMES

Causes of Abnormal Chromosomes

Maternal ageing
Interchromosomal effects
Satellite association
Genetic predisposition to non-disjunction
Ionizing radiation
Infectious agents, e.g. viral infection
Autoimmunity

Chromosomal Aberrations

Balanced structural heterozygosity
- In mitotic cells
  - intrachange
  - interchange
    - simple translocations involving autosomes
    - centric fusion of two acrocentric chromosomes
- In meiotic cells
  - pericentric inversion
  - reciprocal translocation

Unbalanced structural heterozygosity
- Deletion
  - short arm deletion
  - long arm deletion
  - ring form

Autosomal trisomies: the commonest is Down's syndrome

Sex chromosome abnormalities
- Including
  - XO Turner's syndrome
  - XXY Klinefelter's syndrome
  - XXX 'superfemale'
  - XYY 'supermale'

SIGNS AND SYMPTOMS OF METABOLIC DISORDERS

Jaundice associated with Genetic Metabolic Defects

Galactosaemia
Hereditary fructose intolerance
Tyrosinaemia [R]
Alpha-1 antitrypsin deficiency
Hereditary spherocytosis
Crigler–Najjar syndrome [R]
Hypothyroidism
Wolman's disease [R]

Genetic Metabolic Disorders associated with Unusual Odour of Body and/or Urine

Phenylketonuria: musty smell
Maple syrup urine disease: maple syrup
Methionine malabsorption: oast house [R]
Isovaleric aciduria: sweaty feet [R]
Beta-methyl crotonyl CoA carboxylase deficiency: cat's urine [R]

Genetic Metabolic Disorders with abnormal Hair Conditions

Phenylketonuria: hair light in colour
Argininosuccinic aciduria: hair friable and coarse [R]
Menke's syndrome: hair sparse and kinky [R]

Genetic Metabolic Disorders associated with Attacks of Hypoglycaemia

Galactosaemia
Hereditary fructose intolerance
Fructose 1,6-diphosphatase deficiency
Glycogen storage disease Type I
Maple syrup urine disease
Branched chain aminoaciduria [R]
Methylmalonic aciduria [R]
Propionic acidaemia [R]
Pyruvate carboxylase deficiency [R]

Genetic Syndromes associated with Glucose intolerance or Clinical Diabetes Mellitus

Pancreas
- Hereditary relapsing pancreatitis
- Cystic fibrosis
- Polyendocrine deficiency disease
- Haemochromatosis
- Alpha-1 antitrypsin deficiency

Other endocrine
- Isolated growth hormone deficiency
- Hereditary panhypopituitarism
- Phaeochromocytoma
- Multiple endocrine adenomatosis
  - type I
  - type II
- Glucagonoma

Glucose intolerance occurs in
- Glucogen storage disease Type I
- Acute porphyria
- Hyperlipidaemia
- Hypertriglyceridaemia

METABOLIC DISORDERS

Neuroglycopenia – Differential Diagnosis

Psychiatric conditions
- hysteria
- depression
- schizophrenia
- dementia
- hyperventilation

Neurological conditions
- epilepsy
- brain tumour
- carotid or basilar artery insufficiency
- hemiplegia
- motor neuron disease
- peripheral neuropathy
- meningitis

- transient diplopia and strabismus
- multiple sclerosis
- intermittent hearing loss

Endocrine disorders
- hypoparathyroidism
- hyperthyroidism (thyrotoxicosis)
- hypothyroidism
- phaeochromocytoma
- spontaneous hypothermia
- obesity
- porphyria

Cardiovascular disorders
- vasovagal syncope
- orthostatic hypotension
- angina pectoris
- pulmonary oedema

Drugs and toxic substances
- alcoholism
- barbiturates
- morphine
- etc.

Hypoglycaemia in Infancy and Childhood

Newborn
- small-for-dates babies
- smaller of twins, or multiple births
- infants of diabetic mothers
- maternal toxaemia
- maternal hyperthyroidism
- asphyxia at birth
- birth injury
- erythroblastosis, kernicterus
- adrenal haemorrhage
- cold injury
- unknown cause

Older infant
- hyperinsulinaemia
    - beta-cell defect, hyperplasia, neoplasm
    - leucine sensitivity
    - nesidioblastosis
- reduced liver glycogen stores
    - ketotic hypoglycaemia (50% after 1 year)
    - endocrine disorders
        - panhypopituitarism
        - isolated growth hormone deficiency
        - Addison's disease
        - hypothyroidism
- hepatic enzyme deficiency states
    - glycogen storage disease
        - glucose-6-phosphatase deficiency
        - amylo-1,6-glucosidase deficiency
        - phosphorylase defects

disorders of gluconeogenesis
fructose-1,6-diphosphatase deficiency
pyruvate carboxylase deficiency
other enzyme deficiencies
glycogen synthetase deficiency
galactose-1-phosphate uridyl transferase deficiency
fructose-1-phosphate aldolase deficiency

Older children
diabetes mellitus
adrenogenital syndrome

Non-ketotic Insulin-resistant Early-onset Diabetes

May occur in
Muscular dystrophies
Late-onset proximal myopathy
Huntington's chorea
Machado's disease
Herrmann's syndrome
Optic atrophy: diabetes mellitus syndrome
Friedreich's ataxia
Alström's syndrome
Laurence–Moon–Biedl syndrome
Retinopathy: hypogonadism: mental retardation: nerve deafness syndrome
Pseudo–Refsum's syndrome
Progeroid syndromes with glucose intolerance
Cockayne's syndrome
Werner's syndrome
Glucose intolerance secondary to onset of obesity
Prader–Willi syndrome
Achondroplasia
Miscellaneous
Steroid-induced ocular hypertension
Mendenhall's syndrome
Epiphysial dysplasia and infantile-onset diabetes mellitus
Chromosome abnormalities
Trisomy 21
Klinefelter's syndrome
Turner's syndrome

Lactic Acidosis

Type A: associated with tissue anoxia
hypotension
poor tissue perfusion
arterial oxygen desaturation
Type B: no clear evidence of tissue anoxia
Type B_1 diabetes mellitus
renal failure
liver disease
leukaemia

Type B_2 biguanide therapy in diabetes
- parenteral nutrition
  - fructose
  - sorbitol
  - xylitol
  - ethanol
- salicylates
- methanol poisoning

Type B_3 inherited conditions
- Type I glycogen storage disease
- fructose 1,6-diphosphatase deficiency
- Leigh's syndrome
- methylmalonic aciduria

Disturbance of Hydrogen Ion Concentration

Acidosis
Primary excess of acid
- Respiratory acidosis
  - rebreathing
  - hypercapnoea, e.g.
    - emphysema
    - pulmonary fibrosis
    - etc.
- Non-respiratory acidosis
  - metabolic
    - diabetes mellitus
    - starvation
    - lactic acidosis, etc.
    - ammonium chloride ingestion
  - renal failure

Primary reduction of base
- gastrointestinal disorders with loss of base
- renal tubular acidosis
- dilutional acidosis

Alkalosis
Primary acid deficit
- Respiratory alkalosis
  - salicylate poisoning
  - overbreathing
  - high fever
  - hypoxic anoxaemia
- Non respiratory alkalosis
  - metabolic
    - potassium deficiency
    - excessive loss of gastric juice
    - alkali administration, milk-alkali syndrome
  - bone resorption
  - excessive diuresis
- Mixed disturbances: including
  - severe salicylate poisoning
  - toxaemia of pregnancy
  - etc.

Water Intoxication

Ectopic antidiuretic hormone production: tumour, e.g. carcinoma of bronchus
Excess production of antidiuretic hormone
- Post-anaesthesia
- Post-surgery
- Head injury: may be exacerbated by excess fluid therapy

Inadequate diuretic response to water load
- hypopituitarism
- hypoadrenocorticalism

Lung disease
- severe pyogenic pneumonia
- tuberculosis
- pneumothorax
- empyema

Iatrogenic
- potentiation of endogenous antidiuretic hormone
- antidiuretic hormone secretion enhanced by
  - thiazides
  - chlorpropamide
  - carbamazepine
  - clofibrate
- overdosage with pitressin tannate in the treatment of diabetes insipidus

Acute porphyria

Temperature Effects

Hypothermia
- Exposure to cold
  - local effects – frostbite
  - general hypothermia
- Regulatory body control failure
  - in the very young
  - in the very old
  - severe illness
    - myocardial infarction
    - cerebrovascular accident
    - severe infection
  - intoxication
    - alcohol
    - drugs, e.g. chlorpromazine

Hyperthermia
- Exposure to heat
  - heat cramps
  - heat syncope
  - heat oedema
  - heat exhaustion
    - water depletion
    - salt depletion
  - heat stroke
  - burns

Hyperpyrexia
- infection
  - Gram-negative septicaemia
  - rickettsial infection
  - viral infection
  - protozoal infection
  - fungal infection
- Neoplasm
  - hypernephroma
  - Hodgkin's lymphadenoma
  - lymphosarcoma
  - primary and secondary hepatic tumours
  - pancreatic carcinoma
  - gastric carcinoma, etc.
- Autoimmune disease and serum sickness
- Drug fever (probably allergic)
- Cerebral lesion: especially affecting the brainstem
- Tissue damage
- Thromboses
- Haemorrhage
- Malignant hyperpyrexia in susceptible subjects
- Heat stroke
- Thyroid crisis
- Steroid fever
- Acute gout
- Porphyric attack
- (Etiocholanolone in familial Mediterranean fever) [R]

Globulin Abnormality

Multiple myeloma: Types
- IgG
- IgA
- IgD } rare
- IgE } rare

Macroglobulinaemia: IgM

Benign monoclonal gammopathy

Heavy chain disease
- γ-chain disease } rare
- α-chain disease } rare
- μ-chain disease } rare

Light chain disease [R]

Effects of abnormal protein
- Hyperviscosity
- Cryoglobulinaemia
- Cold agglutinin disease
- Amyloid
- Recurrent infections associated with reduced antibody production
- Bence Jones proteinuria

MUSCLE DISORDERS

Signs and symptoms
- pain in muscles on exertion
- muscle pain at rest
- muscle cramps
- myoglobinuria

Neuromuscular disorders
- central nervous system or muscle disorders with an autoimmune aetiology
- neuromuscular disorders associated with malignancy
- disorders of neuromuscular transmission

Muscle disorders
- inherited muscle disorders
- myositis
- polymyositis
- myopathy due to trauma
- drug-induced myopathy
- metabolic disorders associated with myopathy
- endocrine myopathies

SIGNS AND SYMPTOMS

Pain in Muscles on Exertion

Muscle ischaemia
Intermittent ischaemia of
- spinal cord
- cauda equina

McArdle's disease
Phosphofructokinase deficiency
Pain may occur in
- muscular dystrophy (occasional)
- motor neuron disease: early stages
- early spasticity

Muscle Pain at Rest

Tension headache
Low back pain
'Fibrositis'
Muscle cramps
- following unaccustomed exertion
- sodium depletion
- uraemia
- tetany
- drugs
- unexplained

- Flexor spasms
  - spinal cord lesions, e.g. multiple sclerosis
  - associated with spasticity
- Neuralgic amyotrophy: pain in arm and shoulder
- Pain in muscles preceding clinically diagnosable
  - poliomyelitis
  - Guillain–Barré syndrome
- Painful polyneuropathies
  - alcohol
  - porphyria
  - arsenic
  - polyarteritis nodosa
- Tender muscles
  - vitamin B_1 deficiency
  - vitamin B_{12} deficiency
- Diabetic amyotrophy
- Virus infections: myalgia
- Benign myalgic encephalomyelitis
- Coxsackie B myalgia (Bornholm disease)
- Polymyositis tendinosa

Muscle Cramps

- Occurring at rest: usually not muscle disorders
- Occurring following exertion, and relieved by rest
  - benign and low-grade muscular dystrophies
  - metabolic myopathies
    - glycogenoses
    - carnitine palmityl transferase deficiency [R]
    - myophosphorylase deficiency [R]
    - muscle adenylate deaminase deficiency [R]
  - (myoglobinuria may occur)
  - other myoglobinuric syndromes

Myoglobinuria

- Muscle damage
  - ischaemia
  - crush injury
  - high voltage electric shock
  - violent exercise plus heat stroke
  - chronic alcoholism – acute myopathy after drinking bout
  - carbon monoxide poisoning
  - barbiturate poisoning
  - severe trichinosis
  - sea snake bite
  - following succinylcholine injection during halothane anaesthesia
- Fulminant polymyositis
- 'Haff' disease
- Paroxysmal paralytic myoglobinuria of Myer-Betz
- Glycogen storage disease:
  - McArdle's disease (Type V): phosphorylase deficiency

one-third to a half of cases give history of occasional attacks after exercise

Type VIII: phosphofructokinase deficiency [R]

Familial myoglobinuria:

? autosomal recessive

Paroxysmal myoglobinuria:

Type I in males, with onset at puberty to 25 years: Family history in one-third with unaccustomed exercise provoking attack

Type II: onset in childhood frequently in association with acute infection. In attacks there is neutrophilia with raised plasma potassium and uraemia

NEUROMUSCULAR DISORDERS

Central Nervous System or Muscle Disorders with an Autoimmune Aetiology

Central nervous system

Acute disseminated encephalomyelitis

1. Post-bacterial infection
2. Post-viral infection
3. Post-immunization

Acute haemorrhagic leucoencephalitis

Multiple sclerosis

Peripheral nervous system

Acute idiopathic polyneuritis (Landry–Guillain–Barré syndrome)

Sensory carcinomatous neuropathy (non-metastatic complication of carcinoma)

Muscle

Myasthenia gravis

Polymyositis

General

Disseminated lupus erythematosus

Neuromuscular Disorders Associated with Malignancy

Muscle

malignant cachexia

myopathic-myasthenic syndrome of Eaton and Lambert

proximal myopathy without myasthenia

polymyositis and dermatomyositis

Neuropathic muscular weakness

motor neuron disease

primary sensory neuropathy (ganglioradiculitis)

peripheral sensorimotor neuropathy

neuromyotonica

Endocrinal muscular weakness

ectopic production of ACTH in Cushing's syndrome

ectopic production of parathormone in hyperparathyroidism

muscular weakness associated with hypercalcaemia

Disorders of Neuromuscular Transmission

Genetic
- Hereditary myasthenia gravis
  - transient neonatal
  - congenital and juvenile
  - myasthenia with myopathy
- Pseudocholinesterase deficiency (suxamethonium paralysis)

Toxic
- Botulism
- Tick paralysis
- Puff-fish paralysis (tetrodotoxin)
- Magnesium intoxication
- Kanamycin and other antibiotics

Myasthenic syndromes occurring in
- Thyrotoxicosis
- Malignant disease (Eaton–Lambert syndrome)
- Systemic lupus erythematosus
- Polymyositis
- Anterior horn cell disease
- Chronic polyneuropathy
- Mild periodic myasthenia (Alajouanine)

Cholinergic paralysis
- Poisoning with anticholinesterases (e.g. nerve gases)
- Depolarizing drugs
- Black Widow spider venom

MUSCLE DISORDERS

Inherited Muscle Disorders

Glycogen storage disease
- Type 1 (glucose-6-phosphatase deficiency): muscle hypotoma without direct muscle involvement
- Type 2 (acid maltase deficiency):
  - Infantile, Pompe's disease. Rapidly fatal
  - Juvenile type
- Type 3 (debrancher deficiency): Forbes–Cori disease
- Type 5: McArdle's disease [R]
- Type 7: phosphofructokinase deficiency [R]

Lipid myopathy
- Carnitine palmityl transferase deficiency [R]
- Muscle carnitine deficiency [R]

Periodic myopathy
1. Hypokalaemic periodic paralysis. Autosomal dominant. Attacks at rest after exercise or after heavy meal
2. Hyperkalaemic periodic paralysis. Autosomal dominant. Attacks provoked by rest after exercise, prevented by carbohydrate intake
3. Normokalaemic periodic paralysis. Attacks response to sodium chloride

4. Malignant hyperpyrexia
   a. Primary: autosomal dominant. Attacks develop during anaesthesia, or with muscle relaxant
   b. Secondary: occurring in
      central core disease
      congenital myotonia
      Noonan' syndrome
      masseter hypertrophy syndrome
      arthrogryposis
      other rare syndromes
5. Familial myoglobinuria and idiopathic rhabdomyolysis

Inherited myopathy with abnormal mitochondria
- Hypermetabolic myopathy
- Megaconialmyopathy (megaconial) [R]
- Hypotonia with salt craving and periodic muscular weakness
- Kearns Sayre syndrome
- Distal myopathy with hyperglycaemia
- Fascioscapulohumeral syndrome
- myopathy and lactic acidosis

Inherited myopathy with specific structural changes in the fibres
- Central core disease [R]
- Minicore disease [R]
- Nemaline myopathy [R]
- Centronuclear (myotubular) myopathy
  - muscle fibres resemble myotubular of fetal muscle [R]
  - Type I fibre atrophy [R]
- Fingerprint body myopathy [R]

Inherited myopathy with changes in histochemical fibre type

Genetic myopathy with progressive degeneration of muscle fibres (muscular dystrophy)
- X-linked muscular dystrophies
  - Duchenne's muscular dystrophy
  - Becker's muscular dystrophy
  - a benign syndrome of Emery and Dreifuss
  - a rare syndrome confined to females (incompatible with life in males)
- Autosomal recessive muscular dystrophies
  - childhood muscular dystrophy, resembling Duchenne's type [R]
  - limb-girdle muscular dystrophy
  - congenital progressive muscular dystrophy
- Autosomal dominant muscular dystrophies
  - fascioscapulohumeral muscular dystrophy
  - distal muscular dystrophy
  - ocular myopathy
  - oculopharyngeal muscular dystrophy
- Myotonic muscular dystrophy

Inherited myopathy with non-specific changes in fibres
- Benign congenital myopathy
- Non-progressive 'congenital muscular dystrophy'

Inherited disorders with abnormal muscle fibre activity

Congenital myotonia
Thomsen's disease: autosomal dominant
autosomal recessive form
congenital paramyotonia: myotonia occurs on exposure to cold, with attacks of generalized muscle weakness
chondrodystrophic myotonia
myokymia with impaired muscular relaxation
Inherited disorders of the anterior horn cells
Arthrogryposis multiplex congenita
Acute Wernig–Hoffmann disease (SMA type I) (spinal muscular atrophy)
Intermediate type 2 SMA
Wohlfart–Kugelberg–Welander disease (SMA type 3)
Distal SMA
Scapuloperoneal SMA
Fazio–Londe syndrome (Rare. Affecting bulbar and facial muscles)
Juvenile amyotrophic lateral sclerosis
Inherited diseases of muscle connective tissue
Progressive myositis ossificans
Familial myosclerosis

Myositis

Neuromuscular
Progressive muscular dystrophy
Polymyositis and dermatomyositis
Myasthenia gravis
Polyneuritis
Poliomyelitis
Progressive muscular atrophy
Paralytic myoglobinuria
Tumour of muscle
Connective tissue disorders
Rheumatoid arthritis
Systemic lupus erythematosus
Fibrositis
Polymyositis
Dermatomyositis
Diffuse systemic sclerosis
Scleroderma
Sjögren's syndrome
Dermatological disorders
Scleroderma
Seborrhoeic dermatitis
Exfoliative dermatitis
Infection
Bacterial
Streptococcal infections
Staphylococcal myositis
Viral: especially Coxsackie B – epidemic pleurodynia (Bornhölm disease)

Parasitic
- trichinosis
- cysticercosis
- *Taenia solium*
- toxoplasma

Unknown origin
- Sarcoidosis

Polymyositis

Polymyositis
- Acute with myoglobinuria
- Subacute or chronic
  - childhood
  - early adult
  - middle and late adult

Polymyositis with dominant-inheritance muscular weakness
Polymyositis complicating connective tissue disease
Polymyositis complicating malignancy

Myopathy due to Trauma

Physical
- direct injury
- surgical operation
- intramuscular injection
- post-severe exercise
- ischaemia
- electrical injury
- heat
- cold

Toxin
- e.g. tetanus toxin
- botulinus toxin

Drugs
- *See* following list

Drug-induced Myopathy

Focal myopathy which may progress to muscle fibrosis and contracture. Following intramuscular injection, e.g. in addicts

Acute or subacute painful proximal myopathy
- clofibrate
- epsilon-aminocaproic acid
- emetine
- heroin
- alcohol
- vincristine
- isoetherine
- damazol
- cimetidine
- metolazone

lithium
cytotoxics

Weakness which may be periodic with depressed or absent reflexes, caused by drugs causing hypokalaemia
- diuretics
- purgatives
- liquorice
- carbenoxolone
- amphotericin B

Acute rhabdomyolysis
- heroin
- amphetamine
- phencyclidine
- alcohol

Subacute or chronic painless proximal myopathy
- corticosteroids
- chloroquine
- alcohol
- heroin
- perhexiline
- drugs causing hypokalaemia

Myasthenic syndromes
- aminoglycosides
- tetracyclines
- succinylcholine
- D-penicillamine
- propanolol
- practolol
- phenytoin
- chlorpromazine
- procainamide
- trimethadone

Polymyositis/dermatomyositis: D-penicillamine

Myotonic syndromes
- 20,25 -diazocholesterol
- suxamethonium
- propranolol

Malignant hyperpyrexia
- suxamethonium
- halothane
- diethylether
- cyclopropane
- chloroform
- methoxyflurane
- ketamine
- enflurane
- psychotropic drugs

Metabolic Disorders associated with Myopathy

Nutritional myopathy
- protein-calorie malnutrition

vitamin D deficiency, osteomalacia with myopathy
coeliac disease
renal acidosis

Inherited metabolic disorders
myopathy with lysine-cystinuria [R]
myopathy with xanthinuria [R]

Endocrine Myopathies

Thyroid
- Thyrotoxicosis
  - thyrotoxic myopathy
  - myasthenia
  - periodic paralysis
  - exophthalmic ophthalmoplegia
- Hypothyroidism
  - Kocher–Debré–Semelaigne syndrome (cretins)
  - Hoffmann's syndrome: myotonia-like syndrome responding to thyroid (adults)
  - Hypertrophia musculorum vera [R]
- Myopathy with calcitonin-secreting medullary carcinoma of thyroid

Parathyroid
- Hyperparathyroidism: easy fatiguability, waddling gait, spontaneous muscle cramps

Pituitary-adrenal
- Hyperpituitarism
- Hypopituitarism
- Cushing's syndrome with myopathy
- Steroid myopathy
- Addison's disease with myopathy
- Hyperaldosteronism with hypokalaemic periodic paralysis
- ACTH myopathy
- Acromegaly with muscle hypertrophy and paratrophy

OPHTHALMIC SYSTEM

Disturbance of colour vision caused by drugs
Drugs which may be essential with visual system disorders
Strabismus

DISORDERS OF THE EYELIDS

Hordeolum: staphylococcal infection of lid glands
  internal, affecting Meibomian glands
  external ('sty') affecting Zeis's or Moll's glands
Chalazion: sterile granulomatous inflammation of a Meibomian gland
Blepharitis: inflammation of the lid margins
Meibomianitis: chronic inflammation of the Meibomian glands
Positional defects
  Entropion: turning inward of lids
  Ectropion: sagging and eversion of lower lid
Anatomical defects
  Blepharochalosis
  Dermatochalasia
  Epicanthus
Ptosis
  Congenital
  Acquired
    mechanical
    myogenic
    neurogenic

EPIPHORA, WATERING EYES, OVERFLOW OF TEARS

Excess production
  Weeping
  Foreign body
  Ingrowing lashes (trichiasis)
  Conjunctivitis
  Corneal ulcer
  Drugs
    iodides
    bromides
    mercury
  Irritants
    smokes, etc.
    dusts
Imperfect apposition of the lacrimal puncta
  Ectropion, e.g. due to laxity of tissue in old age

- Entropion
- Burns, scars, etc.
- Facial palsy

Obstruction of the lacrimal duct

- Dacryocystitis
  - acute
  - chronic
- Obstruction
  - idiopathic
  - calculus
  - granulomatous disease
  - neoplasm
  - trauma

CONJUNCTIVA

Ocular Hypersensitivity

Type I

- Hay fever conjunctivitis
- Acute atopic conjunctivitis
- Adult atopic conjunctivitis
- Vernal catarrh
- Urticaria
- Angioneurotic oedema

Type II

- Benign mucous membrane pemphigoid

Type III

- Erythema multiforme
- Uveitis with serum sickness

Type IV

- Contact dermatoconjunctivitis
- Drug-induced dermatoconjunctivitis
- Staphylococcal blepharoconjunctivitis
- Inclusion conjunctivitis
- Adenovirus conjunctivitis
- Molluscum contageosum
- Homograft (corneal) rejection
- Keratitis: phlyctenular
- Rosacea keratitis
- Disciform keratitis
- Punctate keratitis
  - staphylococcal
  - adenoviral
  - TRIC agent
- Interstitial keratitis
  - syphilis
  - tuberculosis
- Uveitis
  - syphilis
  - toxoplasmosis
  - tuberculosis
  - helminths

Conjunctivitis

Sun glare
- tropics
- reflection from snow

Trauma
- dust
- irritants in the atmosphere: smoke, etc.
- foreign body

Eyelid affections
- trichiasis
- concretions in palpebral conjunctiva

Drugs

Infection
- bacterial
- viral

Allergy
- hay fever
- phlyctenular conjunctivitis

Rheumatic disorders
- Behçet's syndrome
- Reiter's syndrome
- Relapsing polychondritis

Dry Eye

Reduced tear flow
- old age, inflammation, surgical damage } affecting lacrimal glands

Excess mucus from goblet cells in dry conjunctiva – kerato-conjunctivitis sicca
1. Rheumatoid arthritis, adult form
2. Sjögren's syndrome
3. Erythema nodosum
4. Progressive systemic sclerosis (scleroderma)

Lid defects

Local infection

Red Eye

Watery red eye with vision impaired
- Acute glaucoma
- anterior uveitis (iridocyclitis)
- secondary glaucoma following
  - injury
  - iritis
  - intra-ocular haemorrhage
  - central vein occlusion
  - dislocation of lens
- deep keratitis and disciform keratitis
- corneal ulceration
  - viral

        - herpes simplex
        - herpes zoster
        - adenovirus
        - trachoma
    - bacterial
- Watery red eye without impairment of vision
    - allergic conjunctivitis
    - viral conjunctivitis
    - chronic conjunctivitis
    - mechanical irritants
        - ingrowing lash
        - spastic ectropion
    - episcleritis
    - scleritis
- Sticky red eye without impairment of vision
    - purulent conjunctivitis

SCLERA

Scleritis

- Connective tissue disease
    - ankylosing spondylitis
    - rheumatoid arthritis
    - polyarteritis nodosa
    - relapsing polychondritis
    - Wegener's granulomatosis
    - systemic lupus erythematosus
    - active rheumatic heart disease
- Granulomatous disease
    - tuberculosis
    - syphilis
    - leprosy
    - sarcoid
- Metabolic disorders
    - gout
    - thyrotoxicosis
    - psoriatic arthritis
- Infection
    - onchocerciasis
    - herpes zoster
    - herpes simplex
- Physical damage
    - irradiation
    - thermal burns
    - chemical
        - alkali burns
        - acid burns
    - trauma
        - penetrating injury
- Unknown

Keratotic Scleritis

Adult rheumatoid arthritis
Behçet's syndrome
Wegener's granulomatosis
Polyarteritis nodosa
Relapsing polychondritis

OCULAR COMPLICATIONS OF STEROID THERAPY

(*e.g. following long-term therapy with 20 mg prednisone per day*)

Posterior subcapsular cataract: opacity may develop in chronic uveitis, and steroids increase this tendency
Glaucoma: The response may be genetically determined, with the homozygous condition associated with primary open-angle glaucoma. Dexamethasone more likely than either prednisone or hydrocortisone to cause rise in intra-ocular pressure
Enhancement of infective disease
- fungus infection
- herpetic epithelial keratitis (a clinical disaster)

CORNEA

Corneal Arcus

Arcus
- deposition of cholesterol and its esters, especially in Bowman's and Descemet's membranes, and especially beginning in the upper and lower quadrants
  - idiopathic, harmless, developing at any age during adult life, with increasing incidence with increasing age. 'Arcus senilis'
  - Type II hyperlipidaemia – arcus present in 10% of cases under 30 years of age

Differential diagnosis (depositions in cornea)
- calcium salt deposition, beginning medially and laterally leading to basal keratopathy, especially secondary to sarcoidosis
- copper: Kayser–Fleischer rings in hepatolenticular degeneration (Wilson's disease)
- cystine: in cystinosis
- chloroquine (after long-term therapy)
- familial lecithin: cholesterol acyltransferase deficiency

Arcuate Corneal Opacities

1. Arcus senilis – common after 65 years, appearing first at 6 o'clock and 12 o'clock, consisting of deposition of cholesterol, triglycerides and phospholipids

2. Band keratopathy – in the early stages, arcuate corneal opacities appear near the limbus in the interpalpebral areas at 3 o'clock and 9 o'clock. They are separated by a lucid interval from the limbus, and consist of deposition of hydroxyl apatite
   They may follow –
   - Chronic uveitis, e.g. in juvenile rheumatoid arthritis
   - Hypercalcaemia
     - hyperparathyroidism
     - sarcoid
     - excess vitamin D
     - renal failure
3. Kayser–Fleischer ring: copper aggregates accumulate between the endothelium and Descemet's membrane, extending to the limbus with no lucid interval

Corneal Disease

- Nutritional deficiency
  - (xerophthalmia which can progress to keratomalacia)
  - vitamin A deficiency } interrelated
  - protein-energy malnutrition } interrelated
  - rarely associated with
    - alcoholism
    - neoplasia
    - bizarre diets
- Infection
  - viral
    - herpes simplex
    - herpes zoster
    - adenovirus
  - bacterial
    - usually secondary to
      - trauma
      - debilitating disease
      - nutritional defect
      - poor hygiene
- Systemic disease
  - Sjögren's syndrome (dry eyes, dry mouth and disease process)
  - rheumatoid arthritis
  - lupus erythematosus
  - Wegener's granulomatosis
  - Stevens–Johnson syndrome
  - other connective tissue disorders
- Trauma
  - abrasions
  - laceration
  - chemical injury
- Degenerative: leading to corneal opacity

IRITIS

Infection
- bacteria
  - brucella
  - *Mycobacterium leprae*
- virus
  - herpes simplex
  - herpes zoster
  - mumps
  - Epstein–Barr virus
- treponema: syphilis
- leptospira
- onchocerca

HLA–associated disorders
- ankylosing spondylitis
- Reiter's syndrome
- inflammatory disease of the bowel

Connective tissue disorders, e.g. juvenile rheumatoid arthritis
Granulomatous disorders
Oculoparotid disorders
Mucocutaneous disorders
Mucocutaneous ulceration, skin lesions and polyarthralgia
- Stevens–Johnson syndrome
- Behçet's syndrome
- Reiter's syndrome
- systemic lupus erythematosus
- ulcerative colitis

UVEITIS

Rheumatoid arthritis (juvenile)
Akylosing spondylitis
Behçet's syndrome
Reiter's syndrome
Erythema nodosa
Wegener's granulomatosis
Polyarteritis nodosa
Relapsing polychondritis
Heterochromic uveitis (Fuch's heterochromic cyclitis)
Chronic cyclitis
Lens-induced uveitis
Sympathetic ophthalmia
Tuberculous uveitis
Sarcoidosis
Toxoplasmic uveitis
Histoplasmosis
Toxocariasis
Anterior uveitis
- iritis } more often non-
- iridocyclitis } granulomatous

Posteroir uveitis
- chorioclitis } more often
- chorioretinitis } granulomatous

RETINA

Retinal Vascular Accidents

Central retinal artery occlusion
- embolus – platelet embolus
- hypertension
- arteriosclerosis: embolism of plaque material
- temporal arteritis
- other connective tissue disease
  - blood dyscrasias
  - orbital space-occupying lesion
  - blood loss with hypotension

Branch artery occlusion
- embolus
- hypertension, arteriosclerosis
- rare: arterial spasm following
  - migraine attack
  - quinine
  - ergot derivatives

Central retinal vein occlusion
- hypertension, arteriosclerosis and hyperlipidaemia
- chronic simple glaucoma
- hyperviscosity syndrome
  - polycythaemia
  - leukaemia
  - macroglobulinaemia
- renal failure
- malignancy
- vasculitis
- trauma

Branch vein occlusion: compression of vein at an arterio-venous crossing, in association with hypertension

Disorders of the Retina

Diabetic retinopathy
- background retinopathy
- proliferative retinopathy

Oedema of the retina
- diabetes mellitus
- retinal vein obstruction
- hypertension
- retinal angioma
- retinal telangiectasia
- traction by vitreous or pre-retinal membranes
- inflammation involving vitreous or retina

Retrolental fibroplasia

Retinitis pigmentosa
Peripheral cystoid degeneration
Senile retinosclerosis
Paving stone degeneration of the retina
Lattice degeneration of the retina
Retinal holes
  retinal tears
  retinal holes without an operation
Retinal detachment
Preretinal membranes

Retinal Vasculitis

Systemic lupus erythematosus
Behçet's syndrome
Erythema nodosa
Wegener's granulomatosis
Polyarteritis nodosa
Dermatomyositis

Retinal Vein Occlusion

- Predisposing factors
  - Haematological disease
    - raised blood viscosity (e.g. polycythaemia)
    - raised plasma viscosity (and hence whole blood viscosity) e.g. Waldenström's macroglobulinaemia
  - Disease of arterial vessel wall
    - vasculitis
      - sarcoidosis
      - Behçet's syndrome
  - Pressure on retinal vein
    - pressure from adjacent retinal artery may lead to central vein occlusion
    - at arteriovenous crossings
    - in simple glaucoma

Congenital Conditions associated with Retinal Detachment

Alport's syndrome
Arthropo-ophthalmopathy
Cervenke's syndrome
Dysplasia spondyloepiphysaria congenita
Ehlers–Danlos syndrome
Homocystinuria
Marfan's syndrome
Pierre Robin syndrome
Weill–Marchesani syndrome

Retinitis Pigmentosa

Early autosomal recessive form (Leber's amaurosis congenita)

Late autosomal recessive form
Autosomal dominant form
Sex-linked form
Syndromes associated with pigmentary retinopathy
- Lipidoses
  - Gaucher's disease
  - amaurotic familial idiocy
- Late form of Pelizaeus–Merzbacher disease
- Progressive familial myoclonic epilepsy
- Spinocerebellar degeneration
  - Marie's ataxia
  - Friedreich's ataxia
  - unclassified spastic paraplegia
  - Charcot–Marie–Tooth disease
  - progressive pallidal degeneration with retinitis pigmentosa
  - hereditary muscular atrophy, ataxia and diabetes mellitus
- Specific syndromes with progressive external ophthalmoplegia and retinitis pigmentosa
  - progressive external ophthalmoplegia
  - retinitis pigmentosa, external ophthalmoplegia and heart block
  - retinitis pigmentosa, ophthalmoplegia, and spastic quadriplegia
  - a-β-lipoproteinaemia [R]
  - Refsum's syndrome [R]
- Generalized muscular dystrophy
- Myotonic dystrophy (Steinert's disease)
- Syndromes with hearing loss
  - Hallgren's syndrome
  - Refsum's syndrome [R]
  - Usher's syndrome
  - Retinitis pigmentosa with deafness
  - Cockayne's disease
  - Alström's syndrome
- Syndromes with renal disease
  - familial juvenile nephrophthisis
  - hereditary nephritis, retinitis pigmentosa and chromosomal abnormalities
  - cystinuria
  - cystinosis
  - oxalosis
- Syndromes with skin disease
  - Werner's disease
  - psoriasis
- Syndromes with bone disease
  - Paget's disease
  - osteogenesis imperfecta
  - Marfan's syndrome
  - osteopetrosis
- Others
  - Laurence–Moon–Biedl syndrome

Dresbach's elliptocytosis
Klinefelter's syndrome
Mucopolysaccharidoses
Type I
Type II
Type III
Hooft's disease (hypolipidaemia)

LENS

Cataracts in Infancy and Childhood

Idiopathic (i.e. cause not known): 50% of cases
Inherited: autosomal dominant or X-linked trait, with single cataract [R]
Chromosome disorders: Associated with
Down s syndrome
Trisomy 13
Trisomy 18
Turner's syndrome
Congenital infections
Congenital rubella
Congenital varicella
Congenital herpes simplex
Congenital toxoplasmosis
Congenital cytomegalic inclusion disease
Prematurity
Metabolic disorders
Galactosaemia
Galactokinase deficiency
Hypothyroidism
Pseudohypoparathyroidism
Lowe's syndrome [R]
Dislocated lens of Marfan's syndrome
Dislocated lens of homocysteinuria
Secondary to copper distribution in Wilson's disease
Retinitis pigmentosa
Juvenile rheumatoid arthritis with uveitis
Syndromes associated with cataracts
Alport's syndrome
Cerebrotendinous xanthomatosis
Oxycephaly
Congenital stippled epiphyses (Conrad's syndrome)
Francois–Hallermann–Streiff syndrome
Laurence–Moon–Biedl syndrome
Marinesco–Sjögren syndrome
Myotonic dystrophy (Steinert's disease)
Pseudo-pseudohypoparathyroidism
Norman (pseudo-Turner) syndrome
Norrie's disease
Secondary to –
Glaucoma

Retrolental fibroplasia
Retinal detachment
Endophthalmitis
Ionizing radiation
Trauma
Chronic head banging (in mental retardation)

Occasionally secondary to –
Retinoblastoma
Osteopetrosis
Pierre Robin syndrome
Treacher Collins syndrome
Goldenhar syndrome

Drug-induced
Corticosteroids
Chlorpromazine in children (reversible)
Also described with
ergot
dinitrophenol
naphthalene
triparanol

Dermatoses associated with cataracts
Rothmund–Thomson syndrome
Cockayne disease
Incontinentia pigmentosa
Marshall syndrome
Schäfer's syndrome
Congenital ichthyosis
Siemen's syndrome
Werner's syndrome

Dislocated Lens

Congenital
Marfan's syndrome (majority of these cases probably really homocystinuria)
homocystinuria
Marchesani's syndrome

Acquired
Traumatic: contusion injury
partial
complete

VITREOUS DISORDERS

Vitreous 'floaters'
Asteroid hyalosis
Synchysis scintillans
Massive vitreous retraction
Injury
Inflammation: uveitis
Haemorrhage
retinal tear
systemic hypertension

trauma
vascular accident during oral anticoagulant therapy
central vein occlusion
inflammatory disease

Diabetes mellitus
Non-diabetic vascular disease
Congenital cataract
Spontaneous rupture of cataract
Retinal detachment
Macular pucker
Persistent hyperplastic primary vitreous
Terson's syndrome
Eales' disease
Endophthalmitis

MACULA

Macular Cherry-red Spot

Corneal clouding syndrome of Goldberg–Cotlier
Farber's lipogranulomatosis
Gangliosidosis
GM1 type
GM2 type
Niemann–Pick disease
Sandhoff disease
Sea-blue histiocyte syndrome [R]
Tay–Sachs disease

Disorders of the Macula

Central serous detachment of macula
Detachment of pigment epithelium
New vessels beneath the pigment epithelium and disciform degeneration of the macula
Senile degeneration of Bruch's membrane
Angeoid streaks
Macular hole
Histoplasmosis damage (?)
Hereditary disease
central areolar choroidal sclerosis
autosomal dominant
autosomal recessive
Stargardt–Behr disease: autosomal recessive
Best's vitelliform macular degeneration: autosomal dominant

ORBIT

Exophthalmos (Proptosis)

Acute
emphysema: air from sinus into orbit

- haemorrhage
    - trauma
    - spontaneous
- orbital cellulitis

Pulsating exophthalmos
- carotid-cavernous sinus fistula
- vascular tumour
- aneurysm
- cerebral pulsation due to defect in orbital roof

Unilateral
- Inflammatory
    - cellulitis
    - orbital periostitis
    - pseudotumour of the orbit
    - abscess
    - lacrymal gland inflammation
    - panophthalmitis
    - cavernous sinus thrombosis
    - orbital vein thrombosis
    - tenoscitis (?)
    - gumma
    - tuberculosis
- Vascular
    - haemorrhage
        - trauma
        - spontaneous
    - varicosities
    - aneurysm, including arteriovenous aneurysm
- Trauma
    - fracture
    - haemorrhage
    - muscle rupture
    - emphysema from sinuses
    - aneurysm
- Tumour
    - primary
    - secondary
- Cysts
    - congenital, dermoid
    - parasitic
    - mucocele from local sinus
- Relaxation of retraction of the eyeball
- Paralysis of the extra-ocular muscles
- Infiltrating disease
    - leukaemia
    - lymphoma
- Meningocele
- Encephalocele

Bilateral exophthalmos
- thyrotoxic: Graves' disease
- thyrotropic: malignant ophthalmoplegia

Local lesions affecting both orbits
- thrombosis of the cavernous sinuses

empyema of the accessory nasal tissues
oxycephaly
orbital tumours
leontiasis ossium

Pseudo-exophthalmos
congenital macrophthalmos (bull's eye)
high myopia
lid retraction (Graves' disease)

Enophthalmos

Congenital
Wasting diseases
Paralysis of the cervical sympathetic nerves
Phthisis of the eyeball

Glaucoma

Primary glaucoma

1. Open-angle glaucoma
2. Angle-closure glaucoma { acute / intermittent / subacute / chronic }

Congenital

1. Primary congenital, infantile glaucoma: buphthalmos
2. Glaucoma with congenital anomalies
    a. Pigmentary glaucoma
    b. Aniridia
    c. Axenfeld syndrome
    d. Sturge–Weber syndrome [R]
    e. Infantile glaucoma
    f. Marfan's syndrome
    g. Neurofibromatosis
    h. Lowe's syndrome [R]
    i. Microcornea
    j. Megacornea
3. Secondary glaucoma
    a. Changes in lens
        i. Dislocation
        ii. Intumescence
        iii. Phacolytic
        iv. Exfoliative syndrome (glaucoma capsulare)
    b. Changes in uveal tract
        i. Iridocyclitis
        ii. Tumour
        iii. Essential iris atrophy
    c. Trauma
        i. Massive haemorrhage
            into anterior chamber
            into posterior chamber
        ii. Corneal or limbal laceration with prolapse of iris into wound
        iii. Retrodisplacement of iris root following contusion

iv. Absolute glaucoma: final result

d. Following surgery
   i. Epithelial growth into anterior chamber
   ii. Failure of prompt restoration of the anterior chamber

e. Associated with rubeosis
   Diabetes mellitus
   Central retinal vessel occlusion

f. Associated with pulsating exophthalmos

g. Associated with topical steroids

Phakomatoses

(*Lesions of skin, central nervous system and frequently eyes*)

Neurofibromatosis (von Recklinghausen's disease)
Angiomatosis retinae (von Hippel–Lindau disease)
Sturge–Weber syndrome [R]
Tuberose sclerosis (Bourneville's disease)

Tumours of the Orbit

Primary in Orbit
- Choristoma
  - dermoid cyst
  - epidermal cyst
  - teratoma
- Hamartoma
  - haemangioma
  - neurofibroma
- Mesenchymal
  - adipose
    - lipoma
    - liposarcoma
  - fibrous
    - fibroma
    - fibrosarcoma
  - myomatous: rhabdomyosarcoma
  - cartilaginous
    - chondroma
    - chondrosarcoma
  - oeseous
    - osteoma
    - osteosarcoma
- Neural
  - neurofibroma
  - neurilemmoma
- Epithelial: lacrymal gland tumour
- Lymphoid
  - lymphoma
  - lymphoid hyperplasia
  - inflammatory disease

Secondary

1. From adjacent structure

Intra-ocular
melanoma
retinoblastoma
Cornea and conjunctiva
melanoma
epidermoid carcinoma
Eyelids and face: basal cell carcinoma
Upper respiratory tract
carcinoma
sarcoma
mucocele
Cranial: meningioma
2. Metastases
carcinoma
sarcoma
neuroblastoma
3. Reticuloendotheliosis
juvenile xanthogranuloma
eosinophilic granuloma
4. Metabolic: thyrotoxic exophthalmia
5. Phakomatoses: neurofibromatosis

VISION

Inherited Diseases of the Eye

Colour blindness: affecting 4% of males (with a further 4% mildly affected): red/green defect
Albinism
Ptosis
Corneal dystrophy
Cataract
Aniridia: dominant inheritance
Retinitis pigmentosa
Inherited optic atrophy
Heredomascular dystrophy
Inborn errors of metabolism with associated eye damage
amino-acidurias
lipid disorders
carbohydrate metabolic disorders
mucopolysaccharide disorders
haemoglobinopathies:
sickle cell disease
haemoglobin C (homozygote)
(both may be associated with vitreous haemorrhages)

Amblyopia
(*Uncorrectable blurred vision due to closure of eye with no organic defect*)

Methyl alcohol poisoning
Chronic overindulgence in alcohol and/or ethyl alcohol

Quinine and related compounds
Organic arsenical compounds
Salicylates in very large dosage

Gradual Loss of Vision

Affecting one eye
- Keratitis
- Uveitis
- Glioma of optic nerve
- Sphenoidal ridge meningioma
- Orbital space occupying lesion
- Postoperative oedema at macula (Irvine–Gass syndrome)

Affecting both eyes
- Hereditary corneal dystrophy
- Uveitis
- Glaucoma
  - simple, chronic
  - low tension
  - exfoliative
  - pigmenting
- Cataract
- Tapeto-retinal degeneration
- Macular degeneration
- Cone dysfunction syndrome
- Vascular and haematological retinopathy
- Papilloedema
- Toxic optic neuropathy
- Paget's disease of bone
- Intracranial space-occupying lesion compressing visual pathway
- Drug toxicity

Sudden Loss of Vision

Transient
- obscurations: lasting a few seconds, and occurring bilaterally, usually associated with papilloedema
- amaurosis fugax: usually unilateral, and lasting from minutes to hours, due to
  - atherosclerotic disease of
    - middle cerebral artery
    - carotid artery with platelet emboli
  - glaucoma with high intra-ocular pressure

Permanent
- One eye
  - vitreous haemorrhage
  - retinal detachment
  - retinal artery occlusion
  - retinal vein occlusion
  - central serous retinopathy (especially in young males)
  - optic disc disease
    - ischaemic optic neuropathy
    - optic neuritis

Both eyes
retina: drugs, such as quinine
pigmented epithelium
acute multifocal placoid pigment epitheliopathy
Harada's disease
optic nerve
hereditary optic neuropathy (Leber's disease)
bilateral optic neuropathy
drugs, such as methanol
parasellar
pituitary apoplexy: infarction of pituitary tumour
extension of craniopharyngiomatous cyst
occipital: cerebral blindness

Common Causes of Blindness in the Tropics

May be uniocular in
- measles
- smallpox
- chickenpox

Blindness may be found in
- onchocerciasis and other parasite infections
- virus infections: including trachoma
- yaws
- leprosy
- leishmaniasis
- solar retinopathy
- Burkitt's lymphoma

Nystagmus

Physiological
- Endpoint nystagmus: commonly occurs at the extreme lateral gaze after a latent period of not more than 30 seconds
- Optokinetic nystagmus: this can be elicited by rotation of a drum drawn with alternate black and white lines. The nystagmus is jerky
- Nystagmus follows stimulation of the semicircular canals following rotation (e.g. fairground, fast roundabout)
  caloric stimulation

Pathological
- Congenital
  1. Sensory defect type: associated with congenital impairment of vision
  2. Motor defect type: ? lesion in brainstem
  3. Latent: occurs following occlusion of either eye
- Spasmus nutans: occurs in infants, and is often associated with non-synchronous head nodding
- Neurological damage
  - pendicular or jerky nystagmus
  - ocular flutter

see-saw nystagmus
nystagmus refractorius
Vestibular nystagmus
labyrinthitis
Menière's disease
trauma to labyrinth
lesions of labyrinth
vascular damage
inflammatory disease
neoplasm
lesions affecting the vestibular nuclei
encephalitis
multiple sclerosis
syringobulbia
poliomyelitis
thrombosis of the postero-inferior cerebellar artery
cerebellar tumour: pressure on the vestibular pathways
Gaze nystagmus
drug toxicity
demyelination
vascular disease
neoplasm
Voluntary and hysterical nystagmus: can only be maintained for a few seconds

Limited Elevation of One Eye

*Paresis of superior division of III
*Myasthenia gravis
Unilateral double elevator palsy
*Abiotrophic ophthalmoplegia
*Dysthyroid ophthalmopathy
Myositis
*Amyloidosis
Fracture in the orbital floor
Brown's superior oblique syndrome
Vertical retraction syndrome
'Heavy eye' phenomenon

*May accompany ptosis

Tunnel Vision
(Loss of peripheral visual field)

Papilloedema, advanced
Glaucoma
Posterior cerebral artery occlusion
Retinitis pigmentosa
Syphilitic optic neuritis
Migraine
(Hysteria)
Disseminated choroidoretinitis
Constriction of optic nerve by arachnoiditis

Central Scotoma

Relative
- Central vision loss of ability to distinguish between red and green small objects
- Tobacco
- Alcohol

Absolute
- Multiple sclerosis (central or paracentral in 25% of cases)
- Hereditary optic atrophy (e.g. Leber's atrophy)
- Following retrobulbar neuritis
- Early compression of optic chiasma by pituitary tumour
- 'Eclipse blindness': resulting from direct observation of the sun without any protection
- ? In some cases of lead poisoning

Congenital Colour Vision Defects

Anomalous trichromatism (three primaries to match all spectral colours)
- (Commonest)
- Protanomaly (red)
- Deuteranomaly (green)
- Tritanomaly (blue)

Dichromatism (two primaries to match all spectral colours)
- (2 kinds of cones)
- Protanopia
- Deuteranopia
- Tritanopia

Monochromatism (one primary to match all spectral colours)
- Cone monochromatism
  - (only one kind of cone)
- Rod monochromatism
  - (very rare, with complete lack of cone formation. Associated with photophobia, nystagmus and poor visual acuity)
- Complete typical type
- Incomplete typical type
- Blue monocone monochromatism
- Central cone monochromatism

Night Blindness

Congenital stationary night blindness

Night blindness with changes in ocular function
- Fundus albi punctatus
- Oguchi's disease

Acquired: vitamin A deficiency

Disturbance of Colour Vision caused by Drugs
(rare occurrence)

Dazzling whiteness of objects with delayed light adaptation

troxidone

Yellow vision

sulphonamides
streptomycin
barbiturates

Dazzling effects, or yellow, orange or green vision, hallucinations, flickering lights and mental confusion

digitalis

Drugs which may be associated with Visual System Disorders

Ethambutol: dose-related optic neuritis
Isoniazid
Chloramphenicol
Chloroquin
Arsenicals
Methysergide maleate
DL-penicillamine
Phenothiazines
Phenylbutazone
Larger doses

barbiturates
meprobamate
diphenylhydantoin
alcohol

Strabismus

1. Esotropia ('crossed eyes'): the commonest form
   Non-paralytic (comitant)
   a. Non-accommodative
   b. Accommodative
   c. Combined (a) + (b)
   Paretic (non-comitant)
   Angle of deviant vision varies with the direction of gaze
2. Exotropia: 'divergent' strabismus
   a. Intermittent
   b. Constant
3. Hypertropia: deviation of one eye upwards
   a. Paralytic
   b. Non-paralytic

PAEDIATRICS

GENERAL SUBJECTS

Intra-uterine infection
(*commoner infecting agents*)

Virus
- Rubella
- Cytomegalic inclusion disease
- Variola-vaccinia
- Herpes simplex
- Varicella-Zoster
- Hepatitis B
- Poliomyelitis
- Influenza
- Mumps
- Coxsackie B
- Echo virus
- Herpes hominis (HVH)

Bacteria
- Listeriosis
- *E. coli*
- *Proteus genus*
- Klebsiella
- Streptococcus (haemolytic)
- Staphylococcus
- *Strept. faecalis*
- Mycoplasma

Treponema
- Syphilis

Protozoa
- Toxoplasma
- Malaria

Causes of Perinatal Mortality
(*in order of decreasing incidence in U.K.*)

Intrapartum hypoxia
Congenital malformations
Antepartum hypoxia
Antepartum death with no visible lesion
Intrapartum hypoxia with brain damage
Cerebral birth trauma
Iso-immunization

Major Causes of Death in First Week of Life (in UK)

Respiratory distress syndrome	3·2/1000 live births
Congenital malformations	2·5/1000 live births
Intra-uterine anoxia	1·8/1000 live births
Extreme immaturity (birth weight less than 1 kg)	1·6/1000 live births

Maternal Risk Factors Predisposing to Low Birth-weight Babies

Young mother (under 18 years of age)
Previous induced abortion
Unmarried mother: often also young
Previous sterility
Moderate to severe eclampsia
History of renal disease
History of previous perinatal loss
Bleeding in the first trimester of pregnancy

Cot Deaths

Prolonged apnoea
Nasal obstruction
Laryngeal spasm
Airway obstruction during smooth muscle relaxation in rapid eye movement sleep (REM)
Infections

Respiratory syncytial virus Influenza Other viruses	Bronchitis Pneumonia	50% of cases

'Hypoimmunity' ? lack resistance to certain organisms
Milk allergy ? Bacterial antigen allergy ?
Unsuspected
- Uraemia
- Hypernatraemia
- Clinical illness in the period shortly before death in a very high proportion of cases

Common factors
- Peak age of incidence 2–4 months
- Low income families
- Bottle feeding of infant
- Low birth-weight infants
- Some respiratory tract histological abnormality found at postmortem

Pyrexia of Unknown Origin in Children

Include:
Infections
Overheating with dehydration: excessive fluid loss
- polyuria
- hypercalcaemia
- renal acidosis
- persistent vomiting, diarrhoea etc.

'Drug fever'
Neoplasm, neoplasm during cytotoxic therapy
Collagen-vascular disease e.g. rheumatoid arthritis

Catarrh in Infants

Upper respiratory tract infections
- virus

bacteria
Atopic subjects
Cystic fibrosis
Environment (e.g. smoke)
Obesity
Cleft palate
Immune deficiency states
Congenital heart disease
Down's syndrome
Hypothyroidism

Pain in Lower Limbs in Children

Congenital
- Dislocation, subluxation or dysplasia of hip
- Tarsal coalition
- Accessory tarsal ossicle

Developmental
- Transient synovitis of hip and knee
- Slipped capital femoral epiphysis
- Limb deformities
  - genu valgum
  - ankle valgus
  - pes planus (flat foot)
  - infantile cortical hyperostosis (Laffey's disease)
  - hypervitaminosis A
  - Baker's cyst

Avascular necrosis of bone
- Femoral capital epiphysis (Legg–Calvé–Perthe's disease)
- Tibial tubercule apophysitis (Osgood–Schlatter's disease)
- Calcaneal apophysitis (Haglund's disease)
- Second metatarsal (Freiberg's infraction)
- Osteochondritis dissecans
  - hip
  - knee
  - ankle

Trauma
- Fracture, including stress fracture, pathological fracture
- Dislocation and subluxation
- Joint
  - sprain
  - contusion
  - haemorrhage around, or into joint
- Soft tissue
  - contusion
  - haemorrhage
- Trauma causing
  - synovitis
  - periostitis

Infection
- Septic arthritis
- Osteomyelitis
- Osteitis

- Soft tissues
    - cellulitis
    - abscess
    - ascending lymphadenitis
- Vascular disorders
    - Sickle cell intravascular stasis and thrombosis
    - Haemophilia
    - Anterior and posterior compartment syndromes
    - Haemangioma
    - Lymphangioma
    - Poor peripheral circulation
- Connective tissue disease
    - Rheumatic fever
    - Rheumatoid arthritis
    - Dermatomyositis
    - Scleroderma
- Tumour
    - Benign
        - Osteoid osteoma
        - Fibrous dysplasia
        - Giant cell tumour
        - Osteochondroma
        - Some bone cysts
    - Malignant
        - Osteogenic sarcoma
        - Ewing's sarcoma
        - Soft tissue sarcoma
        - Leukaemia
        - Neuroblastoma

Pain in Foot in Children

- External cause
    - Foreign body in shoe
    - Foreign body in foot
    - Ill-fitting shoe
    - Ingrowing toenail
    - Trauma
        - sprain, bruises, etc.
        - fracture, including stress fracture
        - tendonitis, affecting the Achilles tendon
    - Inflammatory disease
        - osteomyelitis
        - rheumatic fever
        - juvenile rheumatoid arthritis
- Intrinsic cause
    - Structural defect
        - pes cavus
        - hypermobile flat foot with tight heel cord
        - peroneal spastic flat foot (tarsal coalition)
        - osteochondroses
        - accessory navicular (prehallux)

Tumours
osteoid osteoma
Ewing's sarcoma
sarcoma of the synovia

Abnormalities of Micturition in Neonate

Anuria
Empty bladder
Bilateral renal agenesis
Severe dysplastic and afunctional kidneys (maternal oligohydramnios)
After the fifth month of pregnancy the amniotic fluid consists of mainly fetal urine with a normal volume of 500–800 ml
Distended bladder
Boys with prune-belly syndrome and complete atresia of membranous urethra (rare). There is usually an umbilical urinary fistula
Temporary transient acute retention, possibly related to maternal ephedrine or nortriptyline
Urinary ascites (due to prenatal perforation of the urinary tract)
intravesical obstruction (especially by posterior urethral valves
supravesical obstruction
neuropathic bladder due to spina bifida
premature infants (? weak area in the bladder musculature)
associated with hydronephrotic kidney
Painful or Difficult Micturition
Pyelonephritis
Dribbling Micturition (rarely continuous)
Distended bladder
Obstruction
in males: posterior urethral valve
ectopic ureterocele causing infravesical obstruction
in girls: hydrocolpos
stenotic urethral meatus high on the anterior vaginal wall in patient with female hypospadias
Neuropathic bladder
meningomyelocele
sacral agenesis or dysgenesis
(The bladder is expressible by manual compression)
Dribbling from empty bladder
unusually from neuropathic bladder
severe epispadias with short wide posterior urethra and inadequate sphincters. Dribbling occurs when the baby cries or when lifted into a vertical position
ectopic urethra opening into the urethra below the sphincters in the female

Voiding of Urine from Abnormal Sites
- Male
  - with congenital absence of penis: the urethra opens into the anus or just anterior to it
  - double ureter
    - one opening in the normal position
    - one opening onto perineum or at anus
- Girl
  - persistent cloaca: urethra anterior with rectum posterior and vagina between
  - persistent urogenital sinus: urethra opens onto the anterior vaginal wall
- Patent urachus
  - leaks at umbilicus in boys with prune belly syndrome
  - patent urachus may persist in isolation

RESPIRATORY

Hypoxia in the Newborn Infant

Failure of the normal cardiopulmonary adaptation at birth
- apnoea at birth
- transient tachypnoea of newborn (wet lung)
- hyaline membrane disease: idiopathic respiratory distress syndrome of newborn
- persistent fetal circulation of unknown origin
- recurrent apnoea in preterm infants

Congenital malformations

Acquired disorders
- aspiration of meconium
- pneumothorax
- haemorrhagic pulmonary oedema and massive pulmonary haemorrhage
- hydrops fetalis
- pneumonia
- chronic lung disease

Infantile Apnoea at Birth

Prematurity

Multiple pregnancy

Placental insufficiency

Maternal conditions
- essential hypertension
- pre-eclampsia
- diabetes mellitus
- excess maternal sedation
- antepartum haemorrhage

Fetal conditions
- severe erythroblastosis fetalis
- fetal distress
- prolapsed cord

severe fetal acidosis
abnormal delivery
breech
forceps
Caesarean

Respiratory Distress Syndrome

Transient tachypnoea
Meconium aspiration
Pneumonia
Pneumothorax
Pulmonary haemorrhage
Cyanotic congenital heart disease
Diaphragmatic hernia

'Delayed' Respiratory Distress Syndrome in Infants
(*onset more than one week after birth*)

Primary pulmonary lesions
Wilson–Mikity syndrome: immature lung with variable hyperinflation and collapse
chylothorax and congested pulmonary lymphangiectasia
congenital lobal emphysema
cystic fibrosis
histiocytosis X
acute infection
Extra-pulmonary conditions affecting respiration
congenital heart disease (especially about the 10th day when the ductus arteriosus closes completely)
foregut duplication
tracheo-oesophageal fistula
diaphragmatic hernia
asphyxiating thoracic dysplasia

Wheezing in Children

Obstructive lesions of trachea and main bronchi
Foreign body
Vascular ring
Tuberculosis
Mediastinal cysts and tumours
Tracheal webs, tracheal stenosis
Obstructive disease of small airways
Asthma
Acute bronchiolitis
Aspiration syndrome
Non-specific suppurative bronchitis
Cystic fibrosis
Bronchopneumonia

METABOLIC DISORDERS

Complications of Infants of Diabetic Mothers

Hypoglycaemia

Polycythaemia
Hyperbilirubinaemia
Hypocalcaemia
Congenital malformations
Respiratory distress syndrome (rare cause)

Neonatal Hypocalcaemic Convulsions

Maternal hyperparathyroidism
Maternal diabetes mellitus
Untreated maternal coeliac disease
Placental insufficiency
Post-Caesarean delivery
(More common in male infants, born at the end of winter, of mothers over 25 years of age, multipara of Social Classes III, IV, and V, and fed on non-human milk)

Inherited Metabolic Disorders associated with Metabolic Acidosis

Glycogen storage disease Type I
Fructose-1, 6-diphosphatase deficiency
Maple syrup urine disease, and other branch-chain amino-acidurias
Including isovaleric acidemia
Propionic acidemia [R]
Methylmalonic aciduria [R]
Pyruvate carboxylase deficiency [R]
Succinyl CoA ketoacid transferase deficiency [R]
Pyroglutamic acidemia [R]
Glutaric acidaemia [R]
Pyruvate dehydrogenase deficiency [R]

Secondary Hyperlipidaemia in Children

Glycogen storage disease: Type I, III, and VI
Diabetes mellitus
Idiopathic hypercalcaemia
Hypothyroidism
Isolated growth hormone deficiency
Obstructive jaundice

GASTROINTESTINAL DISORDERS

Inherited Disorders associated with Vomiting in the Newborn

Phenylyketonuria
Galactosaemia
Hereditary fructose intolerance
Steroid metabolism disorders
Urea cycle disorders [R]
Organic acid metabolism disorders

Hypervalinaemia [R]
Wolman's disease [R]

Constipation in Children

Low faecal bulk
- undernutrition
- diet high in refined starches or protein

Abnormally hard stools
- high cow's milk intake

Abnormally dry stools
- dehydration
- infantile renal acidosis
- diabetes insipidus
- idiopathic hypercalcaemia

Obstruction
- anorectal stenotic lesions
- tumours
  - intrinsic
  - extrinsic
- Crohn's disease
- Aganglionosis coli

Spinal reflex arc damage
- spinal cord lesions

Voluntary muscles of defaecation damage
- congenital absence of abdominal musculate
- hypothyroidism
- cerebral palsy
- amyotonia congenita
- cerebral palsy
- poliomyelitis
- infectious polyneuritis

Intractable Diarrhoea in Infants

Extra-intestinal infection – e.g. Urinary tract infection

Inflammatory disorders of gastrointestinal tract
- Infectious diarrhoea
- Allergic gastroenteropathy
  - cow's milk protein
  - soy protein
- (Ulcerative colitis)
- Pseudomembranous colitis

Biochemical deficiency states
- Monosaccharide malabsorption
- Disaccharide malabsorption
- Pancreatic insufficiency
- Chronic chloridorrhoea
- Acrodermatitis enteropathica
- a-β-lipoproteinaemia
- Wolman's disease
- Coeliac disease

Anatomical disorders of gastrointestinal tract
- Hirschprung's disease
- Intestinal stenosis, malrotation, or duplication

Primary immunodeficiency disorders – e.g. Wiskott–Aldrich syndrome, Thymic dysplasia

Hormonal disorders
- Addison's disease
- Adrenogenital syndrome
- Thyrotoxicosis
- Zollinger–Ellison syndrome

Others
- Renal tubular acidosis
- Tumours
  - neuroblastoma
  - ganglioneuroma
  - lymphoma
- (Histiocytosis–X)
- (Intestinal lymphangiectasia)

Acute Abdominal Pain in Childhood

Include –

Medical causes
- upper respiratory tract infection
- renal tract infection
- gastroenteritis
- constipation
- non-specific abdominal pain
- etc.

Surgical causes
- appendicitis
- volvulus
- strangulated hernia
- Meckel's diverticulum
- ruptured viscera
- etc.

Carbohydrate Malabsorption in Infants

Primary
- Oligosaccharidase deficiency
  - Lactase
  - sucrase: isomaltase
  - trehalase
- Transport across mucous membrane alteration
  - glucose: galactose

Secondary
- Diarrhoeal disease
- Protein energy malnutrition
- Malabsorption syndrome
- Giardia lamblia infection
- Cystic fibrosis
- Chronic inflammatory disease of gut

Gastro-intestinal surgery
Immune deficiency states
Allergy, e.g. allergy to cow's milk protein
Drugs: neomycin, etc.
Hypoxia

Neonatal Necrotizing Enterocolitis

Precipitating factors
- Infection: associated sepsis
- Endotoxins
- Intestinal ischaemia: especially in premature infants with perinatal asphyxia or umbilical vessel catheterization
- Oral feedings, associated with increased intestinal bacterial endotoxin production
- Intestinal mucosal injury
- Altered host defence. Secretory IgA plays an important part in defence

LIVER DISORDERS

Factors Affecting Physiological Jaundice of Newborn

Increased bilirubin production
Increased enteric reabsorption of bilirubin
- meconium reabsorption
- lack of bacterial degradation of bilirubin in gut
- high glucuronidase activity in newborn gut
- diminished inhibition of glucuronidase in gut

Impaired hepatic uptake of bilirubin
- ineffective liver perfusion
- diminished transfer of bilirubin into liver cells
- competition between bilirubin and other anions
- low calcium intake in the first three days of life

Defective rate of bilirubin glucuronide formation
- low concentration of available glucuronate
- low enzyme activity
- inhibitor of conjugating enzyme system

Defective bilirubin excretion

Factors Aggravating Neonatal Physiological Jaundice

Infection
Haemolysis
Prematurity
Hypoxia
Excess bruising
Dehydration
Drugs conjugating with glucuronic acid
Hypothyroidism
High small intestinal obstruction
Breast milk jaundice

Crigler–Najjar syndrome
Transient familial neonatal hyperbilirubinaemia

Neonatal Jaundice

Increase in unconjugated bilirubin
- Infection
  - septicaemia
  - urine infection
  - meningitis
- Haemolysis
  - Rh incompatibility
  - ABO incompatibility
  - red cell enzyme deficiency states, e.g. G-6-PD
  - red cell membrane defects
    - congenital haemolytic anaemia
    - acquired vitamin E deficiency
  - infection
  - excessive bruising, with excessive reabsorption of blood pigment, e.g. thrombocytopenia
- Polycythaemia
  - twin–twin transfusion
  - excessive placental transfusion
  - infants of diabetic mothers
- Hypoxia
  - placental lesions
  - difficult delivery
  - respiratory distress syndrome
- Dehydration
  - vomiting
  - diarrhoea
  - inadequate fluid intake
- Metabolic
  - premature infant
  - breast milk jaundice
  - meconium retention
  - hypoglycaemia
  - hypothyroidism
  - inherited metabolic disorders
    - galactosaemia
    - fructosaemia
    - tyrosinosis [R]
    - Crigler–Najjar syndrome
    - Dubin–Johnson syndrome
    - alpha-1-antitrypsin deficiency
    - cystic fibrosis
    - sphingomyelin storage disease
    - transient familial neonatal hyperbilirubinaemia
- Surgical
  - duodenal atresia
  - pyloric stenosis
  - Hirschprung's disease

Drugs interfering with bilirubin metabolism
- sulphonamides
- chloramphenicol
- synthetic vitamin K in large doses

Increase in conjugated bilirubin

Bacterial infections
- Predominantly Gram–ve organisms
- Listeria

Virus:
- Cytomegalovirus
- Rubella
- Hepatitis B
- Herpes simplex
- Coxsackie B
- Varicella

Treponema pallidum

Toxoplasma gondii

These agents cause liver damage with intrahepatic obstruction

Cirrhosis in Childhood

Genetic: including

Hepatolenticular degeneration (Wilson's disease)

Carbohydrate metabolism
- galactosaemia
- fructose intolerance
- glycogen storage disease

Amino acid metabolism
- tyrosinosis [R]
- cystinosis

Lipid storage disease
- Niemann–Pick disease
- Gaucher's disease
- cholesteryl ester storage disease

Mucopolysaccharide disease
- Hurler's syndrome
- Byler's syndrome

Gastrointestinal respiratory disorder
- Alpha-1 antitrypsin deficiency
- Cystic fibrosis

Haemopoietic system
- thalassaemia (secondary to excess storage iron)
- sickle cell disease (secondary to excess storage iron)
- hepatic porphyria

Non-Genetic

Neonatal hepatitis

Biliary tract
- extrahepatic biliary atresia
- choledochal cyst
- ascending cholangitis
- cyst fibrosis

Posthepatic disease
- acute viral hepatitis
- chronic active hepatitis
- induced by drug, toxin, poison
- post-radiation

Complicating ulcerative colitis (from ascending cholangitis)

Passive venous congestion of liver
- constrictive pericarditis
- Ebstein's anomaly
- congestive cardiac failure
- Budd–Chiari syndrome

Veno-occlusive disease (Jamaica)

Indian childhood cirrhosis

HAEMATOLOGY

Blood Loss in Newborn

- Haemorrhage before birth or during delivery
  - Feto-maternal
    - spontaneous
    - following version
    - following traumatic amniocentesis
  - Twin-to-twin bleed
  - Feto-placental haemorrhage
- Obstetric accidents, malformed placenta and cord
  - Rupture of umbilical cord
    - normal cord
    - abnormal cord
  - Haematoma
    - of cord
    - of placenta
  - Rupture of anomalous vessels
  - Incision of placenta during Caesarean section
  - Placenta praevia
  - Abruptio placenta
- Iatrogenic bleeding
- Bleeding following trauma
- Internal haemorrhage
  - Rupture
    - of liver
    - of spleen
  - Retroperitoneal haemorrhage
  - Lung haemorrhage
  - Intracranial haemorrhage
- Bleeding immediately after birth
  - Blood disorders
    - plasma coagulation factor defects
      - congenital, haemophilia syndrome
      - acquired, vitamin K deficiency
    - platelet deficiency, thrombocytopenia

Neonatal Polycythaemia

Intra-uterine hypoxia
- Placental insufficiency
  - small infant for gestational age
  - post-mature baby
  - maternal drug therapy, e.g. propanolol

Placental transfusion
- Delayed clamping of cord, with placenta higher than baby
- Feto-fetal bleed
- Maternofetal bleed

Endocrine disorders
- Maternal diabetes
- Fetal adrenal hyperplasia

Congenital anomalies
- Chromosome abnormalities
  - Trisomy 21
  - Trisomy 13
  - Trisomy 18
- Myeloid metaplasia
- Beckwith's syndrome
- Erythroderma ichthyosiforme congestiva

NEUROLOGICAL DISORDERS

Clumsiness in Children

Developmental
Minimal cerebral palsy
Visuomotor and visuospatial defects
Global mental handicap
Hyperkinesis
Minor epilepsies
Neurological disease
Muscle disease

Floppy Infant Syndrome

Paralytic conditions with hypotonia
- Hereditary infantile spinal muscular atrophy
  - Werdnig–Hoffmann disease
  - Benign variants
- Congenital myopathies
  - Structural
    - nemaline myopathy
    - myotubular myopathy
    - congenital fibre type disproportion
    - central core disease
    - mitochondrial abnormalities
    - other abnormalities
    - minimal change myopathy

Metabolic
glycogenoses types II, III, (? IV)
lipid storage myopathy
periodic paralysis
Other neuromuscular disorders
Congenital dystrophia myotonica
Congenital muscular dystrophy
Neonatal myasthenia: congenital myasthenia
Motor neuropathies
hereditary
acquired
poliomyelitis
Guillain–Barré syndrome
other neuromuscular disorders
Hypotonia without paralysis
Central nervous system
Non-specific associated with mental retardation
Birth injury
trauma
intracranial haemorrhage
intrapartum asphyxia, anoxia
Hypotonic cerebral palsy
Metabolic disorders
lipidoses, leucodystrophies
mucopolysaccharidoses
aminoacidurias
Leigh's syndrome
chromosomal abnormalities, including Down's syndrome
Connective tissue disorders
Congenital laxity of ligaments
Ehlers–Danlos syndrome
Marfan's syndrome
Osteogenesis imperfecta
Prader–Willi syndrome
Metabolic
Endocrine including hypothyroidism
organicacidaemia
calcium metabolism
hypercalcaemia
rickets
renal tubular acidosis
Benign congenital hypotonia, Essential hypotonia

JOINTS

Chronic Arthritis in Children (Juvenile Chronic Arthritis)
(*systemic illness with polyarthritis in 4 or fewer joints*)

Juvenile ankylosing spondylitis
Seropositive juvenile rheumatoid arthritis
Seronegative chronic arthritis

Psoriatic arthritis
Amyloidosis

This group of diseases does not include –
arthritis secondary to
infection
bleeding diathesis
neoplasm
psychogenic origins
disease of the skeletomuscular system
specific diseases
rheumatic fever
systemic lupus erythematosus
post-infective arthropathy

SOLID TUMOURS IN CHILDREN

Wilms' tumour: the commonest intra-abdominal tumour in childhood
Neuroblastoma
60% occur in the abdomen
65% associated with increased catecholamine excretion in the urine
Rhabdomyosarcoma: commonest soft tissue sarcoma in children
occurs most commonly in (in order of decreasing frequency)
head and neck
extremities
genitourinary tract
trunk
histological types in order of decreasing frequency
embryonal
alveolar
botryoid
pleomorphic
extraskeletal 'Ewing's tumour'
Hodgkin's disease: the commonest lymphoma in children
histological types in order of decreasing frequency
nodular sclerosing
mixed cellularity
lymphocytic predominant
lymphocyte depleted
Non-Hodgkin lymphoma
nodal
extranodal
non-lymphatic
Osteosarcoma
occurring especially in the metaphysial portions of long bones, especially in the distal portions of the femur
Ewing's sarcoma
bones of trunk, midshaft or metaphysial portions of long bones, especially femur

PHARMACOLOCY AND TOXICOLOGY

BIOAVAILABILITY OF DRUG

Depends on
- tablet disintegration
- dissolution time
- excipients in tablet
- gut lumen pH
- gastric emptying time
- intestinal transit time
- gut surface area
- gut bacteria acting on drug
- state of gout
  - surface area
  - presence of disease process
- mesenteric blood flow
- first pass effect

These factors affect
- Peak plasma concentration of drug after one dose
- Time of peak value

FACTORS AFFECTING CONCENTRATION OF A DRUG OR CHEMICAL IN THE BLOOD

Drug
- dosage
- use and dose
- route of administration
- concentration of toxic agent
- duration of exposure to the substance

Body factors
- age
- body weight
- time of sampling, related to time of dose
- presence of other drugs
- disease state
  - of liver
  - of kidney
  - of other organs
- body water status
- menstruation
- any anatomical abnormalities
- any genetic abnormalities

Estimation
- time of sampling, and duration between sampling and estimation
- mode of storage of sample prior to estimation

Other factors
- gastrointestinal absorption rate
- tissue binding at active and inactive sites
- rate of elimination and inactivation
- storage
  - bone
  - hair
  - nails
  - fat
- induction or inhibition of microsomal enzymes
- synergism or antagonism by other drugs
- tolerance (prolonged use of drugs or drugs with cross-tolerance)
- rate of detoxication
- addictive drug effects

ADVERSE DRUG REACTION

Side effects

Overdose effects

Idiosyncracy
- urticaria
- haematological: in susceptible individual

Adverse Reaction to Drugs (Probably Allergic)

Immediate (2–30 minutes)
- Hypotension
- Shock
- Urticaria
- Asthma
- Laryngeal oedema

Accelerated (1–72 hours)
- Urticaria
- Laryngeal oedema

Late (more than 3 days later)
- Skin eruptions
  - urticaria
  - morbilliform rash
  - diffuse erythema
  - erythema multiforme
  - purpura
  - exfoliative dermatitis
  - Stevens–Johnson syndrome
  - fixed drug eruption
  - contact dermatitis
- Fever
- Arthralgia

Unusual reactions
- haemolysis
- thrombocytopenia
- neutropenia
- aplastic anaemia
- cholestatic jaundice
- acute renal insufficiency

MECHANISMS OF DRUG INTERFERENCE

- Displacement of other substances from plasma protein binding sites
- Enzyme induction
- Inhibition of enzyme metabolism
- Competition for sites of degradation
- Alteration in affinity for receptor sites
- Other side effects
  - Interference with absorption of other substances from the gastrointestinal tract
  - Interference with immunity systems
  - Interference with platelet function

DRUGS INHIBITING DRUG METABOLISM

- Allopurinol
- Chloramphenicol
- Disulfiram
- Isoniazid
- Levodopa and methyldopa
- Hydrazine
- Methandrostenolone
- Monoamine oxidase inhibitors
- Nortryptiline
- Oral contraceptives
- Oxyphenylbutazone and phenylbutazone
- Para-aminosalicylate
- Perphenazine
- Phenyramidol

Sulphaphenazole
Sulthiame

DRUGS CAUSING MICROSOMAL ENZYME INDUCTION

Barbiturates
- amylobarbitone
- barbitone
- cyclobarbitone
- hexabarbitone
- phenobarbitone
- quinalbarbitone

Phenytoin
Carbamazepine
Glutethimide
Chloral hydrate
Dichloralphenazone
Meprobamate
Antipyrine
Phenylbutazone
Antibiotics
- griseofulvin
- rifampicin
- doxycyclin

Alcohol
Halofenate
Spironolactone
Chlorinated insecticides
- endrin
- dicophene (DDT)
- gamma benzene
- haxachloride

Cigarette smoking

POSSIBLE TERATOGENIC RISK ASSOCIATED WITH DRUGS

Cytotoxic drugs, e.g.
- azathioprine, mercaptopurine: increased susceptibility to virus infection in-utero

Barbiturates
- retinal damage in fetus
- multiple abnormalities may occur

Chloroquinine: fetal haemorrhage. Rarely fetal abnormalities
Diazepam and related compounds: newborn withdrawal syndrome
Frusemide: fetal growth retardation
Ganglion blockers: increased susceptibility to virus infection in utero
Glucocorticoids: increased susceptibility to virus infection in utero

Live vaccines used in vaccination: fetal virus infection
Narcotics: respiratory depression and newborn withdrawal syndrome
19-Nor-steroids: virilization of female fetus
Phenytoin, primidone
- fetal abnormalities
- newborn withdrawal syndrome
- ? bleeding

Rauwolfia – newborn depression syndrome
Antithyroid drugs, iodides: fetal goitre

ALCOHOL – CONSEQUENCES OF PROLONGED EXCESSIVE INTAKE

General: Trauma to the intoxicated patient
Metabolic
- Attacks of hypoglycaemia
- Protein deficiency
- Thiamine deficiency
  - peripheral neuropathy
  - Beri-beri heart
- obesity
- lead poisoning: home brewing in soft lead glaze vessels
- Haemochromatosis

Liver
- Alcoholic hypoglycaemia
- Simple hepatomegaly
- Fatty liver
- Alcoholic hepatitis
- Cirrhosis
- Hepatic encephalopathy
- Hepatic myopathy
- Hepatic neuropathy

Gastrointestinal tract
- Gastritis, peptic ulcer, oesophagitis
- Malabsorption with consequent malnutrition and vitamin deficiencies
- Acute and chronic pancreatitis

Heart: Alcoholic cardiomyopathy
Haematopoiesis
- folate deficiency
- sideroblastic anaemia (if iron stores are adequate)

Pregnancy: damage to fetus
- characteristic facial appearance
- prenatal onset growth deficiency
- reduced central nervous system performance, including mental retardation
- increased frequency of major anomalies

Central nervous system
- Acute intoxication
- Withdrawal syndromes
  - acute alcoholic tremulousness

tremulousness with hallucinations
acute alcoholic hallucinosis
epilepsy
delirium tremens
atypical delusional states
Wernicke–Korsakow syndrome
ophthalmoplegia often with nystagmus
ataxia of gait
organic mental syndrome
polyneuropathy
Central pontine myelinolysis
Marchiafava–Bignami's disease (uncommon: related to red wine drinking): there is degeneration of myelin and axons in central portion of corpus callosum
Retrobulbar neuropathy: can be exaggerated in raw cider drinkers, due to increase in cyanide intake derived from apple pips, or in heavy smokers from tobacco
Alcoholic myopathy

DRUGS CAUSING SYSTEMIC LUPUS ERYTHEMATOSUS SYNDROME

Anti-arrhythmic drugs
Antibiotics
Anticonvulsants
Antihypertensives
Anti-inflammatory analgesics
Anti-tuberculous drugs
Beta-adrenergic receptor blockers
Sulphonamides
(The condition may remit following withdrawal of the agent concerned)
Compare with classic SLE and drug-induced SLE
More male patients affected
Lung is involved more frequently
Kidney is not affected
Anti-DNA antibodies are to single-strand denatured DNA and *not* to double-strand native DNA
There is no reduction in complement

SHELLFISH HAZARDS

Contamination
Hepatitis Virus A
Typhoid and other Salmonella
Vibrio cholerae
Esch. coli (gastroenteritis)
Vibrio parahaemolyticus (gastroenteritis)
Shellfish poisoning

FISH AND SHELLFISH POISONING

Vertebrate fish

1. Ichthyosarcotoxic fish: responsible for most cases
   - Ciguatera, Scombroid, Puffer fish — commonest

   Toxins present in muscle, viscera, skin or mucus
2. Ichthyotoxic fish: toxins in gonads. Rare cause
3. Ichthyhaemotoxic fish: toxin in blood. Rare cause

Shellfish poisoning

1. Paralytic shellfish poisoning. Occurs when bivalves* contain toxins derived from diflagellates in warm weather
   - Gonyaulax catanella
   - Gonyaulax tamarensis

   A milder illness occurs due to Gymodinium breve, a dimoflagellate which colours the sea red-brown when numerous
2. Neurotoxic shellfish poisoning due to Gy. breve 'red' tides'

*Bivalves include
- mussels
- clams
- oysters
- scallops

VENOMOUS ANIMALS

Venomous fish

Sting ray (Myliobatoidea): tropical and subtropical seas. Serrated spine on tail, with venom-secreting glands in ventrolateral grooves

Weaver fish (trachinidae): Flat coastal area of the Atlantic and Mediterranean. Dorsal spines with venom glands. The venom is both neurotoxic and haemotoxic

Scorpion fish (Scorpionidae): tropical and temperate seas. Dorsal, pelvic and anal spines with venom glands

Jelly fish

Colonial hydroids (Siphonophora), e.g. Portuguese men-of-war. Tentacles with special organs

Box jellies: Sea Wasps: (Cubomedesae): warmer seas, especially in sheltered bays. Most deaths due to these: death occurs within three hours

Molluscs: (Conus): Pacific and Indian oceans under rocks, on coral or on sandy beaches

Insects

Centipedes: (Chilopoda): appendages of the first body segment are poisonous claws

Millipedes: (Diplododa): Irritant fluid secreted from the the sides of the body which may cause a vesicular dermatitis

Scorpions: The sting is present in the upturned tail. The venom may be neurotoxic or haemolytic in action

Spiders

Latrodectus: Black Widow: Throughout the world, but most common in the United States of America. Causes severe muscle spasms

Loxosceles: USA, Central and South America. Haemolysis may occur

Phoneutria: South America, causing many deaths especially in children

Atrax: Australia and Tasmania. Neurotoxic venom

Venomous snakes

Colubrine snakes: wide bite needed to inject venom. Little local effects. After some hours haemolytic and neurotoxic effects, with respiratory or cardiac arrest

Hydrophinae: sea snakes. Found in shallow waters of Indian and Pacific oceans. The venom is neurotoxic and myotoxic

Elapinae: including cobras, kraits and mambas. The venom is mainly neurotoxic

Viperinae: vipers – worldwide distribution. The venom is cytotoxic and haemolytic

Crotalinae: pit vipers, including rattlesnakes. The venom is cytotoxic, haemolytic and in some cases neurotoxic

PSYCHIATRY

Amnesia
- amnesia
- transient amnesia
- dysamnesic syndrome (Korsakow state)

Anorexia nervosa
Antisocial behaviour
Catatonia
Delirium
Delusions
Dementia
Depressive illness
Euphoria
Abnormal excitement
Hallucinations
Hysterical syndromes
Neurosis
Paranoid psychosis
Psychoses and associated disorders in childhood
Psychiatric disorders in adolescence
Explosive rage
Schizophrenia
Sleep disorders
Suicide
- suicide factors
- risk factors in suicide
- suicide and mental illness
- suicide risk factors in the elderly

Withdrawal

AMNESIA

Toxaemia: from any cause
Brain disease
- meningitis
- encephalitis
- brain abscess
- brain tumour
- specific infections
  - syphilis causing general paralysis of the insane
  - cerebral malaria
- brain injury
- degenerative diseases
  - Huntington's chorea

hepatolenticular degeneration
Pick's disease
Alzheimer's disease
cerebral arteriosclerosis
etc.
post-epileptic convulsions
Neuroses and psychoses

Transient Amnesia

Psychogenic
Migraine
Epilepsy, after convulsion
Transient global amnesia
? due to bilateral temporal lobe ischaemia following vertebrobasilar artery disease
Encephalitis, especially if the temporal lobes are affected

Dysamnesic Syndrome (Korsakow State)

Impairment or loss of recent memory, with preservation of recall of remote memory and cognitive functions
Medial aspects of temporal lobes, with function of the limbic system (hippocampi, hippocampal gyri, mamillary bodies and connections) damaged
Chronic alcoholism (preceded by episodes of Wernicke's encephalopathy)
Arsenic poisoning
Bilateral infarction
Neurosurgical interference
Bilateral invasive tumours
Head injury
Subarachnoid haemorrhage

ANOREXIA NERVOSA

Primary
Secondary
1. Neurotic-manipulative
   phobias
   obsessions
   eccentricity in diet
2. Psychosis
   primary depression
   schizophrenia
   catatonic symptoms
   bizarre delusions about food or about eating
   hypomania with overactivity

(Differential diagnosis: gross physical illness)

ANTI-SOCIAL BEHAVIOUR
(*defined by the cultural setting*)

Juvenile deliquency
- Truancy
- Stealing
- Breaking and entering
- Destruction
- Cruelty

Adult delinquency
- Psychopathic personality
- Sexual perversion
- Drug addiction
- Stealing
- Breaking and entering
- Destruction
- Cruelty
- etc.

Liable to occur
- ? 'pure' criminal
- emotionally deprived
- physically deprived
- brain damage
  - some epileptics
  - some mentally retarded
  - some psychotic
  - dementia
  - head injury, etc.
  - *see* 'explosive rage'

CATATONIA

Psychiatric
- Schizophrenia
- Affective illness
- Neurosis

Neurological
- Damage to basal ganglia
  - arteriosclerotic Parkinsonism
  - following bilateral surgery to globus pallidus to relieve Parkinson's syndrome
  - focal lesions of globus pallidus
- Damage to limbic system and temporal lobes
  - viral encephalitis
  - focal temporal encephalomalacia
  - severe vascular lesions in temporal lobes
  - tumour of septum pellucidum impinging on fornix
- Damage to diencephalon
  - tumour } in region of third ventricle
  - traumatic haemorrhage } in region of third ventricle
  - focal lesion of thalamus

Other causes
- frontal lobe tumour
- focal frontal lobe lesion
- anterior cerebral artery aneurysm
- diffuse brain damage
- diffuse encephalomalacia
- petit mal states
- post-ictal phase in epilepsy
- Wernick's encephalopathy
- tuberose sclerosis
- general paresis
- narcolepsy
- acute phase of encephalitis lethargica

Metabolic
- diabetic ketoacidosis
- hypercalcaemia in hyperparathyroidism
- pellagra
- acute intermittent porphyria
- acute glomerulonephritis (membranous)
- hepatic encephalopathy

Toxic
- organic fluorides
- carbon monoxide poisoning
- psychotomimetic drugs
- excessive alcohol intake
- chronic amphetamine intoxication
- large doses of phencyclidine
- aspirin
- ACTH
- antipsychotic agents
- fluphenazine inanthate

DELIRIUM

Toxic and metabolic
- Liver damage
- Renal failure
- Diabetes mellitus
- Porphyria
- Water intoxication
- Electrolyte disturbance
- Systemic lupus erythematosus

Nutrition defects
- Wernick's encephalopathy
- Nicotinic acid deficiency encephalopathy
- Vitamin B_{12} deficiency

Poisons
- Sedative drugs
- Alcohol
- Organic phosphates
- Salicylates
- Heavy metal poisoning
- Cyanides

Endocrine
- Addison's adrenocortical insufficiency
- Hyperparathyroidism
- Hypoparathyroidism
- Pituitary insufficiency
- Thyroid disease
- Pancreatic islet cell tumour with hypoglycaemia

Infection
- Meningitis
- Encephalitis
- Septicaemia

Cardiorespiratory
- Anoxia
- Myocardial infarction
- Hypertensive encephalopathy
- Cardiac failure
- Pulmonary insufficiency

Brain damage
- Tumour
- Subdural haematoma
- Extradural haematoma
- Head injury
- Brain abscess
- Subarachnoid haemorrhage
- Cerebral embolus
- Cerebral atherosclerosis

Epilepsy

DELUSIONS
(*false belief*)

Depression: delusion of guilt frequent
Elderly people
Paranoia
Paranoid schizophrenia
Progressive cerebral disease
- generalized paralysis of the insane due to syphilis
- severe dementia from a variety of causes

DEMENTIA
(*Global disruption of personality affecting behaviour and intelligence with impairment of learning of new responses, and disorganized emotional response*)

Infective
- Following
  - meningitis
  - encephalitis
  - slow virus: Creutzfeldt–Jakob disease
  - torulosis
  - meningovascular syphilis
  - general paresis
  - etc.

Trauma

Following

head injury { acute / chronic, e.g. professional boxer

major intracranial surgery

epilepsy following birth injury

Metabolic disturbance

Chronic alcoholism

Myxoedema

Hypopituitarism

Post-anoxia

Post-hypoglycaemia

Vitamin B_{12} deficiency

Pellagra

Hepatolenticular degeneration

Heavy metal poisoning (e.g. mercury)

Degenerative conditions

Simple presenile dementia

Senile dementia

Alzheimer's disease (presenile)

Pick's disease (presenile especially affecting the frontal lobes)

Kraepelin's disease

Spinocerebellar degenerations

Paralysis agitans

Demyelination

Muscle sclerosis

Devic's disease

Familial conditions

Huntington's chorea

Progressive myoclonic epilepsy

Lipid storage diseases

Neoplasms

Cerebral tumours

primary

secondary

Carcinoma of bronchus

Progressive multifocal leucoencephalopathy

Carcinomatosis

Vascular disorders

Atherosclerotic dementia

Cerebral haemorrhage

Thromboangiitis obliterans

Cerebral embolism

Fat embolism

Subarachnoid haemorrhage

Subdural haematoma

Disseminated lupus erythematosus

Normal pressure by hydrocephalus: 'occult hydrocephalus'

DEPRESSIVE ILLNESS

Primary

bipolar: manic-depressive (rare)

unipolar
endogenous
psychotic
neurotic
Secondary: systemic medical diseases
disease of the CNS
drug effects
endocrine effects
post-viral infection depression
following injury e.g.
irradiation
cytotoxic drugs
physical trauma
psychiatric disorders
schizophrenia
alcoholism
organic dementias

EUPHORIA

May occur in
Progressive dementia
Frontal lobe disease
General paralysis of the insane
Mania and hypomania
Disseminated sclerosis
Intoxication with drugs
alcohol
tranquillizers

ABNORMAL EXCITEMENT

Acute mania
Delirious mania: in association with infections, intoxications, etc.
Catatonic schizophrenia
Specific drugs, e.g. LSD
Acute epileptic delirium
Aggressive psychopath
Mentally retarded patients may become excessively excited

HALLUCINATIONS
(*Sensory impression occurring in the absence of a corresponding external stimulus*)

Dreaming and the hypnogogic state
Pathological disturbances of sleep
Narcolepsy: sufferers sometimes experience vivid hallucinations, more often visual than auditory. (? relationship with childhood nightmares)

Organic disease of sense organs or central nervous system
- intracranial tumour. With tumour in temporal lobe, there may be hallucinations of taste or smell
- Rabies
- Epilepsy
  - aura before the onset of epileptic convulsions
  - temporal lobe epilepsy
    - hallucinations of taste and smell
    - sense of unreality, *jamais vu*
    - sense of intense familarity, *déjà vu*
- Electric shock – visual hallucinations may occur

Intoxications
- cocaine addiction
- marihuana addiction
- amphetamine addiction
- chronic bromide intoxication
- hallucinogenic agents, e.g. LSD, mescalin
- withdrawal of alcohol, amphetamine, barbiturates
- severe toxic states, e.g. septicaemia

Certain psychoses

HYSTERICAL SYNDROMES

Conversion phenomena: Signs and symptoms referred to any part of the body, e.g.
- aphasia
- anaesthesia
- blindness
- 'coma'
- deafness
- 'fits'
- mutism
- paralysis
- spasms
- tics
- tremor
- etc.

Dissociative states
- amnesia
- automatism
- fugues
- multiple personalities
- trance states
- vomiting
- writer's cramp
- etc.

NEUROSIS

Anxiety neurosis

Hysterical neurosis
- conversion type
- dissociative type

Phobic neurosis
Obsessive-compulsive neurosis
Depressive neurosis
Neurasthenic neurosis
Depersonalization neurosis
Hypochondriacal neurosis
Others

PARANOID PSYCHOSIS

'Functional'
- Reactive psychosis
- Schizophrenia

Associated with organic brain disorder, intoxication, somatic disease
- Presenile dementia
- Senile dementia
- Cerebral tumour
- Huntington's chorea
- etc.

PSYCHOSES AND ASSOCIATED DISORDERS IN CHILDHOOD

Autistic psychosis: early onset infantile autism: Kanner's syndrome
Disintegrative psychosis
- organic
  - lipid storage disorders
  - tuberose sclerosis
  - rubella embryopathy
  - Schilder's disease
  - subacute sclerosing panencephalitis
  - congenital syphilis
  - metachromatic leucodystrophy
  - neurodegenerative diseases
- childhood schizophrenia
  - pseudodefective or autistic regressive type
  - pseudoneurotic or phobic, obsessive, compulsive, hypochondriacal type
  - pseudopsychopathic or paranoid, acting out, aggressive antisocial type

Hyperkinetic syndrome
Affective psychosis
- manic-depressive psychosis. Rare
- depression
  - endogenous. Uncommon
  - reactive. Most cases

Hysteria
Mental retardation
- psychosis
- reactive depression

PSYCHIATRIC DISORDERS IN ADOLESCENCE

Conduct disorder
Neurotic disorder
Suicide
Bereavement problems
Anorexia nervosa
Psychosis developing in adolescence
Psychosomatic disorders
Drug abuse
Sexual difficulties

EXPLOSIVE RAGE

(*More males than females*)

Family history of uncontrolled tempers
Children raised in contact with frequent outbursts of rage
History of temper tantrums in childhood, leading to rage outbursts in adults – prenatal, natal, postnatal injury, anoxia, hypoglycaemia, etc.
Children following minimal brain damage
Hyperkinetic children
Premenstrual tension
Head injury – ? *contre-coup* affecting temporal lobes of cerebrum
Temporal lobe epilepsy – anger and aggression in the post-ictal phase
Severely affected individuals
1. Cerebral palsy
2. Mental retardation
3. Arrested internal hydrocephalus

Viral encephalitis
Post-encephalitis lethargica
Brain abscess
Stroke
Subarachnoid haemorrhage
Pre-senile dementia
Huntington's chorea
Normal pressure hydrocephalus
Cerebral anoxia
Tumours of limbic region
Post-intracranial surgery
Metabolic: post-hypoglycaemia
Rarely: multiple sclerosis

SCHIZOPHRENIA

Unknown aetiology
Rare causes
Brain tumour
Epilepsy

- Head injury
- Drug reactions (e.g. post-LSD)
- Metabolic disorder stress
- Surgical operation stress

Varieties of schizophrenia
- Hebephrenic
- Catatonic
- Paranoid
- ? Schizoaffective schizophrenia
- 'residual schizophrenia'

SLEEP DISORDERS

Non-Rapid Eye Movement sleep } *normally alternate*
Rapid Eye Movement sleep } *through the night*

Primary disorders
- insomnia
- narcoleptic syndrome
- hypersomnia
  - hypersomnia with sleep drunkenness
  - Kleine–Levin syndrome
  - Pickwickian syndrome
- nightmares

Secondary disorders
- functional psychiatric illness
- chronic alcoholism
- metabolic and nutritional disorders
  - uraemia
  - hypothyroidism
  - anorexia nervosa
  - starvation
  - pregnancy
  - hyperthermia

Parasomnias
- sleep walking
- night terrors
- sleep talking
- nocturnal enuresis
- bruxism (teeth grinding)

Sleep-modified disorders: Disorders modifying sleep
- Ischaemic heart disease
- migraine
- duodenal ulceration
- bronchial asthma
- epilepsy
- neuromuscular disorders

SUICIDE

Suicide Factors

Personal
- sex

age
married/single
mode of living
occupation
environment
Previous history
personal: personality
family
cyclothymic
drinking/drugs
early dementia
organic brain disease
Stresses
bereavement
separation/moves
illness
Other symptoms
Circumstances of attempt
any precautions against discovery
preparatory acts
methods used
? previous attempts

Risk Factors in Suicide

Depression with feelings of guilt, self-accusation, self-depreciation, nihilistic ideas, and restlessness
Severe insomnia with intrusion of distressing thoughts and restlessness
Severe hypochondriasis
Previous suicidal attempt
History of alcoholism or drug addiction
Severe physical disability developing in a previously active fit person
Family history of suicide
Sudden financial difficulty or unemployment, with loss of self-esteem
Depression incompletely treated with recovery of initiative and activity, but without relief of the depression

Suicide and Mental Illness

Depressive illness (70%): also terminal, illness, drug dependence, dementia
Alcoholism (15%): also depression, and terminal illness
Schizophrenia (3%)
Phobic anxiety (3%)
Barbiturate dependency (1%)
Acute schizo-affective psychosis
(The percentage incidence will vary depending on the population studied)

Suicide Risk Factors in the Elderly

More males than females
Increasing age
Living alone
Recent bereavement
Physical illness
Moderate depression with sleep disturbance
Hypochondriasis
Recent suicide attempt
Availability of drugs for suicide attempt
Social Class IV and V

WITHDRAWAL

- Physiological
  - reaction to stress
- Pathological
  - depression
  - schizophrenia
  - organic disease
    - extracranial
      - metabolic
        - diabetes mellitus
        - hypoglycaemia
        - uraemia
        - liver coma
        - Addison's disease crisis
        - circulatory collapse
        - severe infection
        - hypothermia
        - hyperthermia
    - intracranial
      - head injury
      - cerebrovascular accident
      - space-occupying lesion
      - infection
        - encephalitis
        - meningitis
      - degenerative disease
      - epilepsy: postictal state
  - intoxication
  - hysteria
- Malingering

RENAL TRACT DISORDERS

Obstruction to urine flow in immediate newborn period
Urine tract infection in childhood
Urinary tract malignancy
Obstruction in urinary tract
Urine retention
Increased susceptibility to urinary tract infection
Lower urinary tract symptoms
Incontinence
Uninhibited bladder contraction
Bladder dysfunction
Retroperitoneal fibrosis
Prostatic cysts

RENAL FUNCTION

Renal Endocrine Functions

Renin production
Prostaglandin metabolism
Erythropoietin production
Vitamin D activation
Glucose synthesis (small amounts only)
Inactivation of
- Gastrin } some
- Insulin }
- Parathormone

Non-Osmolar Factors affecting Renal Water Excretion

Changes in blood volume: 'Volume receptors'
Changes in systemic arterial pressure: 'Baroreceptors'
Hormones
- Catecholamines
- Prostaglandins
- Adrenocortical hormones
- Renin-angiotensin
- Thyroid hormones
- Posterior pituitary antidiuretic hormone

Physical and emotional stress
Chronic renal failure
Metabolic disorders
- Sodium balance
- Water balance
- Protein balance
- Hypercalcaemia
- Hypokalaemia

Sickle cell disease

Pharmacological agents

1. Diuretics
   - Alcohol
   - Diphenylhydantoin
   - Lithium
   - Demeclocycline
   - Tolazamide
   - Glyburide
   - Propoxyphene
   - Colchicine
   - Vinblastine
   - Orthodox diuretics
2. Antidiuretics
   - Antidiuretic hormone (ADH)
   - Nicotine
   - Chlorpropamide
   - Tolbutamide
   - Clofibrate
   - Cyclophosphamide
   - Morphine
   - Barbiturates
   - Vincristine
   - Carbamazepine
   - Acetoaminophen

Diurnal Urinary Flow

Reversal or loss of rhythm

Normal

evening–night: excretion of sodium, potassium, bicarbonate, chloride, gradually falls, and urine pH falls. Urine concentration increases, with increased phosphate excretion, and increased antidiuretic activity

morning: the above process is reversed, with increased excretion of sodium, potassium, chloride, bicarbonate, decrease in urine concentration and rise in urine pH

This normal rhythm persists during –
- Undernutrition
- Water deprivation
- Salt deprivation
- Sustained activity of pitressin
- Temporary disturbance of sleep rhythm

Reversal or abolition of rhythm

Normal person given cortisone

Congestive cardiac failure Nephrotic syndrome Malnutrition	in the presence of oedema. Diuresis may only follow a diuretic if given in the evening, no response to diuretic given in the morning

Reversal of abolition of rhythm may occur in
- Chronic renal failure
- Malignant hypertension
- Renal artery stenosis
- Small bowel insufficiency
- Addison's hypoadrenalism
- Hyperaldosteronism
- Cushing's syndrome
- Head injury

Anuria

Obstructive
- Ligature of both kidneys
- Removal of sole functioning kidney
- Bladder carcinoma blocking both ureters
- Retroperitoneal fibrosis blocking ureteric flow
- Blockage of ureter of sole functioning kidney

Non-obstructive
- *See under* Acute oliguria

Acute Oliguria
(50–400 ml per 24 hours)

Inadequate renal perfusion
- Depletion of body salt and water
- Intravascular volume depletion with little or no external fluid loss
- Findings:
  - Urine specific gravity greater than 1·015–1·020
  - Urine sodium reduced to less than 5 mmol per litre
  - Microscopy: nil exceptional

Obstruction to urine flow
- Prostatic enlargement
- Bilateral ureteric block
- Unilateral ureteric block with single kidney
- Findings:
  - Urine specific gravity varies with body fluid and electrolyte balance

Intrinsic renal disease
- Acute tubular necrosis
- bilateral renal cortical necrosis
- acute glomerulonephritis
- rapid progressive glomerulonephritis
- malignant hypertension
- acute interstitial nephritis
- Findings in acute tubular necrosis:
  - Urine specific gravity varies only slightly about 1·010–1·012 (specific gravity of plasma ultrafiltrate)
  - Microscopy shows evidence of renal tubular damage, with casts, red cells and high protein output

Failure of Urine Concentration

Chronic renal failure
    50% of cases with glomerular filtration rate below 60 ml per minute
Medullary cystic disease (abnormality of juxta-medullary portion)
Obstructive uropathy } affecting collecting ducts
Amyloidosis } affecting collecting ducts
Hypercalcaemia: defect of concentration and not of dilution power. Calcium deposition occurs in ascending loop of Henle and distal rubules plus collecting ducts
Hypokalaemia: Histological changes in proximal tubule cells, with functional changes in distal tubules. Urine can be concentrated to 300–400 mosmol/l
Sickle cell disease: sickle cells in HnS disease sickle in hypertonic solutions even in the presence of adequate oxygen tension, i.e. they sickle and damage to long loops of Henle
Pharmacological causes: Diuretic therapy
Diabetes insipidus
Congenital nephrogenic diabetes insipidus
Psychogenic polydipsia
Starvation
Post-obstruction diuresis
Post-tubular damage diuresis, in recovery phase
Post-renal transplantation

Impairment of Maximal Free Water Formation and/or Excretion

Severe sodium intake restriction
Hypovolaemia
    true
    effective
        congestive cardiac failure
        cirrhosis
        nephrotic syndrome
Adrenal cortical insufficiency
Inappropriate antidiuretic hormone release
Diuretics (prolonged action)

Polyuria

Diminished Anti-diuretic hormone (ADH)
    Impaired ability to secrete ADH
        1. Persistent
            lesions of supra-optico hypothalamus
            diabetes insipidus
        2. Transient
            compulsive water drinking
            ? potassium deficiency

Diminished ADH secretion due to increased water intake with increased thirst

1. Compulsive water drinking
2. Potassium deficiency
3. Lesion of thirst centre
4. Hypercalcaemia

Circulating antibody to vasopressin

Adequate circulating ADH

Impaired tubule response to ADH

1. Congenital
    a. Nephrogenic diabetes insipidus
    b. Multiple defects
        renal tubular acidosis
        Fanconi's syndrome
2. Acquired
    a. Compulsive water drinking
    b. Diabetes insipidus

Fault in production of hypertonic interstitial fluid in renal medulla

1. Impaired sodium transport in loop of Henle
    a. Potassium deficiency
    b. Hypercalcaemia and/or hypercalciuria
2. Disturbed blood flow in vasa recta, or structural damage to loops of Henle
    a. Papillary necrosis
    b. Widespread gradual nephron destruction
    c. Hydronephrosis
    d. Sickle cell disease

Increased solute output per nephron (osmotic diuresis)

1. Normal number of nephrons
    a. Diuretic therapy
    b. Glycosuria, e.g. uncontrolled diabetes mellitus
    c. Salt diuresis following relief of urinary obstruction
    d. Diuretic phase of acute renal failure
2. Greatly reduced number of nephrons
    Chronic renal failure

Polyuria with urine volume of less than 3–4 litres per 24 hours, plus raised blood urea

1. Chronic renal failure
2. Potassium deficiency
3. Hypercalcaemia
4. Fanconi syndrome

Polyuria with urine volume exceeding 5 litres per 24 hours, with normal blood urea –

1. Diabetes insipidus
2. Compulsive water drinking
3. Hypercalcaemia
4. Familial nephrogenic diabetes insipidus

Nephrogenic Diabetes Insipidus

Hereditary
- Sex-linked inheritance
- Sickle cell disease
- Nephronophthisis

Secondary to
- hypercalcaemia
- hypokalaemia
- prolonged and persistent overhydration, e.g. compulsive water drinking
- chronic renal failure
- long term lithium therapy
- obstructive nephropathy

Diuretic Action

Osmotic diuresis
- Water
- Mannitol – osmotically active non-reabsorbable substance
- (Urea)

Inhibition of chloride reabsorption
- Mercurial diuretics inhibit chloride reabsorption in the thick ('diluting') ascending limb of the loop of Henle
- Furosemide acts at the same site, after being bound to plasma protein, it is secreted into the proximal renal tubules by the same organic acid transport system which excreted p-aminohippuric acid
- Ethacrynic acid is converted to active ethacrynic cysteinate and secreted into the proximal tubules, acting to inhibit chloride reabsorption in the ascending loop of Henle

Inhibition of sodium reabsorption
- Acetazolamide inhibits carbonic anhydrase activity in the proximal renal tubules, resulting in excretion of sodium and bicarbonate ions. Inhibits mercurial diuretics, and potentiates thiazides, furosemide and ethacrynic acid
- Benzothiadiazines, e.g. chlorothiazide, inhibit the re-absorption of sodium ions by the proximal renal tubules
- Triamterene, inhibits sodium reabsorption and potassium excretion, and acts after adrenalectomy. Powerful action in combination with thiazides

Aldosterone antagonist
- Spironolactone causes diminution in distal tubule sodium/potassium and hydrogen ion exchange, resulting in increased sodium excretion. Its action is proportional to the level of circulating aldosterone and is inactive after adrenalectomy

RENAL FAILURE

Acute Renal Failure

- Pre-renal
  - Hypovolaemia
    - fluid loss
    - haemorrhage
    - burns
  - Severe infections
    - Gram-negative septicaemia
  - Hypotension
    - myocardial infarction
    - pulmonary embolism
    - major surgery
    - obstetric accidents
    - acute poisoning
    - acute pancreatitis
    - acute liver failure
    - etc.

(sustained reduced blood flow to renal tubules results in renal tubular damage)

- Renal
  - Acute glomerulonephritis
  - Acute ischaemic failure due to pre-renal causes,
  - Direct nephrotoxins
    - Inorganic
    - Organic
    - Antibiotics
    - Drugs
    - Animal
      - horse serum
      - cantharides
    - Vegetable
      - poisonous fungi
  - Disseminated intravascular coagulopathy
    - haemolytic uraemic syndrome
    - progressive malignant hypertension
  - Transplant rejection
- Post-renal
  - Tubular obstruction
    - urate nephropathy
    - myelomatosis
    - sulphonamides
  - Ureteric obstruction
    - calculi
    - fibrosis
    - tumours
    - papillary necrosis
    - retroperitoneal fibrosis
  - Ureteric damage
    - trauma
    - pelvic surgery

Bladder
    Carcinoma blocking, first one ureter, then both
Urethral stone

Acute Nephritis Syndrome

1. Nephritogenic Group A Beta-haemolytic streptococcal infection (esp. Types 4 & 12)
2. Other bacterial and viral infections: relatively uncommon
    - Staphylococci
    - Non-haemolytic streptococci
    - Viruses (including hepatitis B)
    - Secondary syphilis
3. Glomerulonephritis without known infective cause
    - Proliferative
        - focal
        - diffuse
    - Membranous
    - Membranoproliferative
    - IgG–IgA mesangiocapillary glomerulonephritis
    - Chronic sclerosing glomerulonephritis
    - 'Minimal' change
    - Unclassified
4. Multisystem disease associated with widespread multifocal vasculitis
    - Schönlein–Henoch anaphylactoid purpura syndrome
    - Systemic lupus erythematosus
    - Polyarteritis nodosa
    - Wegener's granuloma
    - Goodpasture's syndrome (lung purpura with nephritis)
    - Subacute bacterial endocarditis
    - Shunt nephritis. Membranoproliferative glomerulonephritis in children with infected ventriculo-atrial shunt for hydrocephalus. (Complement plus IgM along capillary wall)
    - Haemolytic-uraemic syndrome
    - Quartan malaria – common in Tropics, followed by nephrosis and chronic renal failure
    - Malignant disease
    - Liver disease

Crescentic Glomerulonephritis

The chances of recovery are greatly reduced if 60–70% of the glomeruli in a biopsy sample show enveloping crescents

severe glomerulonephritis occasionally in severe systemic lupus erythematosus occasionally in Schönlein–Henoch purpura occasionally binding of anti-glomerular basement membrane antibodies (Goodpasture's syndrome)	vascular and glomerular deposition of circulating antibody–antigen complexes

Acute Renal Failure with Jaundice

Gram-negative bacteraemic septicaemia
Leptospirosis (Weil's disease)
Hepato-renal disease
Haemolytic uraemic syndrome (? viral)
Yellow fever
Mismatched blood transfusion
Poisoning
- Carbon tetrachloride
- Paracetamol
- Amanita phalloides ('mushroom' poisoning)

Lung Haemorrhages with Nephritis

Occasionally in severe soluble complex disease
- post-streptococcal glomerulonephritis
- systemic lupus erythematosus
- Schönlein–Henoch (allergic) purpura
- polyarteritis nodosa

Goodpasture's syndrome

Nephrotic Syndrome

Commonest Causes
- Primary renal disease (80% of cases)
  1. Proliferative glomerulonephritis. More adults than children
  2. Minimal change in glomerulonephritis. 3 children: 1 adult
  3. Membranous nephropathy. More adults than children
  4. Focal hyalinosis. Occurs in children

Rare Causes
- Renal vein thrombosis: precipitated by
  - nephrotic syndrome
  - renal amyloid
  - hypernephroma
  - trauma, e.g. catheter
  - severe dehydration (in children)
- Congestive cardiac failure
- Constrictive pericarditis
- Metabolic
  1. Diabetes mellitus
  2. Amyloid
     - primary
     - secondary
       - infection
       - malignancy
     - familial
- Systemic lupus erythematosus
- Malignancy
  - Hodgkin's disease
  - others

Infections
- quartan malaria. *Pl. malariae*
- syphilis, second stage
- leprosy (in erythema nodosum leprosum type)

Drug reactions
- trimethadione, penicillamine, phenindione } drug acts as hapten
- gold, mercury compounds, bismuth } direct tubular toxicity

Toxins: bee strings, etc. (v. rare)
Congenital varieties: steroid resistant

Interstitial Nephritis

Acute
- Acute pyelonephritis
- Drug reactions, e.g. phenindione (rare)
- Leukaemic infiltration of kidney (rare)

Chronic
- Chronic pyelonephritis
- Papillary necrosis
- Analgesic abuse, e.g. phenacetin
- Uric acid nephropathy
- Balkan nephropathy
- Anatomical renal abnormalities
- Nephrocalcinosis, hypercalcaemia
- Hyperoxaluria
- Renal stones
- Sickle cell disease
- Tuberculosis of kidney
- Bacterial infection (rarely caused by infection alone in adults)
- Irradiation
- Heavy metal poisoning
- Urine tract obstruction
- Vesico-ureteric reflux
- Congenital
  - hereditary nephritis
  - medullary cystic disease

Membranous Nephropathy

Extrinsic
- infections: including
  - Hepatitis B (Australia antigen positive)
  - syphilis
- drugs and toxins
  - including gold

Intrinsic
- systemic lupus erythematosus
- tumour

renal vein thrombosis (more likely that renal vein thrombosis is secondary to membranous nephropathy (plasma complement levels increased)
acute proliferative glomerulonephritis (plasma complement decreased)

Papillary Necrosis

Analgesic abuse
Acute pyelonephritis: especially in diabetes mellitus
Obstruction to the urinary tract
Renal tuberculosis
Sickle cell anaemia
Macroglobulinaemia

Renal Failure with Liver Disease

- Hepatocellular disease
  - cirrhosis
  - fulminant hepatic failure
- Obstructive jaundice
- Prolonged hypotension: following
  - severe blood loss
  - cardiogenic shock
  - septicaemia
- Disorders affecting both liver and kidneys
  - polycystic disease
  - congenital hepatic fibrosis
- Toxins affecting both liver and kidneys
  - Carbon tetrachloride
  - Tetracycline (spoilt)
  - Methoxyflurane
  - Rifampicin
- Infections affecting both liver and kidneys
  - Septicaemia, especially Gram-negative organisms
  - Some leptospiral infections
  - Yellow fever
- Metabolic disorders
  - Sickle cell disease
  - Amyloid infiltration of liver and kidneys

Indications for Dialysis

- General
  - Acute renal failure with gross metabolic disturbance
  - Chronic renal failure: to prolong life
  - Polycystic kidneys and renal failure: patient can be stabilized on low protein diet with intermittent dialysis
  - Acute poisoning, if severe
    - Salicylate
    - Medium and short-acting barbiturates

Methanol
Paracetamol
Glutethimide
Meprobamate
Imipramine
Heroin
Paraldehyde
Chloral hydrate
Digoxin
Amphetamine
Cyclophosphamide
Methotrexate
Penicillins
Sulphonamides
Cephaloridine
Chloramphenicol
tetracyclines
oligomycin
isoniazid
Can all be removed by dialysis, if the clinical condition indicates dialysis

Specific: In renal failure
Poor clinical condition and/or nausea, vomiting, fits, diarrhoea, pericarditis, twitching, pulmonary oedema, clouding of consciousness
Plasma potassium exceeding 7 mmol/l
Plasma bicarbonate less than 10 mmol/l
Blood pH less than 7·15
Blood urea exceeding 30 mmol/l
Blood urea rising by more than 15 mmol/l
Severe sodium and water imbalance
Uraemic peripheral neuropathy

Chronic Renal Failure

Mesangio-capillary glomerulonephritis
Proliferative glomerulonephritis with extensive crescents
Membranous nephropathy
Focal hyalinosis
Multisystem disease

Renal Damage which may be caused by Drugs

Shock
Vasculitis
Hypersensitivity glomerular diseases
Tubular degeneration and necrosis
Blockage of tubules by uric acid crystals
Blockage of tubules and glomeruli by haemorrhage

Drug-induced Renal Damage

Analgesic nephropathy: phenacetin

Acute interstitial nephritis: hypersensitivity reaction
- penicillin
- sulphonamides
- polymyxin
- rifampicin

Renal tubular damage
- sulphonamides
- aminoglycosides
- cephalosporins
- polymyxin
- colistin
- amphotericin

Nephrotic syndrome
- trimethadione
- mercury
- gold
- penicillamine
- rarely
  - tolbutamide
  - probenacid
  - perchlorate
  - sequestrene

Others
- lithium salts: may cause nephrogenic diabetes insipidus
- methoxyflurone: vasopressin-resistant polyuria
- vitamin D: hypercalcaemia with renal damage
- methysergide – retroperitoneal fibrosis leading to obstruction and renal failure
- tetracyclines (especially in the old): irreversible Fanconi's syndrome

Involuntary Movements in Renal Failure

Tremor and asterixis
Akinesia and rigidity
Oculogyria and trismus
Torticollis
Choreoathetosis
Myoclonus

KIDNEY AND RENAL PELVIS

Congenital Macroscopic Lesions of Kidney

Renal agenesis
1. Bilateral: always associated with hydramnios
2. Unilateral

Renal hypoplasia
1. Bilateral hypoplasia
2. Unilateral dwarfed kidney

Renal ectopia
- Kidneys liable to develop hydronephrosis and pyelonephritis

Anomalies of fusion

1. Horseshoe kidneys
2. Unilateral fused kidney with crossed renal ectopia. There is an increased liability to the development of hydronephrosis and recurrent urinary tract infection

Duplication of pelvis and ureter

Often associated with ureteric reflux, pain and hydronephrosis, with recurrent tract infection

Cystic disease of kidneys

1. Polycystic kidneys
   a. Rapidly lethal in newborn form
   b. Onset of symptoms in adult form, 40 years, with average duration of life after clinical onset 5–10 years (much individual variation)
2. Solitary cysts
3. Cystic disease of renal medulla–renal failure in adolescence or early adult life, with polyuria and sodium leak
4. Sponge kidney–urinary tract infection with haematuria. The X-ray films from intravenous pyelogram and retrograde pyelogram completely different, as the cysts do not fill from below

Renal Infarction

Renal artery occlusion: 75% follow embolism
Renal vein occlusion: Infarction in the neonate follows renal vein thrombosis
Following trauma in renal region

Renal Artery Stenosis

Atherosclerosis of renal artery
Fibromuscular hyperplasia of renal artery

Renal Calculi

Hot climate with persistent reduced fluid intake
Idiopathic hypercalciuria
Primary hyperparathyroidism
Urine infection
Medullary sponge kidneys (without hypercalciuria)
Hyperoxaluria

- Primary
  - with glycolic aciduria
  - with glyceric aciduria
- Secondary
  - excess oxalate intake with persistent reduced fluid intake
  - increased oxalate absorption associated with steatorrhoea

ethylene glycol (antifreeze) ingestion
excessive ascorbic acid intake in occasional susceptible otherwise normal individuals
pyridoxine deficiency
methoxyflurane anaesthesia

Uricaciduria with increased incidence of urate stones
some gout cases
polycythaemia vera } especially after onset
leukaemia } of chemotherapy

Decreased urine pH resulting in increased incidence of urate stones
gout: some cases
chronic diarrhoea
idiopathic

Contributory Factors to Urinary Stone Formation

Increased crystalloid concentration
Dehydration
Hypercalciuria
Hyperoxaluria
Excess uric aciduria
Cystinuria
Xanthinuria (very rare)
Silica stone (rare: high intake of magnesium trisilicate over long periods)
Alcaptonuria

Low urine pH: increases an existing tendency to uric acid stones

High urine pH: increases an existing tendency to phosphate stones

Deficiency of a crystallization inhibitor
Inhibitors
1. Pyrophosphate
2. Magnesium
3. Citrate
4. Other substances

Urinary tract abnormalities
Urine tract infection
Congenital abnormalities
Medullary sponge kidney
Polycystic kidneys

Others
Nephrotoxic substances associated with stone formation
1. Worcester sauce excess
2. Curry kidney
? Vitamin A deficiency

Nephrocalcinosis

Associated with hypercalcaemia and/or hypercalciuria
Hyperparathyroidism
Sarcoidosis

Renal tubule acidosis
Idiopathic hypercalciuria
Multiple myeloma
Carcinomatosis
Cushing's syndrome
Steroid therapy
Milk alkali syndrome
Hypervitaminosis D

Due to structural or biochemical changes favouring calcium deposition
Medullary sponge kidney
Papillary necrosis

Idiopathic nephrocalcinosis

Other conditions in which nephrocalcinosis may occur
Primary oxaluria [R]
Oxalosis
Renal cortical necrosis
Renal infarction
Renal tuberculosis
Chronic renal failure

Hydronephrosis and Hydro-Ureter

Congenital
Increase in collagen in pelvis
Abnormality in local musculature
Abnormal blood vessels blocking outflow
Urethral valves: transverse urethral folds may persist in male children
Kinks
High insertion of ureter on the renal pelvis
Hydro-ureter–megaureter, with no apparent organic cause
Phimosis or pinhole meatus (very rare cause)

Acquired
Pregnancy: recovery 6 weeks after delivery
Contraceptive pill: rare
adhesions
outflow obstruction
retroperitoneal fibrosis
occasionally secondary to atonicity of normal elasto-muscular tissues of renal pelvis
pelvic-ureteric junction obstruction
gross vesicoureteric reflux
unilateral hydronephrosis with ureteric tumour, stone, or other obstruction

TUBULAR DISORDERS

Renal Cysts

Solitary or multiple
Found incidentally in adult

Polycystic renal disease
1. Infantile
   Autosomal recessive inheritance
   Fatal in weeks
2. Adult
   Autosomal dominant
   Onset of symptoms usually at 20–40 years

Renal Tubular Acidosis Type I
(Classic renal tubular acidosis, Gradient RTA, distal RTA)

Primary
- sporadic
  - infantile
  - adult
- Genetically transmitted: Mendelian dominant

Secondary
- Associated with genetically transmitted disease
  - Galactosaemia (after chronic galactose intake in diet)
  - Hereditary fructose intolerance with nephrocalcinosis (after chronic fructose intake in diet)
  - Ehlers–Danlos syndrome
  - Fabry's disease
- Metabolic disorders
  - Hepatic cirrhosis
  - Idiopathic hypergammaglobulinaemia
  - Hypergammaglobulinaemia purpura
  - Hyperthyroidism with nephrocalcinosis
  - Primary hyperparathyroidism with nephrocalcinosis
  - Sarcoidosis
- Autoimmune conditions
  - Lupoid hepatitis
  - Systemic lupus erythematosus
  - Sjögren's syndrome
- Infection
  - Tuberculosis
- Malignancy
  - Hodgkin's disease
- Renal
  - Pyelonephritis
  - Medullary sponge kidney
  - Renal transplantation
- Drugs
  - Vitamin D-induced nephrocalcinosis
  - amphotericin B

Renal Tubular Acidosis Type II (much less common than Type I RTA)
(Bicarbonate wasting renal tubular acidosis, proximal RTA, Rate RTA)

Without multiple dysfunctions of proximal renal tubules
- Primary
  - Infantile

Adult
Secondary
Sulphonamides
With multiple dysfunctions of proximal renal tubules
Primary
Sporadic
Genetic
Genetically transmitted systemic disease
Hereditary fructose intolerance (after short-term ingestion of fructose)
Cystinosis
Wilson's disease, hepatolenticular disease
Lowe's syndrome [R]
Tyrosinosis [R]
Metabolic disorders
Hypercalciuric rickets
Vitamin D deficiency (?)
Protein metabolism disorders
Multiple myeloma
Sjögren's syndrome
Amyloidosis
Idiopathic immunoglobinuria
Renal disorders
Nephrotic syndrome
Medullary cystic disease
Following renal transplantation
Drugs and chemicals
6-mercaptopurine
methyl-5-chrome
outdated tetracycline
cadmium
lead

Renal Complications in Myeloma

Hypercalcaemic nephropathy
Renal tubular obstruction
Renal amyloid (5–10% of cases)
Urate nephropathy during cytotoxic therapy
Pyelonephritis

URINE

Urine Pigmentation

Red–brown
Haemoglobinuria
Red
Myohaemoglobinuria
Porphyrins
Phenolphthalein in alkaline urine
Eosin

Phenindione
Beetroot pigment
Clofazimine (lamprene) in leprosy therapy
Aniline dyes
Blackberries
Pink
Rifampicin
Orange
Concentrated normal urine
Urobilin
Bilirubin
Urochrome increased in fever
Yellow
Mepacrine
Milky yellow
Chyluria
Green–green/blue
Methylene blue
Indigo compounds
Ps. aeruginosa infection of urinary tract
Blue–black
Melaninuria
Homogentisic acid (alkaptonuria)
Methaemoglobinuria
Cloudy
Bacteria
Leucocytes
Urates in acid urine
Oxalates in alkaline urine
Phosphates in alkaline urine
Smoky
Erythrocytes (traces of blood)
Colourless
High output of dilute urine

Haematuria

Some causes
Urethral lesions
Urethritis
Foreign body
Papilloma or carcinoma
Prostatic lesions
Bladder
Papilloma
Carcinoma (other tumours rarer)
Infection: bacterial, Schistosoma
Calculus
Varices (bleeding following sudden release of pressure)
Ureter
Calculus
Papilloma
Carcinoma

(Ureterocele)
Renal pelvis
Infection
Calculus
Papilloma, angioma (and rarer benign tumours)
Carcinoma (and other rarer malignant tumours)
Renal damage
Medullary sponge kidney
Papillary necrosis
Polycystic disease of kidney
Renal tract infection
bacterial
(viral – varicella, rubella, mumps)
Acute glomerulonephritis
Immunological damage to kidney
primary persistent glomerulonephritis
connective tissue diseases, e.g.
SLE anaphylactoid purpuric nephritis
Familial and congenital urinary tract lesions, e.g. congenital hereditary nephritis
Drug-induced haematuria
anticoagulants, e.g. warfarin, heparin
cantharides
sulphonamides
streptokinase overdose
etc.
Associated with general disease
plasma clotting factor defects
haemophilia: Factor VIII
Christmas disease: Factor IX
rarely Factor V, or Factor VII
von Willebrand's disease: Factor VIII plus platelet plasma defect
platelet defects
thrombocytopenia
platelet function defects
Acute fevers
yellow fever
malaria
smallpox
Uraemia
Liver disease (terminal)
(Temporarily after severe prolonged exercise in normal subjects)

Causes of Haematuria in Children

Nephritis: acute glomerulonephritis
Immunological disorders
primary persistent glomerulonephritis
anaphylactoid purpuric nephritis Schölein–Henoch syndrome)
Pyelonephritis and cystitis

Congenital anomalies
Renal vein thrombosis
Trauma
Tumours of the renal tract
Drug action
Renal calculi

Haemoglobinuria

Following intravascular haemolysis
Exercise
very strenuous
march haemoglobinuria
Severe burns
Crush injury
Mismatched blood transfusion
Venom from some snake bites
Chemicals
arsine
betanaphthol
carbolic acid
hydroquinone derivatives
naphthalene
potassium chlorate
phenylhydrazine
Vegetable toxins: 'mushroom' poisoning
Blackwater fever in malaria
Paroxysmal cold haemoglobinuria
Paroxysmal nocturnal haemoglobinuria
(Transurethral prostatectomy with bladder washout with water)
Haemolysis if red cells in urine occurs if the urine specific gravity is less than 1·007)

Haematospermia
(*75% of cases occur in the 5th, 6th and 7th decades*)

Genito-urinary disorders
Benign prostatic hypertrophy
Prostatic calculi
Prostatic varicosity
Spermatocele
Varicocele
Hydrocele
Renal calculi
Other conditions
Cardiovascular disease
Alcoholism

Chyluria

Dilated aberrant lymphatic channels in the abdomen
Scarring and fibrosis causing blockage of lymphatic tracts in the abdomen, especially around the kidneys and ureters

Genito-urinary disease
- tuberculosis
- hydrocele
- carcinoma of renal pelvis
- ureteric stone
- filariasis

URINARY TRACT

Enuresis

This condition occurs almost exclusively in children

Developmental delay
Disorder of learning
(Deep sleep pattern – no longer considered valid)
Social, Family, Sexual, Psychogenic } factors
Physical factors
- Neurogenic factors, which may disappear at puberty. In the normal adult there is control by inhibition of the micturition centre via the pyramidal tracts, and this control may not be fully developed in childhood
- Minor factors
  - phimosis
  - balanitis
  - small urinary meatus
  - vulvitis
  - constipation
  - intestinal worms
- Enuresis may be associated with –
  - pyelitis
  - cystitis
  - diabetes insipidus

Failure of Urine Formation in Immediate Newborn Period

Restriction of oral fluids
Postnatal intravascular hypovolaemia
Bilateral renal agenesis
Cortical necrosis
Tubular necrosis
Bilateral renal vein thrombosis
Congenital nephrotic syndrome
Congenital pyelonephritis
Congenital nephritis

Obstruction to Urine Flow in Immediate Newborn Period

Imperforate prepuce
Urethral strictures

Urethral diverticulum
Hypertrophy of verumontanum
Neurogenic bladder
Ureterocele
Renal tumour

Urinary Tract Infection in Childhood

Haematogenous spread to urinary tract
Urethral ascent of infecting bacteria
Vesicoureteric reflux
Chronic pyelonephritis
Calculus
Diverticula

Urinary Tract Malignancy

Kidney
- hypernephroma (adenocarcinoma)
- nephroblastoma (Wilms' tumour)

Renal pelvis, Ureter, Bladder } papillary tumour
- papilloma (usually benign)
- transitional cell tumour

Males
- Prostate
  - epithelial carcinoma
  - scirrhous carcinoma
- Testis
  - seminoma
  - teratoma
  - interstitial cell tumour (Leydig cell)

Obstruction in the Urinary Tract

Renal pelvis or ureter – unilateral or bilateral
- calculus
- blood clot
- tumour
  - carcinoma
  - papilloma
- retroperitoneal fibrosis
- aortic aneurysm
- infections, including tuberculosis
- pelvi-ureteric obstruction

Bladder and urethra
- prostate
  - benign hypertrophy
  - carcinoma
- median bar hypertrophy (Marion's disease)
- urethral stricture
- carcinoma of urethra

Urine Retention

Postoperation
Urological
- Urethral stenosis or inflammation

Neurological
- Traumatic paraplegia
- Multiple sclerosis
- Cerebral metastases
- Cerebrovascular accident
- Sacral agenesis

Rectal
- Faecal impaction
- Severe colitis

Psychiatric
Males
- Prostatic obstruction

Females
- Postpartum
- Gynaecological
  - pelvic mass
  - prolapse
  - pessary
  - vulval haematoma

Patients complain of
- frequency
- urgency
- some with overflow incontinence

Increased Susceptibility to Urinary Tract Infection

Urine stasis
- mechanical obstruction to flow
- neurological damage
- reflux of urine
- incomplete emptying of bladder

Foreign body: e.g. stone
Persisting inflammation of urinary tract following cystitis due to
- chemicals
- infections
  - bacterial
  - fungal
  - viral

Impaired local or general immunity to infections

Lower Urinary Tract Symptoms

Urinary tract infection
No bacteriological evidence of urinary tract infection
- Urethral syndrome
  - anxiety
  - (full bladder with voluntary withholding of micturition)

bacterial infection
of paraurethral glands in female
of prostate in male
protozoa: Trichomonas
yeasts–candida
fungus–chlamydia (TRIC agent)
viruses
trauma: sexual intercourse
hypersensitivity to toilet preparations
cold weather and inadequate clothing
urethral stricture
postmenopausal oestrogen withdrawal urethral atrophy

Incontinence

Incontinence with normal nerve supply to bladder
Irritative bladder lesion
severe urinary tract infection
tuberculous cystitis
interstitial cystitis (Hunner's ulcer)
post-irradiation bladder (contracted bladder)
bilharzial infection of bladder
bladder tumours
Outflow resistance
prostatic obstruction
bladder neck obstruction
Normal bladder with normal outflow: multiparous women with weak pelvic floor
Abnormal outflow
Post-prostatectomy – after removal of too much urethra – the external urethral sphincter is unable to maintain continence
incomplete removal of prostate leading to sphincter closure prevention
stricture preventing sphincter closure
Upper Motor Neuron Lesions
Lesions of the spinal cord above the voiding arc (S2–4) result in spastic neurogenic bladder
Lower Motor Neuron Lesions. Lesions to the spinal cord at S2–4, cauda equina, or to nerve roots which interrupt the reflex arc result in Atonic Neurogenic Bladder
Trauma
Tumours
Intravertebral disc herniation
Meningomyelocele
Poliomyelitis
Tabes dorsalis
Psychogenic Enuresis
Complications of Neurogenic Bladder
Infection
Hydronephrosis
Calculus formation

Renal failure
Sex problems
Sphincter incompetence
Congenital urethral defect
fractured pelvis – urethral trauma
epispadias
bladder neck resection in women
carcinoma of prostate in urinary sphincter

Uninhibited Bladder Contractions

Neurological disorders
Cortical
Subcortical
Suprasacral spinal lesions
Outflow obstruction in males
Bladder dysfunction
Prostatic obstruction
Distal sphincter neuromuscular dysfunction
Stricture of urethra
Idiopathic
Urge incontinence in females
Enuresis

Bladder Dysfunction

Reflex pathways interrupted
Detrusor activity cannot take place. The bladder is emptied by straining, or by increased abdominal pressure
Obstruction
1. Overdistension: Bladder nerve fibres are damaged, and there follows secondary paralysis of the bladder
2. Subacute or partial obstruction results in hypertrophy of bladder muscle, including the muscle at the bladder neck, resulting in secondary obstruction
3. Spasm of external sphincter

Infection
1. Initial frequency
2. In very severe infection, the bladder may be paralysed

(N.B. Risk of septicaemia following the passage of a catheter)

Retroperitoneal Fibrosis

Idiopathic (the most frequent)
Malignancy: tumour growth spreads over the posterior abdominal wall, and may entrap the ureters
Methylsergide therapy
In this condition no ureteric peristalsis is seen on retrograde cinepyelography

Prostatic Cysts [R]

Retention cysts: small, acinar, occurring in senile enlargement
Congenital cysts
- from prostatic utricle with enlargement of the verumontanum projecting into the bladder
- Müllerian cysts lying in the midline between the prostate and the rectum
- Wolffian cysts lying laterally between the prostate and the rectum

Malignant cysts: very occasional collections of necrotic tissue and blood
Parasites
- Bilharzia
- Echinococcus

RESPIRATORY SYSTEM

Dry pleurisy with normal chest X-ray
Dullness to percussion over lower lung

Mediastinum

Mediastinal mass

Diaphragm

Paralysis of
eventration of
fixation of
elevation of
depression of
tumours
hernia

CHEST

Deformities of the Chest

- Congenital
    - incomplete fusion of the sternum
    - funnel chest or pectus excavatum
    - absence of pectoral muscles
- Deformities associated with disease
    - rickets (Harrison's sulcus)
    - pigeon breast: caused by
        - rickets
        - chronic bronchopulmonary infections
    - barrel chest
        - may occur normal in people of stocky build
        - pulmonary emphysema
    - associated with scoliosis
        - congenital
        - paralytic
            - poliomyelitis
            - syringomyelia
        - associated with diseases of the spine
    - local changes
        - general expansion of one side of chest
            - spontaneous pneumothorax
            - intrathoracic tumour
            - unilateral obstructive emphysema
        - general contraction of one side of chest
            - chronic empyema
            - tuberculous pleural effusion
            - chronic pulmonary tuberculosis
            - chronic lung abscess

pneumonia
atalectasis
bronchiectasis
local lesion
lesions of skin
infections
tumours
etc.

Emphysema of the Chest Wall

Injury to the lung
Ulcerative or traumatic lesions affecting
the oesophagus
stomach
Escape of air into tissues during therapeutic pneumothorax to collapse lung
Infection by gas-producing organisms involving muscle of the chest wall

LUNGS

Congenital Lung Abnormalities

Primary agenesis
bilateral complete agenesis
unilateral agenesis
congenital absence of bronchi, alveolar, tissues and blood supply
rudimentary bronchus from trachea but no pulmonary tissue investing its tip
poorly developed main bronchus with investing fleshy mass of ill-developed pulmonary tissue
Pulmonary hypoplasia
Accessory bronchi, accessory lungs and sequestrated lungs
Lung cysts
congenital
1. central
peripheral
2. lymphangiomatous cyst
3. cystic change in an intracellular sequestrated or accessory lung and endogenous cysts
4. congenital cystic adenomatoid malformation
acquired
tension cysts in infancy
infection
hypoplastic bronchus
compression of bronchus by large pulmonary artery
foreign body
emphysematous bullae and giant air cysts of adult life
healed abscess
parasitic cysts
hydatid
Paragonimiasis

Congenital absence of pulmonary artery
- complete absence of main trunk
- absence of one main pulmonary artery
- hypoplasia of one or more pulmonary arteries or of a lobar branch
- post-valvular stenosis of pulmonary artery
- aberrant pulmonary artery

Congenital absence of pulmonary veins
- failure of the stem of the common pulmonary vein to become incorporated into the atrium
- failure of the pulmonary vein to join up normally with the lung venous plexus, or having established union then becoming atretic
- drainage of pulmonary veins or common pulmonary vein into right atrium
- drainage of right pulmonary veins into the superior vena cava, azygos or right innominate veins
- drainage of left pulmonary veins into a persistent left superior vena cava, coronary sinus or anomalous vertical pulmonary vein
- persistent connections between pulmonary veins and adult portal vein
- drainage of pulmonary veins of right lung into the inferior vena cava (scimitar syndrome)

Congenital pulmonary lymphangiectasis

Congenital tracheo-bronchomegaly

Pulmonary Sequestration

(? aberrant lung bed with arterial blood supply direct from aorta)

The left lower lobe is affected most frequently. The abnormal portion of lung is not in communication with the normal lung

Intralobular
- Asymptomatic
- Recurrent lung infections
- Dysphagia
- Haematemesis
- Congestive cardiac failure

Extralobular
- Asymptomatic
- Presentation similar to intralobular form
- Associated with congenital diaphragmatic hernia

Pulmonary Collapse

Bronchial carcinoma

Bronchial adenoma

Other tumours in chest, e.g. Hodgkin's lymphadenoma

Enlarged lymph glands

Tuberculous bronchostenosis

Inhaled foreign body

Mucus plugs

Pulmonary Oedema

Altered permeability of pulmonary bed
- infections: pneumonia
  - bacterial
  - viral
- inhaled toxic agents
  - phosgene
  - ozone
  - oxides of nitrogen
- circulating toxins
  - alloxan
  - alpha-naphthylthiourea
  - snake venom
- vasoactive substances
  - histamine
  - kinins
  - prostaglandins
- diffuse capillary leak syndrome
  - endotoxinaemia
  - idiopathic capillary leak
- disseminated intravascular coagulopathy: e.g. post-infection immune complex disease, heat stroke
- immunological reactions
  - drug idiosyncrasy
    - nitrofurantoin
    - busulphan
    - methotrexate
  - allergic alveolitis
  - leucocyte sensitivity states
- radiation pneumonia
- uraemia
- near-drowning
- aspiration pneumonia
- smoke inhalation
- adult respiratory-distress syndromes, e.g. post-traumatic pulmonary insufficiency

Increased pulmonary capillary pressure
- cardiac
  - coronary heart disease
  - mitral valve disease
    - stenosis
    - regurgitation – acute pulmonary oedema may develop following sudden rupture of chordae tendinae in
      - infarction
      - endocarditis
  - aortic valve disease
    - stenosis
    - regurgitation
  - left ventricular failure, left ventricle muscle disease
- pulmonary
  - pulmonary veno-occlusive disease

congenital stenosis of origin of pulmonary veins
pulmonary venous fibrosis with high pulmonary blood flow
acquired pulmonary venous stenosis
mediastinal granuloma
fibrosing mediastinitis
mediastinal masses
acute renal failure
overinfusion

Raised left atrial pressure
hypertension
ischaemia
valvular heart disease

Decreased osmotic pressure
hypoalbuminaemia
renal disease
liver disease
protein losing enteropathy
nutritional disorders

Lymphatic insufficiency: e.g. blockage by tumour

Increased negative interstitial pressure
high negative pressure
aspiration pulmonary oedema
aspiration pneumothorax

Mixed or unknown mechanisms
high altitude pulmonary oedema
neurogenic pulmonary oedema
narcotic overdose, e.g. heroin
pulmonary embolism
pulmonary parenchymal disease
eclampsia
cardioversion
postanaesthesia
cardiopulmonary bypass
? neurogenic
microemboli
release of toxic substances
cerebral injury

Pulmonary Exudates

Haemodynamic causes
Overhydration
Overtransfusion with fluids
Shock lung
Raised left atrial pressure (exceeding 25–30 mmHg)
left ventricular failure
mitral valve disease
left atrial myxoma
Sudden withdrawal of large volume of pleural fluid (avoided if less than 1 litre withdrawn at first aspiration)

Capillary damage
- Infections
  - Pneumonia
    - bacterial
    - viral
- Non-infectious causes
  - noxious fumes
    - nitric oxide (NO_2)
    - mustard gas
    - phosgene
    - halogens
    - welding with molten metals
    - ammonia
    - nickel carboxide
    - cadmium
    - ozone
  - inhaled gastric acid: Mendelson's syndrome
  - uraemia
- Cytotoxic drugs
  - bleomycin
  - busulphan
  - cyclophosphamide
- Hypersensitivity
  - systemic lupus erythematosus
  - Goodpasture's syndrome
  - nitrofurantoin sensitivity
- Lowered colloidal osmolality. Protein-losing states rarely cause exudation alone, unless there is also increased capillary permeability
- Unexplained
  - increased intracranial pressure
  - high altitude

Pneumonia

Primary: in a previously healthy subject
Secondary
1. Pre-existing disease
   - airways obstruction
   - diffuse pulmonary fibrosis
   - bronchiectasis
   - bronchial carcinoma
2. Associated with influenzal epidemic
3. Aspiration from oropharynx in neurological or gastro-intestinal disease
4. Abnormal depression of antibacterial defences
   - in systemic disease
   - during steroid therapy
   - during immunosuppressive therapy

Pneumonia–Specific Infections

Pneumococcal pneumonia
Staphylococcal pneumonia

Mycoplasma infection
Q-fever
Psittacosis
Legionnaires' disease

Fungus Infection of Lung

Actinomycetes
- Actinomycosis: e.g. *Actinomyces israelii*
- Nocardiosis: e.g. *Nocardia asteroides*

Yeasts and Yeast-like fungi
- Moniliasis: e.g. *Candida albicans*
- Torulosis: e.g. *Cryptococcus neoformans*
- Geotrichosis: e.g. *Geotrichum candidum*

Filamentous fungi
- Aspergillosis: e.g. *Aspergillus fumigatus*
- Phycomycosis: e.g. *Mucor*

Dimorphic fungi
- Histoplasmosis: e.g. *Histoplasma capsulatum*
- Coccidioidomycosis: e.g. *Coccidioides immitus*
- North American Blastomycosis: e.g. *Blastomyces dermatitidis*
- South American Blastomycosis: e.g. *Paracoccidioides brasiliensis*

Sporotrichosis: e.g. *Sporotrichum schenkii*

Diseases of Interstitium of Lung
(alveolar walls and the space between them)

Infective
- pneumonia and bronchopneumonia
- miliary tuberculosis
- miliary fungus infection
- bronchiectasis

? origin
- sarcoidosis
- idiopathic pulmonary haemosiderosis
- Goodpasture's syndrome
- intrinsic fibrosing alveolitis (Hamman–Rich syndrome)

Dust diseases, drugs, etc.
- extrinsic fibrosing alveolitis, e.g. Farmer's lung, bird fanciers' disease, etc.
- drugs and poisons
- pneumoconiosis
  - pneumoconiosis
  - progressive massive pulmonary fibrosis
  - silicosis

Connective tissue disease
- rheumatoid arthritis
- Sjögren's syndrome
- systemic lupus erythematosus
- systemic sclerosis
- polyarteritis nodosa

Wegener's granulomatosis

Pulmonary eosinophilia
- simple pulmonary eosinophilia
- prolonged pulmonary eosinophilia
- asthmatic pulmonary eosinophilia: asthma complicated by recurrent lung consolidation and blood eosinophilia
- tropical eosinophilia

Tumours
- secondary carcinoma
- lymphatic carcinomatosis
- reticuloses
- leukaemia

Diffuse Lung Fibrosis

Occupational dust disease
Allergic dust disease (allergic extrinsic alveolitis)
Infections
Connective tissue disease
Vascular disorders
Rare conditions

Occupational Lung Diseases

Silica
- Free silica causing silicosis
  - Mining
    - gold, tin, copper, mica — with associated quartz
  - Quarrying
  - Tunnelling
  - Stone cutting, dressing, polishing, cleaning, masonry
  - Abrasives manufacture
  - Glass manufacture
  - Fillers
  - Abrasive blasting
  - Foundry work
  - Ceramics
    - china ware, porcelain, stove ware, earthenware
    - refractory ceramics
  - Boiler scaling
  - Vitreous enamelling

  Causing or favouring development of –
  - Tuberculosis
  - Cor pulmonale
  - Bronchitis
  - Emphysema
  - Spontaneous pneumothorax
  - Segmental and middle lobe collapse
  - Rheumatoid syndrome
  - Progressive systemic sclerosis
  - Carcinoma of lung
- Mixed dust fibrosis
  - foundry workers
- Diatomite pneumoconiosis

Kaolin (china clay)
- paper, china, paints, etc. } industries

Ball clays and stoneware clays
Fuller's earth
Bentonite
Mica

Beryllium disease

Acute
- contact dermatitis
- conjunctivitis
- rhinitis
- tracheitis
- bronchitis
- pneumonitis

Chronic: sarcoid-like lung disease
- interstitial cellular infiltration
- granuloma formation
- conchoidal bodies

leading to –
- cor pulmonale
- spontaneous pneumothorax
- (carcinoma of lung)

Pneumoconiosis due to coal and carbon

Coal, Graphite, Lamp black, Carbon black } leading to {
- discrete simple pneumoconiosis
- centrilobular emphysema with dust
- progressive massive fibrosis
- 'rheumatoid' coal pneumoconiosis (Caplan's syndrome)

Asbestos
- Diffuse interstitial fibrosis of lungs
- Pleural fibrosis and plaque formation
- Malignant mesothelioma of pleura or peritoneum, especially after exposure to crocidolite, also amosite and crysotile
- Possibly bronchial carcinoma without asbestosis
- Skin corns

Talc pneumoconiosis: (hydrated magnesium silicate)
- Paints
- Pharmacy
- Ceramics
- Roofing industry
- Rubber industry
- Refractory industry
- Textile industry

Cadmium
- Acute poisoning
- Chronic poisoning: emphysema

Noxious gases
- Nitric oxide
  - metal welding and cutting, effects apart from nitric oxide depends on the metal being worked
  - forage tower silos
- Ozone
- Chlorine
- Phosgene
- Metal fume fever
- Polymer fumes
- Hard metal disease
  - tungstate carbide
  - aluminium lung disease
- Manganese pneumonitis
- Ionizing radiation
  - uranium, thorium, radon, hemolite, fluorspar } mining

Fumes and vapours
- Toluene diisocyanate
- Complex platinum salts
- Aluminium soldering flux

Extrinsic Allergic Alveolitis

Farmer's lung (mouldy hay): *M. faeni, Thermoactinomyces vulgaris*
Bagassosis (mouldy sugar cane): *Thermoactinomyces sacchari*
Mushroom worker's lung (compost): *M. faeni, T. vulgaris*
Malt worker's lung (mouldy barley and malt): *Aspergillus clavatus* and *fumigatus*
Maple bark stripper's disease (infected maple bark): *Cryptostroma corticale*
Suberosis (mouldy cork bark): *Penicillium frequentans*
Bird breeder's lung (droppings of pigeons, budgerigars, parrots, hens)
Wheat weevil disease (Weevil infested wheat and flour): *Sitophilus granarius*
Pituitary snuff taker's lung: (pituitary snuff powder)
Ventilatory pneumonitis:
Byssinosis
- cotton, flax, hemp, jute, sisal } A form of asthma with lung airways as 'targets' of a bronchospasm-provoking factor initiated by inhalation of the dust

Drugs associated with Pulmonary Fibrosis

- Bleomycin
- Busulphan

Chlorambucil
Cyclophosphamide
Melphalan
Methotrexate
Vincristine
Paraquat

Rare

Nitrofurantoin: leading to pulmonary infiltration
Sulphasalazine
Oxygen (prolonged use)
Hexamethonium
Mecamylamine
Pentolinium
Gold salts

Infections associated with Diffuse Pulmonary Fibrosis

Bacteria
- Tuberculosis
- Others

Viral: influenza
Fungal: aspergillosis
Generalized chronic bronchial disease
Fibrocystic disease

Pulmonary Manifestation of Connective Tissue Disease

Rheumatoid arthritis
- pleural lesions
- intrapulmonary rheumatoid nodules
- fibrosing alveolitis
- rheumatoid pneumoconiosis
- pulmonary arteriolar vasculitis

Ankylosing spondylitis: pulmonary fibrosis (uncommon, predominantly in males)

Systemic lupus erythematosus
- pleurisy
- pneumonic illness
- breathlessness: the lungs become stiff and smaller

Systemic sclerosis
- pulmonary fibrosis
- pulmonary arteriolar vasculitis resulting eventually in pulmonary hypertension and right ventricular failure
- pleurisy (uncommon)
- aspiration pneumonia

Polyarteritis nodosa: the lung is involved in one-third of patients necrotizing arteritis

Polymyositis
Chronic active hepatitis
Sjögren's syndrome
Löffler's syndrome
Wegener's granulomatosis

Diffuse Lung Fibrosis associated with Vascular Disorders

Thromboembolic disease
Obstruction of pulmonary veins
Pulmonary veno-occlusive disease
Pulmonary venous hypertension
Pulmonary purpura with nephritis (Goodpasture's syndrome)
Idiopathic pulmonary haemosiderosis

Rare Causes of Diffuse Pulmonary Fibrosis

Diffuse interstitial pulmonary fibrosis (Hamman–Rich syndrome)
Desquamative interstitial pneumonitis
Histiocytosis X
Cholesterol pneumonitis
Pulmonary alveolar proteinosis
Pulmonary alveolar microlithiasis
Primary amyloidosis
Leiomyomatosis
Neurofibromatosis
Radiation damage

Chronic Diffuse Radiographic Pulmonary Shadows

Infection:
- Bacteria
  - especially tuberculosis
- Mycoses
  - coccidiomycosis
  - histoplasmosis
  - blastomycosis
  - allergic aspergillosis
- Virus
  - chickenpox
- Parasites
  - Schistosomiasis

Dusts
1. Inorganic
   - coal
   - silica
   - beryllium
   - asbestos
   - iron
2. Organic (with allergic response)
   - farmer's lung
   - bird fanciers
   - malt workers
   - mushroom workers
   - bagasse workers
   - maple strippers
   - pituitary snuff takers

- Malignancy
  - Metastatic carcinoma
  - Lymphangitis carcinomatosa
  - Alveolar cell carcinoma
  - Lymphoma
  - Leukaemia
- Sarcoidosis
  - Cryptogenic fibrosing alveolitis
  - Drug-induced pulmonary alveolitis
    - busulphan
    - bleomycin
    - hexamethonium
    - nitrofurantoin
    - oxygen
- Connective tissue disease
  - Rheumatoid arthritis
  - Systemic lupus erythematosus
  - Polyarteritis nodosa
  - Idiopathic haemosiderosis
- Honeycomb lung appearance
  - Mesodermal dysplasia
  - Tuberose sclerosis
  - Neurofibromatosis
  - Idiopathic histiocytosis
  - Cystic fibrosis
  - Secondary haemosiderosis
  - Alveolar proteinosis
  - Alveolar microlithiasis
  - Aspiration pneumonitis
  - In association with bronchitis and bronchiectasis

Solitary Pulmonary Mass seen on X-ray

Bronchogenic carcinoma
Metastatic tumour
Bronchial adenoma
Hamartoma
Granuloma
Abscess
Arteriovenous malformation
Anomalous pulmonary vein
Hydatid cyst
Infected bulla
Bronchial cyst
Sequestration
Pulmonary infarct
Haematoma
Mucoid impaction
Rheumatoid nodule
Wegener's granuloma

Lung Abscess

Bronchogenic: aspirational

Haematogenous
Specific necrotizing pneumonia
Infected lung cyst
Transdiaphragmatic pulmonary abscess

Pulmonary Cavity

- Solitary
  - Cavitating Pneumonia
    - Primary bacterial pneumonia
      - tuberculosis
      - staphylococcus
      - klebsiella
      - pseudomonas
      - non-specific
    - Underlying bronchial occlusion
      - tumour
      - foreign body
      - bronchiectasis
    - Aspiration pneumonia
    - Fungal pneumonia
    - Underlying pulmonary abnormality
      - bronchiectasis
      - sequestration
      - bronchial cyst
  - Bronchogenic carcinoma
  - Metastatic carcinoma
  - Lymphoma
  - Pulmonary infarct
  - Wegener's granuloma
  - Rheumatoid nodule
  - Post-traumatic haematoma
  - Hydatid cyst
  - Progressive massive fibrosis
- Multiple
  - Metastases
  - Pyaemic abscesses
  - Pulmonary infarcts
  - Rheumatoid nodules
  - Wegener's granulomas
  - Hydatid cysts

Pulmonary Cysts

- Alveolar cysts
  - blebs
  - bullae
  - pneumatocele
- Translucent lung: main pulmonary artery or a lobar branch absent
- Bronchopulmonary cyst
- Cystic bronchiectasis
- Post-infection cyst

Tumours of the Lung

- Malignant
  - Bronchial carcinoma
    - squamous cell 50%
    - oat cell 17%
    - adenocarcinoma 16%
    - large cell carcinoma 17%
  - Aetiology
    - smoking
    - radioactive gases
    - asbestos
    - arsenic
    - nickel
    - chromate
    - atmospheric pollution
    - newspaper printing
    - gas retort workers
    - racial factors
    - pulmonary fibrosis
  - Alveolar cell carcinoma: less than 1%
  - Pulmonary lymphoma
  - Secondary tumours of lung, from primary tumours elsewhere in body
- Potentially malignant
  - bronchial adenoma
- Benign
  - hamartoma

RESPIRATION

Airways Obstruction

- Increased airways resistance
  - small airways
    - chronic
      - chronic bronchitis
      - some asthmatics
      - ? cause
    - reversible
      - asthma
  - large airways, intrathoracic
      - tracheal stricture
      - neoplasm
      - compression
- Diminished elastic recoil
  - reduced lung volume
    - pneumothorax
    - pleural effusion
  - parenchymal changes
    - emphysema
    - ageing
    - prolonged overinflation (severe asthma)

- Increased rigidity of the airways
    - chronic bronchitis
    - emphysema
    - polychondritis affecting the small airways only
    - asthma

Acute Respiratory Failure

- Acute illness
    - Shock lung
    - Drug overdose
    - Left-sided heart failure
    - Pneumonia
    - Asthma
- Chronic illness
    - Chronic bronchitis
    - Emphysema
    - Kyphoscoliosis
    - Cystic fibrosis
- Iatrogenic
    - Sedation (excessive)
    - Prolonged oxygen therapy

Respiratory Failure

- Obstruction of upper airways
    - sudden
        - inhaled foreign body
        - faciomaxillary injuries
        - angioneurotic oedema
        - oropharyngeal infections
            - epiglottis
            - quinsy
        - external compression on trachea
            - goitre
            - strangling
        - laryngeal stenosis
            - croup
            - abductor paralysis
    - coma
- Disorders affecting chest wall and pleural cavity
    - Neurological causes
        - Brainstem
            - compression
            - infarction
            - trauma
            - inflammatory disorders
            - anoxia
            - drugs
        - Cervical cord: high transection
        - Anterior horn cell disease
            - poliomyelitis
            - motor neuron disease

spinal muscular atrophy
Peripheral neuropathy
acute polyneuritis (Guillain–Barré syndrome)
acute porphyria
toxic neuropathies
chronic polyneuritis
Disorders of neuromuscular transmission
myasthenia gravis
myasthenic syndrome
botulism
muscle relaxant
Muscle disease
Duchenne dystrophy
limb girdle dystrophy
dystrophia myotonica
polymyositis
acid maltase deficiency (glycogen storage disease)

Hypoventilation

Dysfunction of lungs, obstruction of airways, weakness of respiratory muscles
Lung disease
chronic obstructive lung disease
asthma
upper airway obstruction
severe diffuse lung disease
Thoracic dysfunction
kyphoscoliosis
obesity-ventilation syndrome
myasthenia gravis
poliomyelitis
myotonic dystrophy
Guillain–Barré syndrome
etc.
Decreased drive to breathing
idiopathic hypoventilation
sedative drugs
myxoedema
metabolic alkalosis
central nervous system disease
(bilateral glomectomy)
etc.

Cheyne–Stokes Respiration

Reduced sensitivity of respiratory centre in medulla to carbon dioxide and reduction in arterial PCO_2. Respirations begin with hardly perceptible respiratory movements, gradually increasing until each respiration exceeds the normal volume, dying away again to end in a period of apnoea before the next cycle

Normal subjects
- high altitude
- following deliberate hyperventilation
- elderly subjects ? due to cerebral vascular disease

Pathological
- ventricular failure
- bronchopneumonia
- diseases of the central nervous system
  - cerebrovascular disease
  - cerebral haemorrhage
  - cerebral thrombosis
  - cerebral tumour
- Uraemia
- drugs suppressing respiration
  - morphine
  - barbiturates

Wheezing in Children

Bronchitis
Asthma
Respiratory tract obstruction
Acute viral bronchiolitis
Pertussis infection
Post-nasal drip (from tonsillar and adenoidal enlargement)
Cystic fibrosis
Recurrent aspiration pneumonitis
- gastro-oesophageal reflux
- palatal paralysis
- rare H-shaped tracheo-oesophageal fistula

Primary pulmonary tuberculosis

Central Alveolar Hypoventilation

Bulbar poliomyelitis
Brainstem encephalitis
Medullary tumour
Medullary infarction
Motor neuron disease
Sarcoidosis of the central nervous system
Inborn metabolic defects
Riley–Day syndrome
High cervical cordotomy

Indications for Tracheostomy

To relieve laryngeal obstruction caused by
- trauma
- inflammation
- oedema
- foreign body
- extension of neck infection
- carcinoma

To facilitate removal of secretions from tracheobronchial tree
- in severe bronchial infection
- in unconscious patient

To relieve respiratory failure where endotracheal inhibition is successful and long periods of artificial ventilation are necessary
To reduce the dead space
To prevent overspill from the pharynx
During laryngeal surgery
Elective operative procedure
Post-trauma: flail chest injury

Lower Respiratory Tract Infection

Acute bronchiolitis
Acute bronchitis
- bacterial
- viral
- fungal
- mycoplasma pneumonia

Bronchiectasis

Post-pneumonia infective bronchiectasis
- follicular
- saccular

Collapse (atalectatic) bronchiectasis
- acute
- chronic

Congenital bronchiectasis

Pulmonary vascular disease

Congenital heart disease: any intracardiac shunt
Acquired
- Heart disease
  - mitral stenosis
- Lung disease
  - chronic bronchitis and emphysema
  - industrial lung disease
  - sarcoidosis
  - connective tissue disease
    - systemic lupus erythematosus
    - scleroderma
  - cryptogenic fibrosing alveolitis
  - fungus infection of the lung
- Obliterative pulmonary hypertension
  - primary hypertension

secondary to
acute pulmonary embolism
recurrent pulmonary thrombo-embolism

Acute Respiratory Insufficiency after Trauma – Shock Lung

Shock
Sepsis
Trauma: non-thoracic
Circulation
overtransfusion
overhydration
disseminated intravascular coagulopathy (DIC)
fat embolism
Oxygenation
hypoxia affecting the central nervous system
oxygen toxicity following prolonged pure oxygen respiration
Drug overdose
Metabolic disorder

Drug-induced Respiratory Disease

Hypoventilation and ablation of cough reflex resulting in pulmonary oedema
barbiturates
narcotics, etc
Hypoventilation: follows therapy with 30% oxygen
Bronchial asthma: beta-receptor blockers, e.g. propanolol
Allergic asthma (Type I immediate reaction)
penicillin and other antibiotics
aspirin-induced
allergic
response to local neural reflexes
Pulmonary eosinophilia with

fever cough sputum dyspnoea crepitations	nitrofurantoin sulphonamides aspirin

Some cases of polyarteritis nodosa and systemic lupus erythematosus: thought to be drug-induced allergic disease due to Type III hypersensitivity
Desquamative alveolitis
busulphan in chronic myeloid leukaemia
hexamethonium
these may produce a condition resembling pulmonary oedema leading to pulmonary fibrosis
Aggravation of pre-existing lung disease
antibiotics therapy resulting in superinfection with resistant bacteria and/or fungi
corticosteroids
may provoke pneumothorax

cause a flare-up of quiescent tuberculosis
'Primary' pulmonary hypertension following therapy with appetite suppressives
Inhaled liquid paraffin leading to lipoid pneumonia
Iodism resulting from
- iodides from bronchography
- iodides in cough mixtures

Allergic alveolitis: pituitary snuff
Congestive atelectasia: resulting from prolonged oxygen inhalation
Pulmonary fibrosis
Pulmonary embolism associated with contraceptive pill (linked to oestrogen)
Pulmonary haemosiderosis associated with penicillamine therapy
Pleural fibrosis and localized effusions associated with methysergide therapy
Tobacco smoking
- carcinoma of lung
- chronic bronchitis

Drug-induced Asthma

Simple irritation of respiratory tract, e.g. disodium cromoglycate inhalation alone
Direct pharmacological action, e.g. Propanolol blocking both beta-1 receptors in the heart and beta-2 receptors in the bronchial tree. Stimulation of beta-2 receptors results in bronchial dilatation
Indirect pharmacological action, e.g. aspirin in approximately 2% of asthmatics (especially late asthmatics) ? interferes with prostaglandin synthesis. E prostaglandins dilate, and F prostaglandins constrict the bronchioles
Allergic reactors: Atopic subjects with IgE antibodies develop an immediate reaction. In the presence of IgG antibodies, they develop a delayed reaction, e.g. to penicillins

Occupational Asthma

Common agents

pollens
fungi
animal danders
	reaction to small amounts
	    atopic subjects
	reaction to large amounts
	    furrier's
	    grain handler's
	    baker's
	    farmer's etc.

Organic dusts
- feathers
- wool
- furs
- wheat grain
- spores of

M. faeni
A. fumigatus
B. subtilis enzymes ('biological' washing powders)
A. clavatus (maltase and alkalase)
cotton
gum acacia
Karagay gum
red cedar wood
antibiotic production
penicillin
streptomycin
small mammals – exposure to material contaminated with serum and urine
Chemical agents (acting as haptens)
piperazine
ethanolamine
epoxy resins
platinum salts
isocyanates

Pulmonary Eosinophilia

With asthma
1. Atopic subject
   with *Aspergillus fumigatus*
   with unknown agent
2. Non-atopic subject
   with *Aspergillus fumigatus*
   unknown agent (some cases progress to polyarteritis nodosa)
   with multiple positive prick tests to 'extrinsic' agents
   with immediate positive skin test to *Aspergillus fumigatus*

Without asthma
Non-atopic subject
1. Fungus – especially *A. fumigatus* with positive precipitating antibody test
2. Helminths including –
   ascariasis
   toxocara
   filaria

with complement fixation test or immunofluorescent antibody test positive (including tropical eosinophilia)

3. Drugs
   nitrofurantoin
   antituberculous drugs
   gold salts
   antibiotics

(often with other features of drug hypersensitivity)

4. Unknown, cryptogenic: a few patients progress to polyarteritis nodosa

Drugs reported associated with pulmonary eosinophilia

- aspirin
- furazolidone
- imipramine
- isoniazid
- mephenesin
- methotrexate
- nitrofurantoin
- para-aminosalicylate
- streptomycin
- sulphasalazine
- sulphonamides

Pulmonary Embolism

Predisposing factors
- Previous thrombosis
- Increasing age
- Trauma, surgery
- Immobility
- Carcinoma
- Heart disease
- Vessel wall changes (atherosclerosis)
- Changes in blood flow locally
- Changes in blood
  - increased haematocrit (increasing blood viscosity)
  - thrombocytosis
  - fibrinolytic activity depressed
  - increased fibrinogen and/or globulin, causing increase in blood viscosity
- Genetic factors
  - congenital antithrombin III deficiency
  - homocystinuria

Cardiopulmonary Collapse

- Acute myocardial infarction
- Pulmonary embolism
  - acute
  - chronic
  - complicating pre-existing pulmonary hypertension
  - complicating pre-existing cardiac failure
- Lung collapse (massive)
- Tension pneumothorax
- Acute cardiac tamponade
- Massive internal haemorrhage

Hypertrophic Pulmonary Osteoarthropathy

- Carcinoma of lung: 80% of cases
- Mesothelioma
- Bacterial endocarditis
- Intrathoracic suppuration

Differential diagnosis
- Thyroid pseudoclubbing
- thyroid acropachy

PLEURA

Pneumothorax

'Spontaneous'
Secondary to
- Spontaneous mediastinal emphysema: rupture of air cyst on lung surface, especially at apex of upper lobe
- Asthma
- Heavy work
- Trauma: especially fracture of rib: intact chest wall with punctured lung

Lung disease
- tuberculosis
- diffuse cystic disease
- obstructive airway disease with/without emphysema
- silicosis
- lung abscess
- hydatid cyst
- neoplasm

During intermittent positive pressure ventilation

Serous Fluid in the Pleural Space

Exudates
- Inflammation
  - pneumonia
  - lung abscess
  - tuberculosis
  - epidemic myalgia
  - subdiaphragmatic infection
  - fungal infection
  - acute pancreatitis
- Malignant disease
  - secondary pleural metastases especially from lung, breast, and ovary primary
  - primary pleural tumour
    - mesothelioma
      - localized fibrous
      - diffuse malignant
  - reticulosis
    - Hodgkin's lymphadenoma
    - lymphoma
- Trauma
  - contusion
  - ruptured oesophagus
- Pulmonary infarction
  - pulmonary embolism
  - infarction in situ
- Connective tissue disorders
  - rheumatoid arthritis
  - acute rheumatic fever

systemic lupus erythematosus
polyarteritis nodosa
Lymphatic deficiency
with lymphoedema and yellow finger nails
Complicating ascites
hydrothorax and cirrhotic ascites
Meigs' syndrome (usually right-sided effusion)
Transudates
Cardiac failure
constrictive pericarditis
Fibrosing mediastinitis
Hypoproteinaemia associated with –
severe malnutrition
cirrhosis of the liver
renal disease

Dry Pleurisy with Normal Chest Radiograph

Tuberculosis
Epidemic myalgia
Rheumatoid arthritis
Systemic lupus erythematosus
Pulmonary embolism
Pulmonary infarction in situ

Dullness to Percussion over Lower Lung

Pleural effusion
Pneumonia
Atelectasis of lung
Solid intrathoracic tumour
Cysts, e.g. hydatid
Diaphragmatic hernia
Gross abdominal distension

MEDIASTINUM: MEDIASTINAL MASS

Anterior mediastinal mass
Retrosternal thyroid
Dermoid (teratoma)
Thymic mass (thymoma, cyst)
Lymphoma
Aortic aneurysm
Sternal tumour
Pericardial cyst
Morgagni hernia
Ectopic thyroid
Ectopic parathyroid
Tortuous innominate artery
Middle mediastinal mass
Bronchogenic carcinoma
Lymphoma

- Sarcoidosis
- Primary tuberculosis
- Fungal disease
- Bronchogenic cyst

Posterior mediastinal mass
- Neurogenic tumours
  - neurilemmoma
  - ganglioneuroma
  - neuroblastoma
  - phaeochromocytoma
  - meningocele
- Paravertebral abscess
- Paravertebral tumour extension
- Oesophageal lesion
- Aortic aneurysm

DIAPHRAGM

Paralysis of Diaphragm
- Interruption of phrenic nerve
  - Injury
  - Surgery
    - irreversible
    - reversible
      - crush
      - infiltration with local anaesthetic
  - Pressure on nerve by tumour in thorax
  - Rarely
    - mediastinal abscess
    - leaking aortic aneurysm
    - polyneuritis
    - poliomyelitis
    - post-viral pneumonia

Eventration of Diaphragm
- Abnormal atrophic leaf of the diaphragm, which is immobile
- congenital, with intact phrenic nerve
- acquired – following longstanding paralysis

Fixation of Diaphragm
- pleural infections } slight movements detectable
- haemothorax } on X-ray screening

Elevation of Diaphragm
- increased abdominal pressure
  - pregnancy
  - tumour
  - flatulence
  - subphrenic abscess
- contracted thoracic contents
  - atelectasis
  - pulmonary fibrosis

Depression of Diaphragm
- large effusion in pleural cavity
- massive pulmonary tumour (unilateral)
- severe emphysema leading to bilateral depression

Tumours
- Benign
  - cysts
  - lipoma
  - fibroma
  - neurofibroma
  - chondroma
- Malignant
  - sarcoma

Hernia
- Congenital (rare) – through
  - foramen of Morgagni
  - foramen of Bochdalek
  - deficiency in central tendon
  - abnormally large oesophageal hiatus
- Acquired (commoner)
  1. Less common:
     - rolling hernia
     - Paraoesophageal hernia, in which cardio-oesophageal junction remains intact
  2. More common:
     - sliding hernia. The competence of the cardia is disturbed